The Acoustic Environment of Care Homes

Case Studies from China

This book examines the indoor acoustic environment of China's care homes. Chapter 1 provides a brief introduction to the current situation in China's care homes. This includes the distribution, size, demand, and future development direction of these facilities. The chapter then presents an in-depth introduction and analysis of the indoor environment of these facilities, especially the acoustic environment. In Chapter 2, a case study and site investigation are described, and these are used to analyze the current state of the acoustic environment in these facilities, including the sound pressure level (SPL) and reverberation time (RT). Chapter 3 details the perceptions of the elderly regarding the acoustic environment of care homes and the correlation between the sound environment and other physical environments at the facilities. Chapter 4 presents the impact of the acoustic environment on the well-being of elderly residents and an analysis of the effects of different sound sources on the activities of the elderly. The effects of the acoustic environment on physiological indices of the elderly under different sound sources in care homes are analyzed in Chapter 5. Finally, in Chapter 6, certain improvement strategies for the indoor acoustic environment of care homes are proposed based on the analysis.

This book is a comprehensive exposition of research on the acoustic environment of care homes in China and is useful reading for researchers in acoustics, architecture, design, engineering, and healthcare facilities. It could also be used as a scientific introduction for readers interested in this field.

Jingyi Mu is Associate Professor and doctoral supervisor at the School of Architecture and Design, Harbin Institute of Technology. Visit Scholar of UCL Institute of Environmental Design and Engineering, The Bartlet, University College London (UCL). She specializes in research on architectural environments for elderly care facilities and healthy environment of public buildings.

Jian Kang is Professor of Acoustics and Soundscape at the UCL Institute of Environmental Design and Engineering, The Bartlet, University College London (UCL). He is Fellow of Royal Academy of Engineering, a Member of Academia Europaea – The Academy of Europe, an International Member (Academician) of the Chinese Academy of Engineering, and President of the International Institute of Acoustics and Vibration (IIAV).

The Acoustic Environment of Care Homes

Case Studies from China

Jingyi Mu and Jian Kang

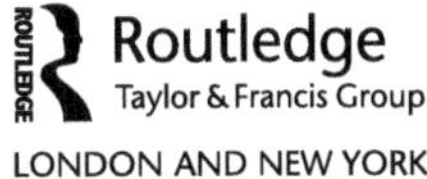

LONDON AND NEW YORK

First published 2025
by Routledge
4 Park Square, Milton Park, Abingdon, Oxon OX14 4RN

and by Routledge
605 Third Avenue, New York, NY 10158

Routledge is an imprint of the Taylor & Francis Group, an informa business

British Library Cataloguing-in-Publication Data
A catalogue record for this book is available from the British Library

ISBN: 978-1-032-50212-0 (hbk)
ISBN: 978-1-032-52568-6 (pbk)
ISBN: 978-1-003-40723-2 (ebk)

DOI: 10.1201/9781003407232

Typeset in Times New Roman
by Apex CoVantage, LLC

Contents

Preface

The global population is rapidly aging, posing significant challenges to local healthcare and elderly care services. According to the World Health Organization, the proportion of the world's population aged 60 and over is projected to double from 12% to 22% between 2015 and 2050. In this context, enhancing elderly care services and actively addressing the challenges of an aging society have become important topics of concern for countries worldwide.

As the most populous country, China also faces serious elderly care issues. Data shows that by the end of 2020, China's elderly population had reached 264 million, accounting for 18.7% of the total population. Currently, China's population is rapidly aging and is expected to enter a super-aged society around 2030. Consequently, the government has implemented a series of policies to promote the development of elderly care services.

Care homes, as important carriers of elderly care services in China, play a crucial role in improving the quality of life for the elderly. However, there is a significant imbalance between supply and demand in China's care homes, and there are considerable differences in their spatial and environmental quality, making it difficult to meet the health needs of the elderly. Therefore, this book will conduct an in-depth study of the current environmental status of care homes in China.

Research indicates that the physical environment of care homes significantly affects the well-being and physical and mental health of the elderly. Existing research has yielded rich results in areas such as thermal and lighting environments, but there is relatively little research on the acoustic environment. However, adverse acoustic environments can disrupt the daily lives of the elderly and even lead to serious health problems such as sleep disorders, hearing loss, tinnitus, and cardiovascular diseases. Therefore, this book will delve into the indoor acoustic environment of care homes.

In terms of content structure, this book first examines the development background of Chinese care homes and the current status of the acoustic environment. Based on this foundation, it analyzes the multifaceted impact of the acoustic environment on the physiology, psychology, behavior, and well-being of the elderly from different perspectives and proposes strategies for improving the acoustic environment of care homes.

This book aims to provide a comprehensive overview of the acoustic environment of Chinese care homes for students, scholars, and professionals in related fields. Through this book, we hope to stimulate readers' thinking on the development of elderly care services, promote the improvement of elderly architectural spatial environments and service quality, and have a positive impact on the health and well-being of the elderly. We hope this book will become an important reference for the field of elderly architectural design, providing valuable support and guidance for academic research and architectural practice.

Acknowledgments

Writing this book has been a challenging yet meaningful process, completed thanks to the generous support and selfless dedication of countless individuals. Here, we sincerely express our heartfelt gratitude to all those who have contributed to this book.

Firstly, we extend our deepest thanks to the staff of the 38 care homes where the research was conducted. Their active cooperation allowed us to delve deeper into the living conditions of the care homes and the environmental needs of the elderly, adding valuable insights to this book.

We would like to especially thank the elderly participants who took part in the surveys and experiments. Their active engagement and sharing of the current state of life in care homes enabled us to gain a deeper understanding of the spatial environment of these facilities. Their wisdom and experiences have provided rich material and profound insights for this book.

We offer our deep appreciation to all members of the research team, including Qin Zhe, Feng Yimeng, Zhang Zhenlin, Li Xuewen, Zhang Cheng, Li Peiyu, Yang Huanhuan, and Liu Yufei. Their dedication to the study of geriatric architecture has played a positive role in the writing of this book. Their hard work and selfless dedication have ensured its successful completion.

We would like to express my deep gratitude to my friends and family. Their understanding and encouragement helped me through the lows of the research and book writing process, and their confidence was the source of my strength to undertake this research.

Lastly, we would like to extend my heartfelt thanks to the publishing team at Routledge. Their tremendous efforts in proofreading, editing, and publishing ensured the high-quality completion of this book. Without their support and assistance, this book would not have been able to reach its readers.

Thank you to everyone who has contributed to and supported this book. Your support and help are deeply appreciated. The completion of this book is the result of our collective efforts and represents our responsibility and contribution to society. In the future, we will continue to strive to contribute to the development of the geriatric care industry.

1 Development and classification of care homes in China

1.1 Current situation of aging in China

Currently, China's population is facing an increasingly severe aging issue. According to data from the Seventh National Population Census [1], the population aged 60 and above in China totals 264 million, accounting for 18.70% of the total population, while those aged 65 and above make up 13.50% (Table 1.1). As per the definition provided by the World Health Organization, a country is considered to have entered an "aging society" when the proportion of elderly individuals aged 65 and above reaches 7%, and it is categorized as a "deeply aging society" when this proportion reaches 14%. Presently, China has essentially transitioned into a deeply aging society and is projected to enter a super-aging society by around 2030. Against this backdrop, China's elderly care issues are increasingly prominent, attracting widespread societal attention.

Since the 18th National Congress of the Communist Party of China, the government has accelerated the implementation of various measures to address population aging. The "14th Five-Year Plan for National Economic and Social Development and Long-Term Goals for 2035" explicitly proposes the "implementation of a proactive national strategy to address population aging," elevating the response to population aging to a level critical for the country's long-term stability [2]. Consequently, China's elderly care industry continues to advance.

1.1.1 Policy

China's population aging issue is becoming increasingly severe, with elderly care services emerging as a focal point of societal concern. As the core carriers of China's elderly care service system, care homes play a crucial role in enhancing the quality of life for the elderly. China has also introduced a series of policy guidelines to promote the construction and development of care homes. The "13th Five-Year Plan for the Development of the National Elderly Programme and the Construction of the Elderly System" (Guo Fa [2017] No. 13) proposes to "promote the quality and efficiency of care homes, and comprehensively improve the quality of care homes," and the "14th Five-Year Plan for the Development of the National Elderly Programme and the Elderly Care System" (Guo Fa [2021] No. 35) further points

DOI: 10.1201/9781003407232-1

Table 1.1 Age composition of the population in successive censuses [1]

Year	*Percentage of population by age group(%)*			
	0-14	*15-59*	*60+*	*65+*
1953	36.28	56.40	7.32	4.41
1964	40.69	53.81	6.13	3.56
1982	33.59	58.79	7.62	4.91
1990	27.69	63.64	8.57	5.57
2000	22.89	66.78	10.33	6.69
2010	16.60	70.14	13.26	8.87
2020	17.95	63.35	18.70	13.50

out that it is necessary to "strengthen the role of the public care homes in providing a basic level of protection and to improve the support system for the elderly's health."

It can be observed that, under the concept of building a Healthy China, the state has raised higher demands for the development of care homes. However, many existing care homes have uneven service quality, and there are significant issues in spatial environments [3], making it challenging to meet the health needs of the elderly. Therefore, it is necessary to research the spatial environments of care homes, explore optimization strategies for healthy spatial environments, and promote the improvement of elderly health levels and quality of life.

1.1.2 Types of facilities

According to the <Code for planning of city and town facilities for the aged> (GB50437–2007), the <Standard for design of care facilities for the aged> (JGJ450–2018), and the <Code for design of residential building for the aged> (GB50340–2016) in China, care homes can mainly be categorized into: retirement homes, geracomiums, apartments for the aged, and nursing homes for the aged. Their specific definitions are as follows:

Retirement homes: Institutions that provide collective residence and elderly care services for the elderly.

Geracomiums: Non-profit organizations providing elderly care services, mainly catering to the elderly with limited means.

Apartments for the aged: Specialized buildings for elderly couples or single elderly individuals to live independently, equipped with relatively complete living service facilities and supplies, generally concentrated in elderly communities or built-in ordinary residential areas. [4]

Nursing homes for the aged: Facilities providing comprehensive services, including residence, medical care, health care, rehabilitation, and nursing for elderly individuals who are unable to care for themselves. [5]

1.1.3 Scale and location

The spatial distribution of care homes and beds in China is highly uneven, primarily concentrated in the central and eastern regions (Table 1.2). Among them, Henan, Heilongjiang, Anhui, and Sichuan provinces have the highest numbers of care homes, while Jiangsu, Shandong, Henan, and Anhui have the densest elderly care bed numbers. The number of care homes and beds in the western and northern regions is relatively low. At the same time, there is no significant difference in the elderly dependency ratio and the number of elderly care beds per thousand elderly individuals among provinces. Provinces with higher numbers of elderly care beds per thousand elderly individuals mainly include Inner Mongolia, Fujian, Jiangsu,

Table 1.2 Relevant data on nationwide pension

Name	*Region*	*Number of care homes*	*Number of beds*	*Number of beds per 1000 elderly population*	*Elderly population dependency ratio*
Beijing	NC	785	11.02	27.2	20.76
Tianjin	NC	610	5.63	21.5	24.28
Hebei	NC	3099	23.27	28.5	23.77
Shanxi	NC	1477	9.07	24.7	20.66
Inner Mongoria IM	NC	707	8.11	42.3	20.4
Liaoning	NEC	3191	18.9	21.8	28.77
Jilin	NEC	3075	14.34	26.8	24.84
Heilongjiang	NEC	3386	19.03	28	24.44
Shanghai	EC	922	14.56	27.4	26.09
Jiangsu	EC	2245	44.3	37.5	26.29
Zhejiang	EC	2082	25.86	29	20.67
Anhui	EC	3368	36.65	35.5	23.86
Fujian	EC	1257	12.05	41.3	17.56
Jiangxi	EC	2198	18.68	33.9	19.42
Shandong	EC	2557	41.39	30.8	25.56
Henan	CC	5566	39.84	29.1	22.67
Hubei	CC	2494	28.76	37.5	23.85
Hunan	CC	3063	25.35	31.1	24.53
Guangdong	SC	2415	24.66	26.6	13.34
Guangxi	SC	1332	9.41	29.8	20.3
Hainan	SC	276	0.95	8.3	16.19
Chongqing	SWC	1810	12.51	28.9	27.26
Sichuan	SWC	4852	31.61	24.3	27.12
Guizhou	SWC	839	8.33	25.4	18.71
Yunnan	SWC	1059	9.42	17.6	16.77
Tibet	SWC	106	1.08	36.3	8.49
Shaanxi	NC	1245	10.92	26.4	21.42
Gansu	NC	632	3.37	33.5	19.8
Qinghai	NC	182	0.73	23	14.7
Ningxia	NC	142	2.74	33.8	14.9
Xinjiang	NC	1266	5.74	27.8	11.86

Note: NC = North China, NEC = Northeast China, EC = East China, CC = Central China, SWC = Southwest China, NC = Northwest China.

Table 1.3 Correlation analysis between aged care homes and regional economic data

Relevance	*Number of beds*	*Beds per 1,000 elderly population*	*Elderly population aged 65 and above*	*Elderly dependency ratio*	*Number of CHs*	*GDP*	*Per Capita G·N·P*
Number of beds	1						
Beds per 1,000 elderly population	0.274	1					
Elderly population aged 65 and above	0.939**	0.162	1				
Elderly dependency ratio	0.568**	0.011	0.545**	1			
Number of CHs	0.797**	0.061	0.783**	0.576**	1		
GDP	0.784**	0.234	0.813**	0.256	0.440*	1	
Per Capita G·N·P	0.156	0.167	0.064	0.204	−0.188	0.439*	1

Note: CH = Care home, GDP = Gross domestic product.
* Significant results.

and Hubei, while provinces with lower bed numbers are mainly concentrated in the central, northern, and southern regions, such as Hainan, Yunnan, Tianjin, and Liaoning. In terms of the elderly dependency ratio, western regions generally have lower ratios (such as Tibet, Xinjiang, and Qinghai), indicating lower elderly care pressure, while eastern regions have no significant differences in the elderly dependency ratio. Among them, Liaoning, Chongqing, Sichuan, Jiangsu, and Shanghai have the highest dependency ratios, indicating greater elderly care pressure.

Table 1.3 presents a correlation analysis of care homes and regional economic data in China. It can be observed that there are correlations between the number of elderly care beds and the elderly population, the elderly dependency ratio, the number of care homes, and regional gross domestic product (GDP), with the elderly population showing the most significant correlation. Additionally, the number of care homes also exhibits significant correlations with the number of beds, elderly population, and elderly dependency ratio, albeit with a relatively low correlation with regional GDP. Overall, the number of care homes and beds is positively correlated with the elderly population, elderly dependency ratio, and regional GDP, indicating that the development of care homes may be influenced by both local elderly care demands and economic development levels.

1.2 Pension model in China

1.2.1 Home care

Home care is a traditional elderly care model in China, where elderly individuals are taken care of by their spouses or children at home. Throughout history, Chinese society has placed a strong emphasis on family values, with caring for the elderly considered a responsibility and obligation of family members. Both policy and morality in ancient times supported this notion [6]. Additionally, research indicates that interaction between elderly individuals and their children in a home care setting can provide the elderly with more emotional support and promote their psychological well-being [7]. As a result, many elderly individuals prefer home care. Currently, approximately 90% of elderly individuals in China receive care at home from their children.

The Chinese government has shown increased support for the home care model. A basic framework for elderly care services has been established, with home care as the foundation, community care as the support, and institutional care as the supplement. Local governments in places like Shanghai and Beijing have introduced models such as "9073" or "9064," where 90% of elderly individuals receive home care, 7% *or* 6%receive community-based care, and the remaining 3% *or* 4%are in institutional care.

1.2.2 Community pension

Community pension represents an improvement over home care, based on family care but with services provided by the community. These services include daily care, medical rehabilitation, legal assistance, and emotional support. This model has emerged due to changes in family structures in modern Chinese society. According to the "2023 China Statistical Yearbook," the average household size in China is 2.76 people per household [8], indicating a gradual weakening of traditional family care. Moreover, due to the previous one-child policy, many families can only have one child, resulting in children having to balance caring for both their parents and their own children. Thus, community pension serves as an important supplement to family care.

In modern society, community pension has become a significant trend in elderly care services. This model not only provides basic facilities for elderly individuals but also reduces the caregiving burden on family members significantly, allowing elderly individuals to receive more specialized care services [9] and enhancing their quality of life effectively.

1.2.3 Institutional endowment

Institutional endowment involves sending elderly individuals to specialized facilities for care. Many families opt for this model when elderly individuals are older or experience symptoms of disability or dementia, requiring specialized care and assistance from institutions. These institutions can be either for-profit or non-profit. Non-profit institutions include welfare homes and geriatric care homes, which primarily rely on government subsidies. However, due to limited funding in some areas, these institutions may lack adequate infrastructure to meet healthcare standards, failing to fully satisfy the needs of the elderly. In recent years, with rising living standards and an increasing elderly population, private for-profit care homes have proliferated. These institutions offer comprehensive services such as daily living assistance, medical care, recreational activities, and emotional support, effectively meeting the diverse needs of the elderly.

1.3 Impact of policy on the development of Chinese pension agencies

1.3.1 China's development policy for pension agencies in the past decades

China's pension policies have evolved over more than 70 years, gradually forming a basic pension insurance system where the government, enterprises, and individuals share responsibilities, effectively improving the quality of life for the elderly (Table 1.4). Since the founding of the People's Republic of China, pension policies have undergone four stages of development: initial exploration, preliminary establishment during the early stages of reform and opening up, rapid development in the early 21st century, and overall advancement in the new era [10]. Initially, urban areas in China relied on government relief and corporate pension systems, with families and enterprises responsible for providing care for urban elderly individuals. In rural areas, traditional family care continued, supplemented by the "Five Guarantees" policy for destitute elderly individuals.

During the early stages of reform and opening up, China's pension policies entered a phase of preliminary exploration. Urban enterprise employees' social insurance pension policies were established during this period [11], while rural social pension insurance policies also began to develop. In the 21st century, China's pension service policies have become more systematic, with home care and community care gaining prominence. Since entering the new era of socialism with Chinese characteristics, China's aging population has continued to deepen, prompting ongoing improvements and maturation of pension policies. Under top-level designs, China has established a diversified pension service system based on home care, supported by community care, and supplemented by institutional care, with initial developments in medical and smart aging.

During the evolution of pension policies in the 21st century, there has been a continual increase in policy quantity and improvement in content. The focus has shifted from "basic security" to "healthy aging," expanding from serving "low-income elderly" and "elderly without family support" to encompassing all elderly individuals. The emphasis has transitioned from purely material security to providing both material and spiritual support. Overall, since the beginning of the new century, China's pension services have gradually shifted towards high-quality development [12].

1.3.2 Contradictions in the development of pension institutions

1.3.2.1 Accelerated aging leads to difficulty in meeting massive elderly care needs

By the end of 2020, China's elderly population had reached 264 million, accounting for 18.7%of the total population. Currently, China's aging population is rapidly increasing, leading to a massive demand for elderly care services.

Table 1.4 Key pension policy documents

Issue time	*Policy name*
1994.01	Regulations on the Work of Rural Five Guarantees Subsistence Programme
1996.08	Law of the People's Republic of China on the Protection of Rights and Interests of the Elderly
2000.08	Decision of the CPC Central Committee and the State Council on Strengthening the Work of the Elderly
2001.07	Circular of the State Council on the Issuance of the Outline of the Tenth Five-Year Plan for the Development of the Elderly in China
2006.01	Regulations on the Work of Rural Five Guarantees Subsistence Programme
2006.04	Opinions of the State Council on Strengthening and Improving Community Service Work
2011.09	Circular of the State Council on the Issuance of the Twelfth Five-Year Plan for the Development of the Elderly in China
2011.11	Circular of the State Council on the Issuance of the Twelfth Five-Year Plan for National Population Development
2012.07	Circular of the State Council on the Issuance of the National Twelfth Five-Year Plan for Basic Public Service System
2012.12	Law of the People's Republic of China on the Protection of the Rights and Interests of the Elderly (2012 Revision)
2012.10	Circular of the State Council on the Issuance of the Twelfth Five-Year Plan for Health Care Development
2013.09	Several Opinions of the State Council on Accelerating the Development of the Elderly Service Industry
2013.09	Several Opinions on Promoting the Development of Health Service Industry
2015.04	Law of the People's Republic of China on the Protection of the Rights and Interests of the Elderly (amended in 2015)
2016.10	Outline of the "Healthy China 2030" Plan
2016.12	Circular of the State Council on the Issuance of the 13th Five-Year Plan for Health and Health Care
2016.12	Circular of the State Council on the Issuance of the National Population Development Plan (2016–2030)
2017.01	Circular of the State Council on the Issuance of the 13th Five-Year Plan for National Education Development
2017.02	Circular of the State Council on the Issuance of the 13th Five-Year Plan for the Development of the National Ageing Programme and the Construction of the Pension System
2018.09	The Central Committee of the Communist Party of China and the State Council issued the Strategic Plan for Rural Revitalisation (2018–2022).
2018.12	Law of the People's Republic of China on the Protection of Rights and Interests of the Elderly (2018 Amendment)
2019.06	Opinions of the State Council on the Implementation of Healthy China Action
2013.09	Opinions of the State Council on Accelerating the Development of the Elderly Service Industry
2017.02	The "13th Five-Year Plan" for the Development of the National Elderly Programme and the Construction of the Elderly System
2020.09	Measures for the Administration of Nursing Care Institutions
2021.03	Outline of the Fourteenth Five-Year Plan for National Economic and Social Development of the People's Republic of China and the Vision for 2035
2021.12	National Plan for the Development of the Elderly and the Elderly Service System in the Fourteenth Five-Year Plan
2023.05	Opinions on Promoting the Construction of a Basic Elderly Service System

Table 1.5 Prevalence of self-reported physician-diagnosed chronic diseases among persons aged 60 and over [13]

Type of disease	*Rate (%)*	*Type of disease*	*Rate (%)*
Hypertension	39.1	Stroke	4.6
Dyslipidemia	17.2	Kidney disease	7.9
Diabetes	11.1	Digestive diseases	24.1
Cancer	1.4	Mental problems	2.0
Lung disease	14.2	Memory disorders	3.8
Liver disease	4.8	Arthritis/Rheumatoid	38.0
Heart disease	20.2	Asthma	6.0

Additionally, elderly individuals often face more health threats. According to data from the Peking University China Health and Retirement Longitudinal Study Group [13], 78.9%of elderly individuals report being diagnosed with at least one chronic disease (Table 1.5). The diseases with the highest prevalence rates include hypertension, dyslipidemia, pulmonary diseases, heart diseases, digestive system diseases, and arthritis/rheumatism.

This indicates that China's large, rapidly growing, and structurally complex elderly population poses a severe challenge to elderly care services. Due to the inadequate construction of China's pension security system and insufficient service capabilities, there is a gap in pension services, and it is unable to meet the demands of rapid aging.

1.3.2.2 Imbalance between supply and demand in pension institutions

There is a significant urban-rural imbalance in the spatial distribution of pension institutions. Compared to urban areas, rural areas have many empty-nest elderly individuals but often lack pension institutions, making it difficult to meet elderly care needs. Furthermore, the distribution and density of pension facilities and beds are heavily influenced by local economic levels. In developed areas like Beijing and Shanghai, high-quality pension institutions are in high demand, while in underdeveloped areas, there is a severe problem of vacant beds in pension institutions. This situation partly results from limited financial resources at the local government level, which makes it challenging to invest more in pension institutions and add service facilities, thereby failing to meet the needs of the elderly in terms of medical services and hardware facilities. Additionally, weak consumption capabilities among local elderly individuals make it difficult for them to afford the financial expenses of residing in pension institutions. Traditional beliefs and the lack of personalized services in pension institutions also have a significant negative impact.

1.3.2.3 Contradictions between small family sizes and traditional views on elderly care

Since the 1970s-1980s, China has implemented the one-child policy, allowing each family to have only one child. Most of the children born during that time have now reached the stage of marriage and childbearing. Consequently, the family structure mostly exhibits an "inverted pyramid" shape, known as the "4–2–1" model (four elderly, one couple, one child) [6]. This has led to a situation where middle-aged individuals often face the dual pressure of caring for both the elderly and children. Consequently, many families opt for community or institutional elderly care. However, influenced by traditional views, most elderly individuals prefer to be cared for at home, enjoying the intimacy and sense of belonging, and rejecting the collective elderly care model. This perspective faces significant challenges and constraints in modern society. On the one hand, middle-aged individuals face significant life pressures, making it difficult for them to find time and energy to care for the elderly. On the other hand, rapid social changes have led to significant differences in ideologies, lifestyles, and habits between young and elderly people. Living together inevitably leads to conflicts, affecting family harmony. Against this backdrop, community and institutional elderly care in China also face enormous demand.

1.3.2.4 Shortage of nursing professionals

Both community-based and institutional elderly care in China face a shortage of nursing professionals. Data shows that there are currently only over 500,000 elderly care nurses in China, facing a shortage of over a million. The main reasons for the shortage of nursing staff are their long working hours, high intensity, and low income. Nursing work is tedious and demanding, with high pressure, but salaries are generally low, leading many young people to reject careers in elderly care nursing. Furthermore, the elderly care nursing workforce in China also exhibits characteristics of low educational and skill levels, low social status, and older age. Due to the scarcity of professional nursing staff, the quality of nursing services varies greatly in many regions, posing significant challenges to elderly care services.

1.3.3 Analysis of the contradiction between supply and demand for pension institutions

This paper selects 10 representative cities in China to analyze the supply-demand contradiction of care homes. These cities are mainly provincial capitals, with significant differences in economic levels, distribution areas, and developmental histories, providing comprehensive reflections on the distribution patterns of care homes and existing supply-demand issues in various cities across China. The selected cities include Shanghai, Tianjin, Hohhot, Harbin, Xi'an, Changsha, Kunming, Guangzhou, Shenzhen, and Sanya.

In these cities, Shanghai and Tianjin are municipalities directly under the central government, economically developed, and have a relatively large number of care homes. Changsha, Xi'an, Kunming, Hohhot, and Harbin are provincial capitals in China, distributed in different regions of the country, with varying economic levels. Among them, Kunming and Hohhot have a relatively high population of ethnic minorities, and their lifestyles and elderly care models may differ from those of the Han Chinese population. Guangzhou, Sanya, and Shenzhen are all located in the southern region of China, with Guangzhou being a provincial capital with a long history; Shenzhen is a newly developed city that achieved rapid economic development in the 1980s with support from the state and government; Sanya is a tourist city, with care homes mainly consisting of holiday apartments and health care centers. Due to different urban characteristics, these three cities also have different elderly care models. Therefore, based on the previous analysis, this paper takes these 10 representative cities as examples to analyze the distribution of care homes, with specific details provided in Table 1.6. Additionally, since some cities have districts, counties, and ethnic autonomous counties under their jurisdiction, with significant differences in economic development levels among different regions, this section mainly focuses on the municipal districts of each city.

1.3.3.1 Spatial distribution of care homes and number of beds

The data for this subsection is obtained from the following sources: (1) Care home data, collected using Python software to scrape data from elderly care websites. The data includes building names, addresses, bed numbers, fee ranges, and types of institutions. Simultaneously, the list of care homes published by various

Table 1.6 Selected cities' characteristics

Name	*Administrative ranking*	*Region*	*Land area(km²)*	*Gross domestic product (100 million yuan)*	*City scale*	*Permanent population (1,0000 persons)*
Shanghai	municipality	East China	6340.5	44652.8	Megacity	2475
Tianjin	municipality	North China	11926.34	16311.34	Megacity	1363
Hohhot	provincial capital	North China	17188.2	3329.1	Type I Large City	355.1
Harbin	provincial capital	Northeast China	53076.4	53516638	Supercity	943.17
Xi'an	provincial capital	Northwest China	10096.81	11486.51	Megacity	1299.59
Changsha	provincial capital	Central China	11818	13966.11	Megacity	1042.06
Canton	provincial capital	South China	7434.4	28839	Megacity	1881.06
Shenzhen	–	South China	1997.47	32387.68	Megacity	1766.18
Sanya	–	South China	1921	847.1	Type II Large City	106.59
Kunming	provincial capital	Southwest China	21012.53	7541.37	Supercity	860

municipal governments' websites includes building names, addresses, bed numbers, and opening times. The data obtained from these two sources is collated, duplicates are removed, and an integrated list of care homes in each city is obtained. (2) Economic and elderly population data for each city. Mainly based on the statistical yearbooks of provinces and cities for 2022/2023, combined with data from the seventh national census bulletin to obtain relevant data for different districts of each city.

The study introduces the geographic spatial analysis method of GIS to explore the aggregation and distribution of care homes and bed numbers in the aforementioned 10 cities. The kernel density analysis method in GIS can be used to calculate the unit density of point and line elements in the neighborhood, effectively reflecting the spatiotemporal distribution characteristics of various elements [14]. Therefore, in this study, this method is used to analyze the care homes in each city visually, and the results are shown in Figure 1.1.

From Figure 1.1, it is discernible that care homes in Shenzhen predominantly inhabit the southern region of the city, with a notable concentration in the Futian and Yantian districts. The distribution of eldercare beds is primarily situated in the southwest, encompassing areas such as Bao'an, Nanshan, Futian, and Luohu districts. In Sanya, care homes are largely situated in the southern part of the city, with a sparse scattering of facilities in the eastern regions. The spatial distribution of care homes and bed capacities in this city aligns with locations primarily in the

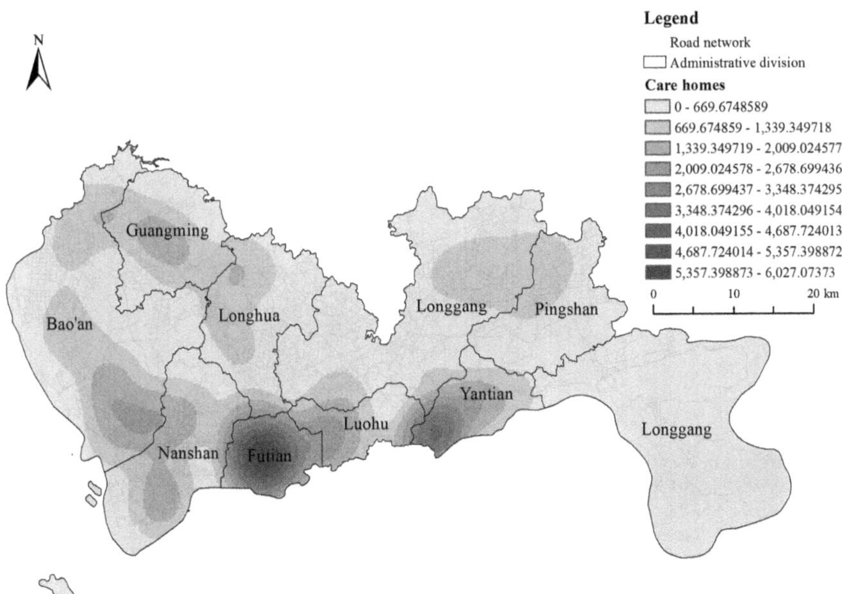

a) Distribution of care homes in Shenzhen

Figure 1.1(a-t) Spatial distribution of care homes and beds in municipal districts by city

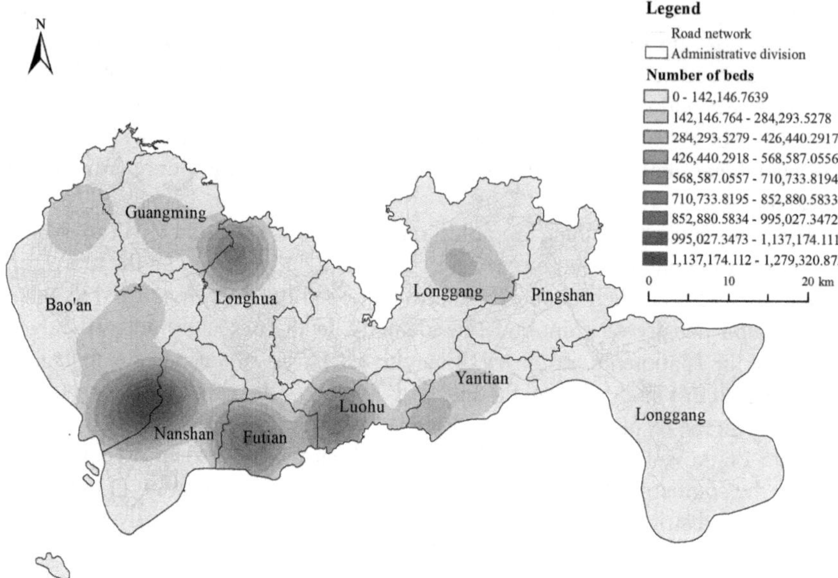

b) Distribution of elderly bed number in Shenzhen

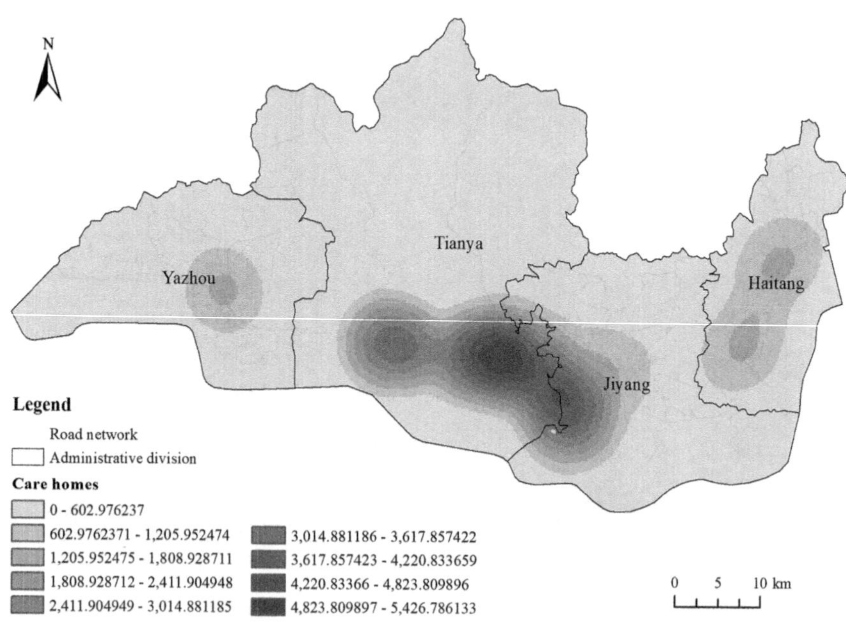

c) Distribution of care homes in Sanya

Figure 1.1(a-t) (Continued)

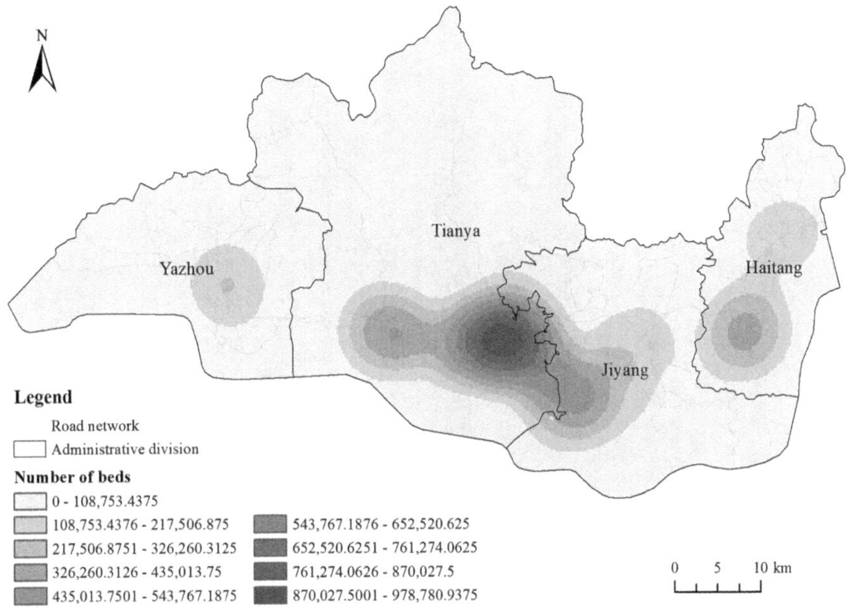

d) Distribution of elderly bed number in Sanya

Figure 1.1(a-t) (Continued)

southern expanse of Tianya district and the western precincts of Jiyang district. Care homes and bed numbers in Guangzhou are predominantly dispersed in the southwest, with a concentration in Liwan, Yuexiu, Haizhu, Tianhe, and Baiyun districts.

In Kunming, a city with a substantial ethnic minority population, aside from the urban core, there are also county-level cities and autonomous counties designated for ethnic minorities. Owing to the inclusion of counties within its urban fabric, Kunming's urban landscape is bifurcated in Figure 1.1g: the northeastern segment is represented by Dongchuan district, which hosts relatively few care homes, whereas the southwestern sector comprises the principal urban area, including Guandu, Chenggong, and Panlong districts. The figure reveals that the distribution of care homes and bed numbers in Kunming is congruent, with a concentration at the nexus of Wuhua, Panlong, Guandu, and Xishan districts.

Care homes and bed numbers in Xi'an are primarily situated in Lianhu, Xincheng, Beilin, and Yanta districts, with additional dispersion in Baqiao, Weiyang, and Chang'an districts. In Tianjin, care homes are predominantly clustered in the central urban area, specifically in Nankai, Hedong, Hebei, Heping, Hexi, and Hongqiao districts, with comparatively fewer facilities in Beichen, Dongli, and Xiqing districts, exhibiting similar patterns in bed distribution.

Shanghai, topping the 2022 Chinese city GDP ranking, also boasts a leading position in terms of the number of care homes. Consistent with the aforementioned

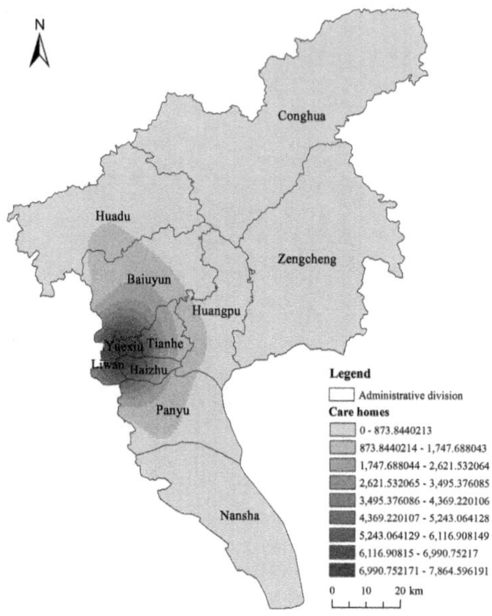

e) Distribution of care homes in Canton

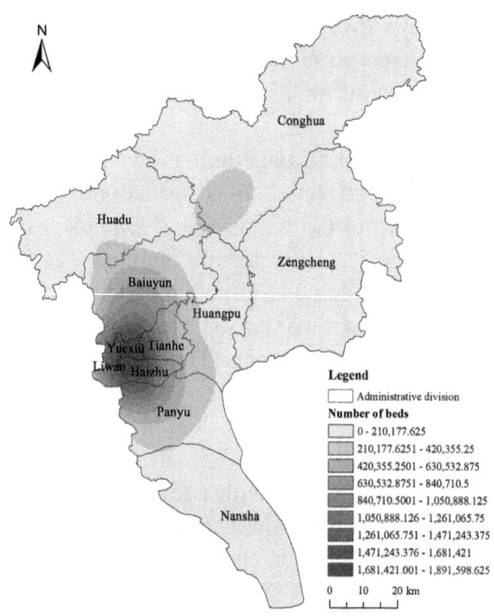

f) Distribution of elderly bed number in Canton

Figure 1.1(a-t) (Continued)

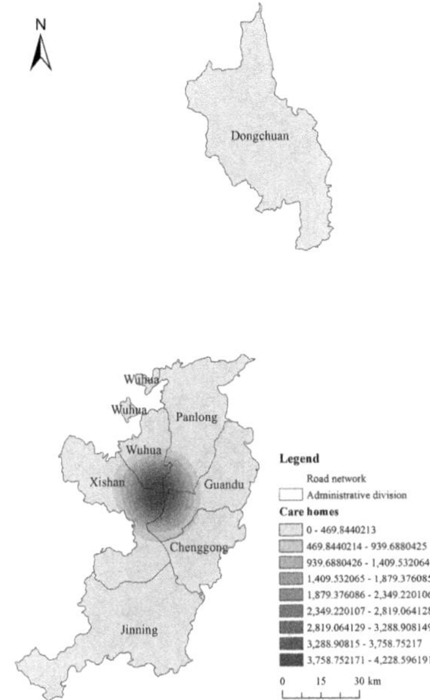

g) Distribution of care homes in Kunming

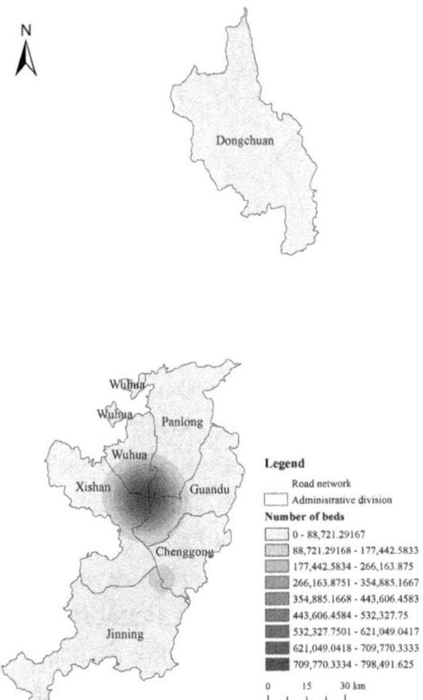

h) Distribution of elderly bed number in Kunming

Figure 1.1(a-t) (Continued)

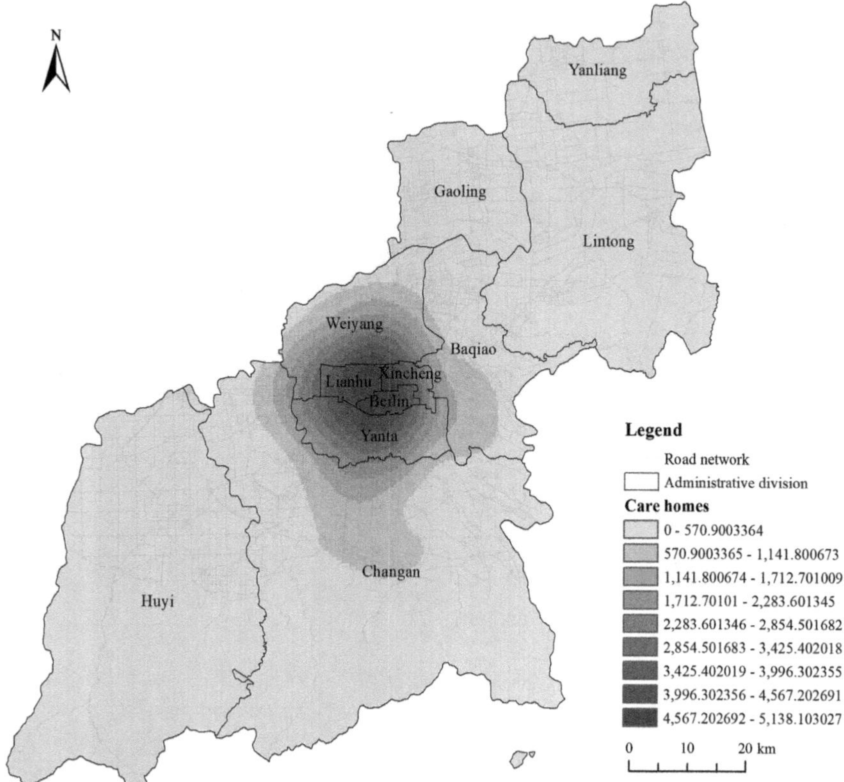

i) Distribution of care homes in Xi'an

Figure 1.1(a-t) (Continued)

cities, care homes and bed numbers in Shanghai are concentrated in economically robust areas such as Jing'an, Hongkou, Huangpu, Putuo, Xuhui, Yangpu, and Changning districts, with some presence in Baoshan, Jiading, Minhang, and Pudong New Area, and a lesser extent in other areas.

In contrast to the aforementioned patterns, the distribution of care homes and bed numbers in Changsha, Hohhot, and Harbin diverges. In Changsha, care homes are predominantly situated in the southeastern quadrant of the urban expanse, at the confluence of Kaifu, Furong, Yuelu, and Tianxin districts, whereas bed numbers are primarily dispersed in the central and southeastern regions, with a concentration in Wangcheng, Furong, and Tianxin districts, accompanied by some presence in the northern reaches of Yuelu and the southern precincts of Kaifu district. Hohhot, the capital of the Inner Mongolia Autonomous Region, renowned for its sizable

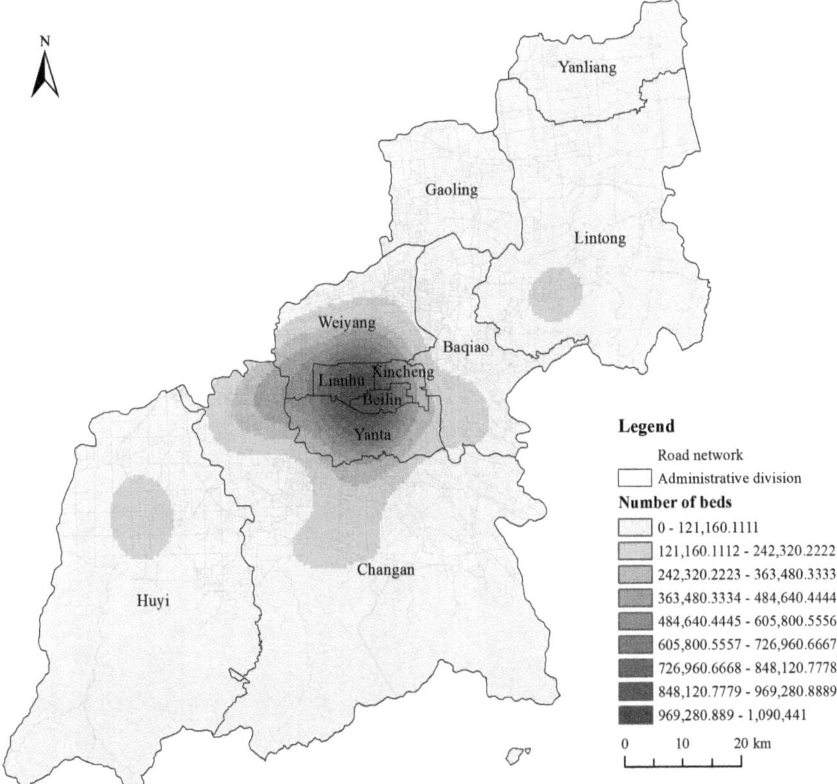

j) Distribution of elderly bed number in Xi'an

Figure 1.1(a-t) (Continued)

ethnic minority populace, encompasses a comparatively diminutive urban jurisdiction consisting of four districts, four counties, and one Tumed Left Banner. From Figures 1.1q-r, it is evident that care homes in Hohhot are predominantly arrayed along the western flank of the urban area, with a notably dense concentration at the confluence of Yuquan and Huimin districts, augmented by some distribution in the central zone. Elderly care beds are primarily situated on the western side and within the central precinct of the urban area, with a focus in Yuquan and the northern sector of Saihan districts, complemented by some presence in the southern regions of Huimin and Xincheng districts. Harbin, nestled in China's frigid northeastern territory, exhibits a concentration of its care homes in the central urban area, particularly dense at the nexus of Xiangfang, Nangang, Daoli, Songbei, and Daowai districts. Elderly care beds are predominantly distributed in Songbei

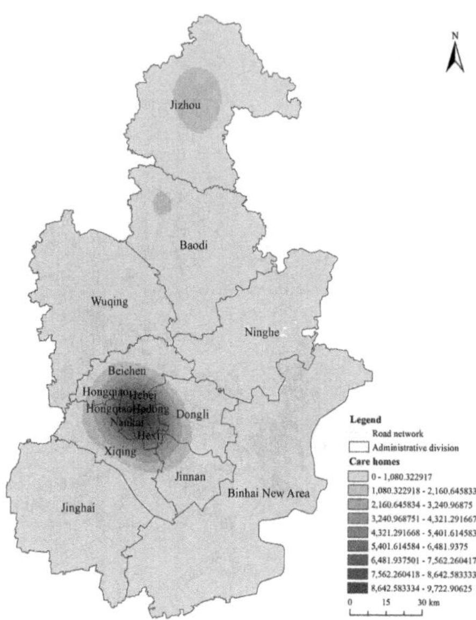

k) Distribution of care homes in Tianjin

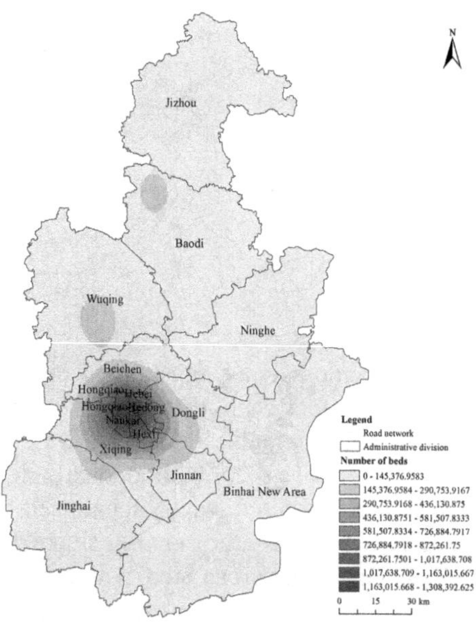

l) Distribution of elderly bed number in Tianjin

Figure 1.1(a-t) (Continued)

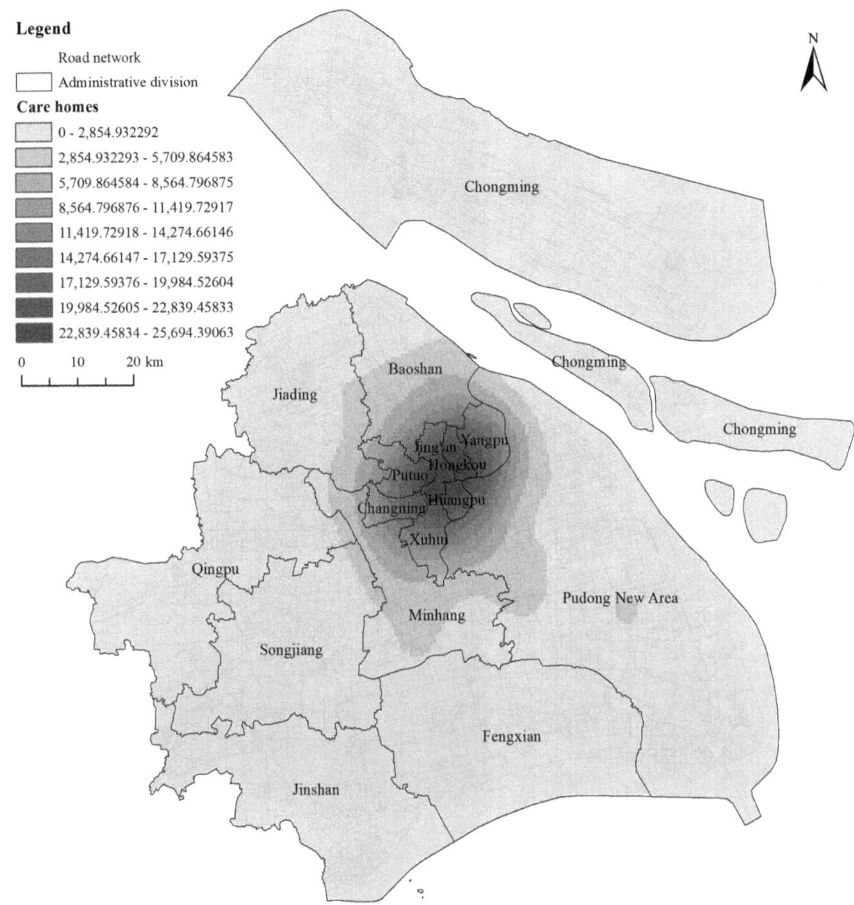

m) Distribution of care homes in Shanghai

Figure 1.1(a-t) (Continued)

district, followed by Daoli, Nangang, Xiangfang, and Daowai districts, with additional dispersion in Shuangcheng and Acheng districts.

In summary, the core areas of care homes and bed distribution exhibit a general consistency across various cities (such as Guangzhou, Kunming, Sanya, Shanghai, etc.), albeit with some cities manifesting significant disparities in the distribution of these two elements (such as Hohhot, Shenzhen, Changsha, Harbin). Furthermore, care homes and bed numbers are predominantly concentrated in economically developed areas characterized by dense road networks, underscoring the pivotal role of economic level in the establishment and scale of care homes.

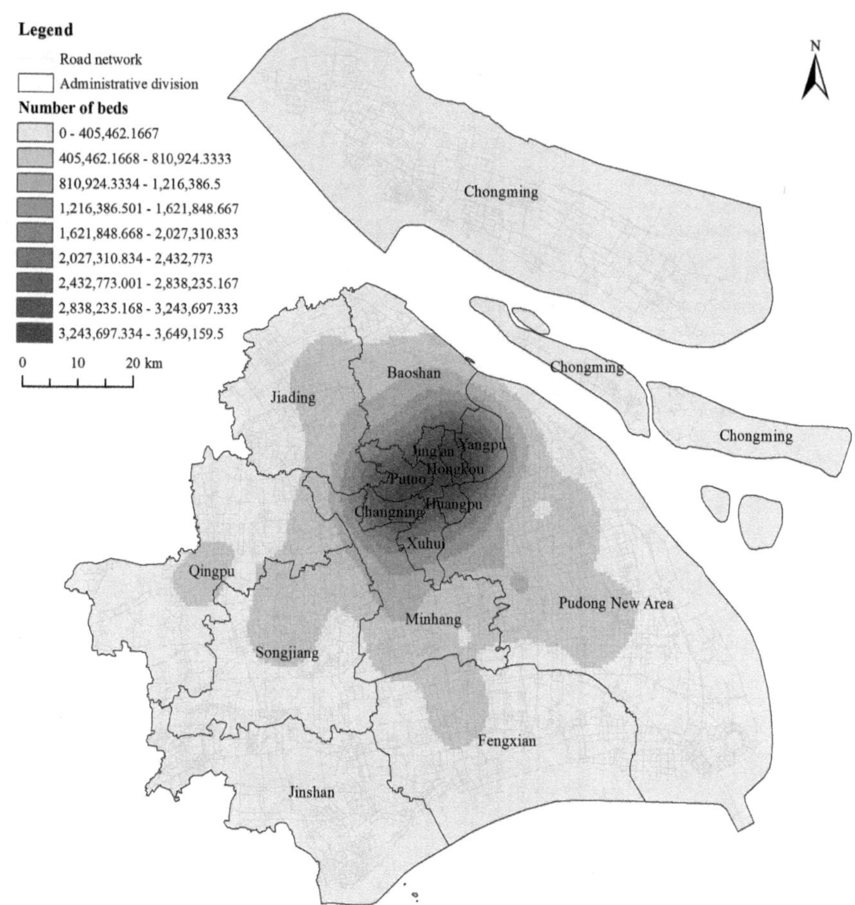

n) Distribution of elderly bed number in Shanghai

Figure 1.1(a-t) (Continued)

1.3.3.2 Analysis of factors influencing care homes construction and supply-demand issues

The determinants influencing the construction of care homes and the analysis of supply and demand issues are scrutinized. Employing SPSS 27.0to investigate the correlation between the number of care homes across various cities and other variables (Table 1.7), it is discerned that the number of care homes exhibits the strongest association with the number of beds in select cities, such as Shanghai, Hohhot, and Xi'an, whereas, in other cities, no correlation exists between these two metrics. Additionally, in certain cities, care homes demonstrate a positive

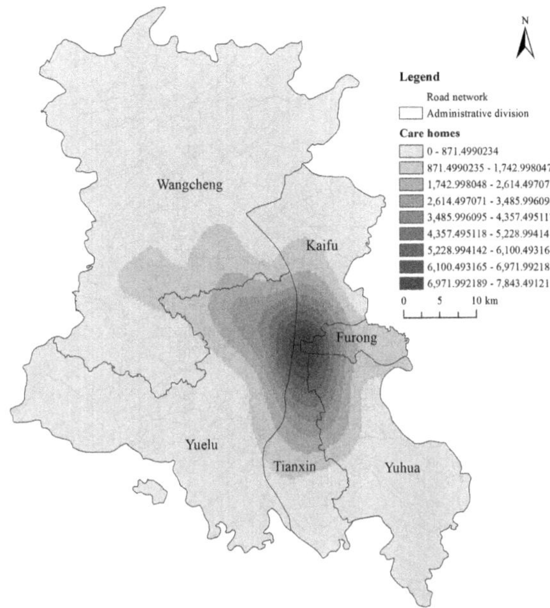

o) Distribution of care homes in Changsha

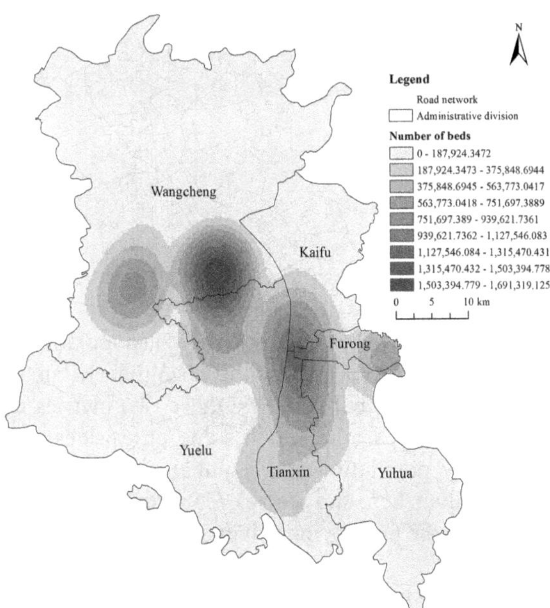

p) Distribution of elderly bed number in Changsha

Figure 1.1(a-t) (Continued)

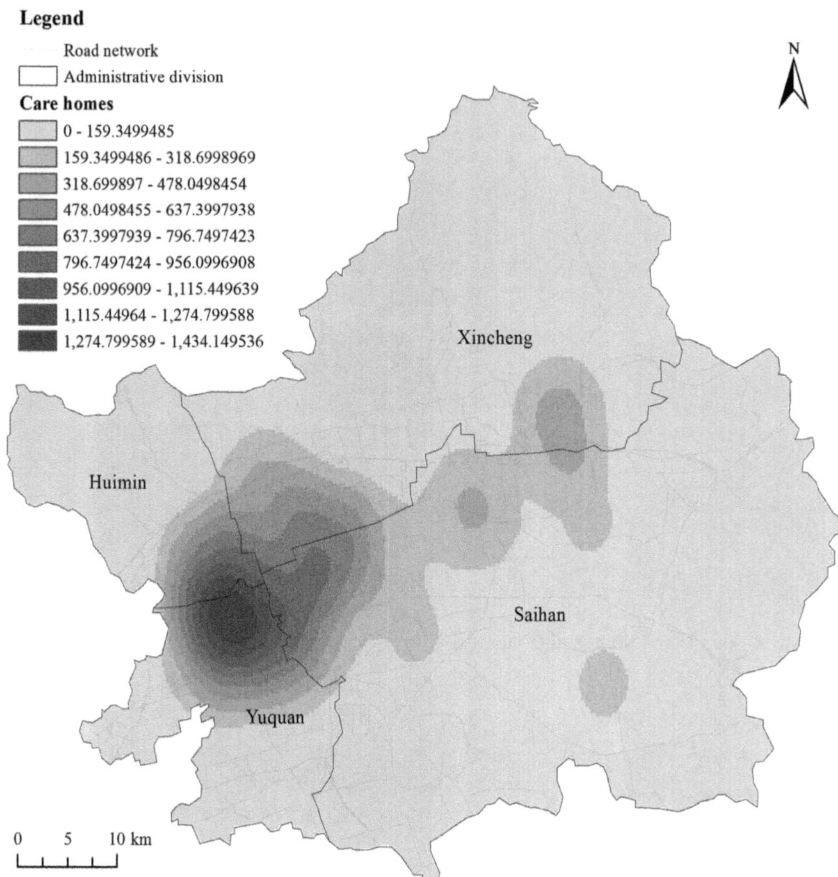

q) Distribution of care homes in Hohhot

Figure 1.1(a-t) (Continued)

correlation with indicators of the elderly population (population number/population density/population proportion), including Shanghai, Xi'an, Guangzhou, and Changsha, yet in a greater number of cities, these two metrics do not correlate. Intriguingly, the number of care homes in some cities does not correlate with indicators of the elderly population and regional economic development level (e.g., Tianjin, Harbin, Shenzhen, and Sanya). Consequently, further investigation is warranted to elucidate the underlying drivers of urban care homes construction and development.

Subsequently, utilizing SPSS 27.0 to analyze the correlation between the number of eldercare beds within each city's urban areas and other variables (Table 1.8), it is observed that the correlation between the number of eldercare beds and the

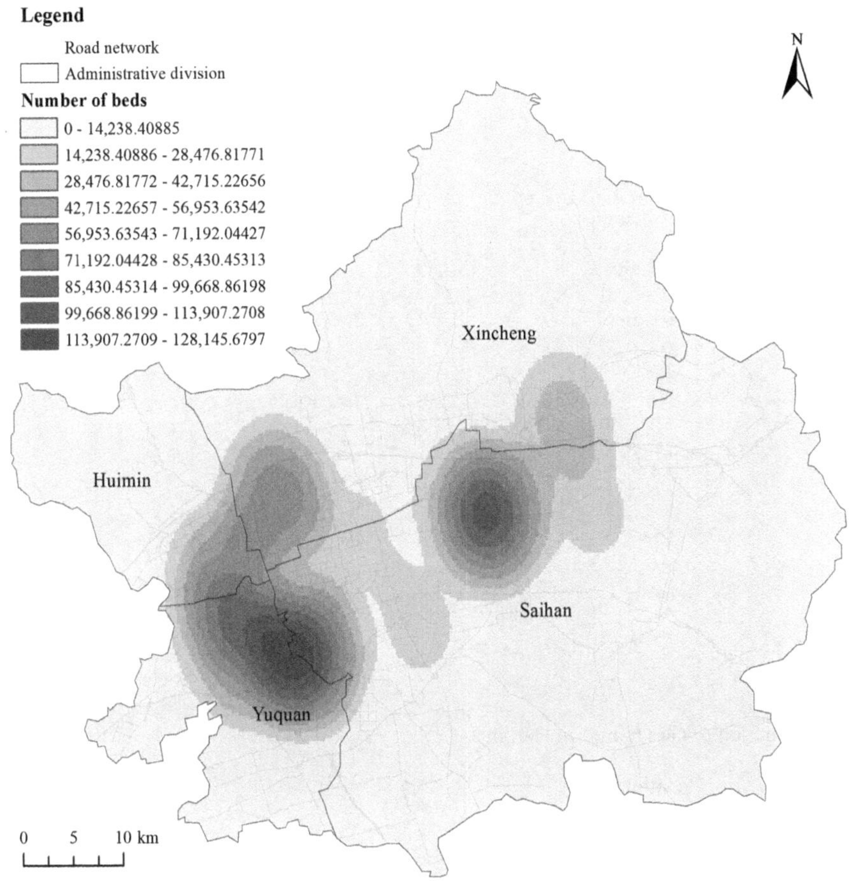

r) Distribution of elderly bed number in Hohhot

Figure 1.1(a-t) (Continued)

number of care homes is most pronounced. In comparison to the analysis outcomes presented in Table 1.7, the correlation between the number of beds and the level of regional economic development has diminished, with Shanghai showcasing the most robust correlation in this context. Moreover, the correlation between the number of eldercare beds and indicators of the elderly population has also waned, with only Shanghai and Guangzhou evidencing a significant correlation between the number of beds and the elderly population. These findings may suggest that the eldercare service development in these two cities is more advanced and, to a certain extent, mirrors the prevalent issue of imbalance between bed capacity and the elderly population in China.

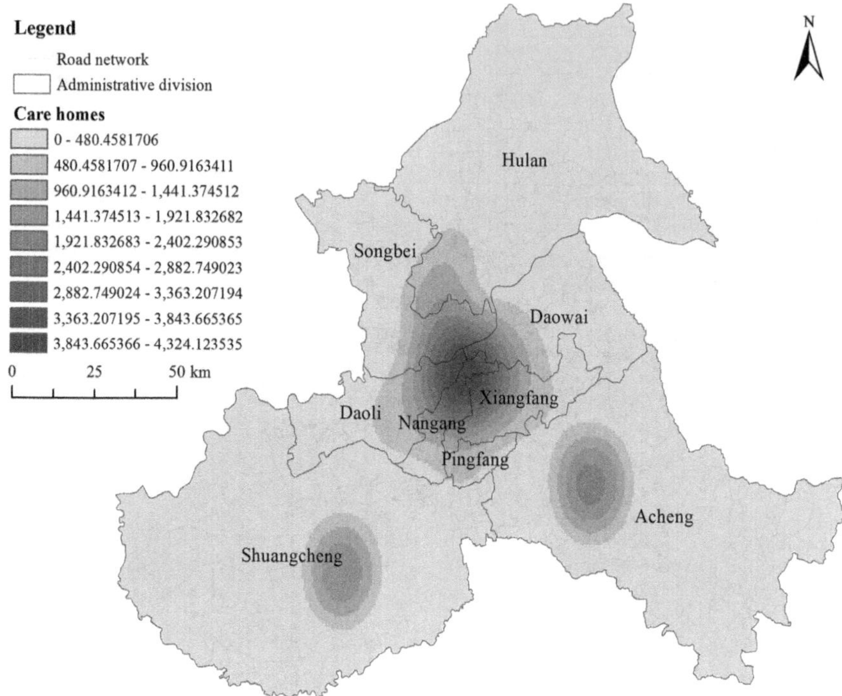

s) Distribution of care homes in Harbin

Figure 1.1(a-t) (Continued)

1.4 Conclusion

As the phenomenon of population aging intensifies, China confronts a burgeoning demand for eldercare services, rendering elderly care a salient societal concern. With the progressive refinement and maturation of pertinent eldercare policies, China has cultivated a diversified eldercare service framework, predominantly anchored in home care, community support, and institutional supplementation. Care homes, as an integral facet of China's eldercare services, are pivotal in elevating the quality of life for the elderly. Nevertheless, China currently grapples with a pronounced imbalance between supply and demand in care homes, with extant institutions and bed capacity predominantly concentrated in the central and eastern regions, such as Jiangsu, Shandong, Henan, and Anhui, while the number of care homes in the western, northern, and southwestern regions remains comparatively low.

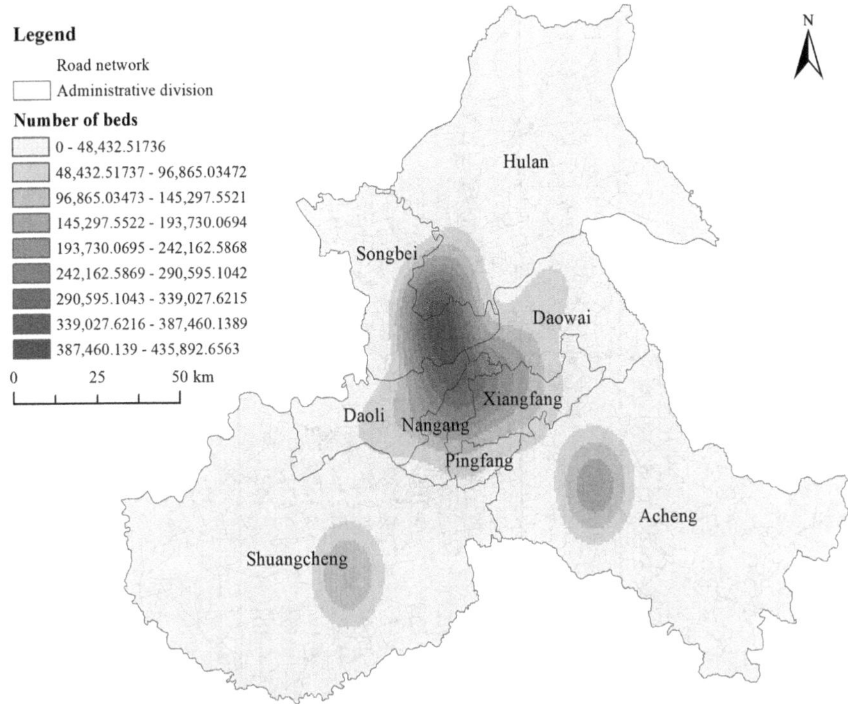

t) Distribution of elderly bed number in Harbin

Figure 1.1(a-t) (Continued)

Furthermore, the construction and evolution of care homes across various regions are frequently impeded by the level of regional economic development. Upon analyzing national care homes and economic data through SPSS software, it is revealed that the number of care homes and beds exhibits a positive correlation with regional GDP and the number of elderly populations. However, when scrutinizing data from disparate urban areas within the same city, it is observed that, in the majority of instances, there is no correlation between the number of nursing homes/beds and the number of elderly populations/regional GDP. This may indirectly underscore significant supply-demand imbalance issues within China's urban care homes. Additionally, during field investigations, it was noted that the caliber of eldercare services varies, accompanied by subpar spatial environmental quality, thereby complicating the fulfillment of the elderly's living and health needs. Consequently, there exists a necessity to investigate the spatial environment of care homes to foster the enhancement of elderly health and living standards.

Table 1.7 Correlation analysis of the number of care homes in municipal districts of cities with other factors

City	*Elderly population*	*Percentage of elderly population*	*Density of elderly population*	*GDP*	*Primary industry*	*Secondary industry*	*Tertiary industry*	*GDP per capita*	*Number of beds*
Shanghai	0.933**	−0.056	−0.117	0.937**	0.371	0.739**	0.919**	0.284	0.891**
Tianjin	0.477	0.292	0.073	−0.036	0.18	−0.02	−0.053	−0.305	0.587*
Hohhot	0.905	0.179	−0.708	0.865	0.972*	0.986*	0.618	0.646	0.651
Harbin	0.641	0.208	−0.143	0.135	0.423	−0.204	0.144	−0.522	0.497
Xi'an	0.448	−.847**	−0.14	0.809**	−0.343	0.958**	0.673*	0.28	0.802**
Changsha	0.721	−0.456	−.823*	0.049	0.66	0.224	−0.395	−0.771	0.563
Canton	0.915**	0.421	0.514	−0.013	−0.365	−0.322	0.128	−0.23	0.670*
Shenzhen	0.449	0.311	0.332	0.42	−0.192	0.135	0.446	0.314	0.823**
Sanya	0.638	−0.156	−0.06	0.544	0.554	0.121	0.545	−0.029	0.991**
Kunming	0.627	–	0.381	0.681	−0.481	0.417	0.770*	0.682	0.878**

Note: GDP = Gross domestic product.
* Significant results.

Table 1.8 Correlation analysis between the number of elderly beds and other factors in the municipal districts of each city

City	*Elderly population*	*Percentage of elderly population*	*Density of elderly population*	*GDP*	*Primary industry*	*Secondary industry*	*Tertiary industry*	*GDP per capita*	*Number of beds*
Shanghai	0.915**	−0.204	−0.221	0.864**	0.381	0.821**	0.815**	0.01	0.891**
Tianjin	0.468	−0.003	0.048	−0.018	−0.072	0.002	−0.034	−0.239	0.587*
Hohhot	0.318	−0.603	−0.066	0.292	0.56	0.723	−0.012	0	0.651
Harbin	0.219	−0.162	−0.174	0.34	−0.058	0.248	0.315	0.247	0.497
Xi'an	0.408	−0.547	−0.41	0.483	0.163	0.652*	0.358	−0.158	0.802**
Changsha	−0.093	0.01	−0.328	−0.445	0.953**	−0.188	−0.772	−0.466	0.563
Canton	0.805**	−0.105	0.001	−0.016	−0.062	−0.129	0.039	−0.421	0.670*
Shenzhen	0.632	0.053	0.148	0.527	−0.331	0.388	0.411	0.056	0.823**
Sanya	0.657	−0.265	−0.043	0.603	0.441	0.237	0.601	0.045	0.991**
Kunming	0.699	–	0.505	0.713	−0.296	0.368	0.838*	0.638	0.878**

Note: GDP = Gross domestic product.
* Significant results.

References

[1] Ning JZ. Main data of the Seventh National Population Census[J]. *China Statistics*, 2021, 36(5):4–5.

[2] Bian S, Wang YJ. Research on the level of regional system coordination in the construction of active aging society in China[J/OL]. *Journal of Xi'an Jiaotong University (Social Sciences)*, 2023 (Aug. 30), 1–20. (In Chinese)

[3] Li LZ. Space management in elderly facilities from stakeholder perspectives[D]. Southeast University, 2017. (In Chinese)

[4] GB50340–2016. *Code for design of residential building for the aged*[S]. Beijing: China Architecture & Building Press, 2017.

[5] GB 50437–2007. *Code for planning of city and town facilities for the aged*[S]. Beijing: China Plan Publishing House, 2019.

[6] Jiao YW. Study on perfecting the system of China's community & home-based elder care service in the new era[D]. Jilin University, 2023. (In Chinese)

[7] Barnay T, Juin S. Does home care for dependent elderly people improve their mental health?[J]. *Journal of Health Economics*, 2016, 45:149–160.

[8] National Bureau of Statistics of the People's Republic of China. *China statistical yearbook*[M]. Beijing: China Statistics Press, 2023.

[9] Mu JY. The evaluation and optimization strategy of suitable ageing of urban residential communities in cold regions from the perspective of community micro renewal[D]. Harbin Institute of Technology, 2022. (In Chinese)

[10] Du Y. Research on the changes of China's elderly care service policy since the founding of new China[D]. Donghua University, 2021. (In Chinese)

[11] Chen M. The course of China's caring for the aged policy change and the path to perfection[D]. Jilin University, 2018. (In Chinese)

[12] Han Y, Fu JP. Policy supply of elderly care services: Evolution, governance framework, future direction[J]. *Lanzhou Academic Journal*, 2020, (09):187–198. (In Chinese)

[13] Zhao Y, Hu Y, Smith JP, Strauss J, Yang G. (2014). Cohort profile: The China Health and Retirement Longitudinal Study (CHARLS). *International Journal of Epidemiology*, 2014, 43(1):61–68.

[14] Zhao F, Cai J, Zhang C, et al. Spatiotemporal characteristic of Biantun toponymical landscape for the evolution of Biantun culture in Yunnan, China[J]. 2021. *Scientific Reports*, 2021, 11:23791.

2 The acoustic environment of care homes

2.1 Case study and site survey

2.1.1 Introduction

As the global aging population continues to expand, the existing eldercare system is increasingly challenged to meet the escalating needs of the elderly [1]. Enhancing and optimizing the spatial environment of care homes has progressively attracted attention. In accordance with the (JGJ450–2018) [2], care homes are expected to provide environments that are conducive to fostering the health of the elderly. Health has emerged as one of the fundamental criteria for assessing the spatial environment of care homes.

As an integral facet of the physical environment, the acoustic environment holds significant sway over the physical and mental health of the elderly. The aforementioned standards also delineate specific requirements for the indoor and outdoor acoustic environment of care homes, encompassing aspects such as the site environment noise limit, indoor and outdoor noise level regulations, adjacent room air noise limit, occupant-centric performance-based indicators like reverberation time, and advocate the utilization of natural environmental soundscapes to augment the comfort of the elderly living environment.

The architectural acoustic environment is inextricably linked to the well-being of residents and exerts a profound influence on their living comfort and health [3]. Nevertheless, there exists a discrepancy between China's current architectural acoustic environment standards and the actual experiences of the elderly. Furthermore, extant research underscores strong correlations between the acoustic environment and variables such as building scale and type. Under identical sound backgrounds, individuals may encounter divergent experiences and satisfaction evaluations within rooms of varying types or spatial configurations [4]. However, research on the acoustic environment of care homes amidst multiple influencing factors remains relatively sparse. Consequently, this paper will delve into the acoustic environment of care homes from perspectives including seasonal variations, functional types, building scale, and geographical regions [5], thereby advancing the health and well-being of the elderly.

DOI: 10.1201/9781003407232-2

2.1.2 Site choose

The acoustic environment of care homes exerts a profound influence on the physical and mental health of the elderly. This paper will employ on-site investigation and acoustic environment simulation methodologies to scrutinize the indoor acoustic environment of care homes. In terms of on-site acoustic environment monitoring, four representative cities in China's frigid regions – Harbin, Changchun, Shenyang, and Dalian – were selected for a year-long investigation. In accordance with the <Code for thermal design of civil building> (GB50176–2016) [6], these cities are situated in the northeastern quadrant of China, characterized by protracted and severe winters. These locales harbor a substantial elderly population, coupled with relatively modest economic conditions and a significant exodus of young individuals. Consequently, population aging has emerged as a pivotal challenge confronting these regions.

In the study, 34 care homes of varying scales and types were chosen for a year-long on-site investigation to ascertain the current indoor acoustic environment status of care homes in northeastern China [5]. These care homes were categorized based on indicators such as geographical location and scale (Table 2.1). To examine the impact of different seasons on indoor acoustic environments, the entire investigation was conducted across three seasons.

The surveyed care homes are equipped to provide accommodation, leisure, and rehabilitation services for the elderly. Table 2.2 enumerates the specific conditions of the surveyed care homes, encompassing building area, number of beds, and construction time. Based on their number of beds, the investigated care homes were stratified into small-scale (≤150), medium-scale (151–300), large-scale (301–500), and extra-large-scale (>500).

In acoustic environment research, a simulation method was also incorporated. Since simulation enables researchers to analyze indoor environments without perturbing the extant building environment, issues can be identified promptly, and corresponding improvement strategies can be proposed to enhance the quality of

Table 2.1 Classification of survey sites based on city, test season, scale and participant satisfaction

	Classification	*Number of questionnaire*	*Proportion (%)*
City	Changchun	346	23.7
	Harbin	485	33.3
	Shenyang	420	28.9
	Dalian	206	14.1
Season	Winter	402	27.6
	Summer	390	26.8
	Transition	665	45.6
Scale	Small	352	24.2
	Medium	280	19.2
	Large	625	42.9
	Super large	200	13.7

Table 2.2 Details of the surveyed care homes

Name	*City*	*Building area*	*Number of beds*	*Construction date*	*Rebuild*	*Price range*
Nansha Home for the Elderly	Dalian	4500	130	2008	no	1000–2000
Red Flag Welfare Center	Dalian	8800	260	2004	yes	1999–3199
Warm Garden Residential Aged Care Facility	Dalian	9200	300	2006	no	660–1336
Yihaizhu Apartment for the Elderly	Dalian	9000	360	2012	no	2600–5800
Jiaojinshan Retirement Center	Dalian	10000	300	2016	no	2500–3200
Jinzhou District, Social Welfare Home	Dalian	29000	750	1999	no	700–900
Songshan Residential Aged Care Facility	Dalian	9269	100	2011	no	6000–10000
longevity House Apartment for the Elderly	Dalian	4200	168	2009	yes	1600–3000
Ganjingzi District Happy Home for the Elderly	Dalian	2700	60	2010	yes	700–2300
Harbin Institute of Technology Group Apartment for the Elderly	Harbin	6050	150	2003	yes	500–1000
Harbin Runfu Apartment for the Elderly	Harbin	110000	2000	2014	no	1800–4500
Harbin Ankang Social Welfare Home	Harbin	66000	1500	2003	no	1800–3500
Harbin Kaifeng Edge Residential Aged Care Facilities	Harbin	2800	135	2015	no	1580–2680
Harbin The First Social Welfare Home	Harbin	15200	550	1998	no	500–1000
Harbin Institute of Technology Activity Center	Harbin	18000	450	2008	no	1200–2500
Harbin Chun Hua DE Shan Apartment for the Elderly	Harbin	8000	500	2017	no	800–4000
Xiangfang District: Fu Lao Nian Apartment	Harbin	3000	150	2018	no	2000–6000
Xinsongmayue Mountain aged care Apartment	Harbin	18000	292	2016	no	4000–7000
Harbin Kunlun Garden Apartment for the Elderly	Harbin	8000	200	2015	no	1300–1500
Dadong Elderly Service Center	Shenyang	10000	300	2002	no	500–1000
Shenyang Ai Da Apartment for the Elderly	Shenyang	11000	250	2012	no	1800–3000
Shenyang Huanggu District Social Welfare Home	Shenyang	9000	140	2004	yes	360–760
Shenyang Shenhe District: Rehabilitation Center for the elderly	Shenyang	4600	120	2001	yes	540–800
Shenyang Colorful Sunshine City Retirement Center	Shenyang	130000	3500	2014	no	2500–5800

(*Continued*)

Table 2.2 (Continued)

Name	*City*	*Building area*	*Number of beds*	*Construction date*	*Rebuild*	*Price range*
Shenyang Bo Yuan Old Care Center	Shenyang	5000	180	2009	yes	1500–2600
Shenyang Dawn Residential Aged Care Facilities	Shenyang	6000	265	2004	yes	700–1500
Changchun Qinqinyuan Apartment for the Elderly	Changchun	7677	200	2016	yes	6000–10000
Changchun Jian Yin Qi Xiang Yuan Retirement Center	Changchun	1600	60	2014	yes	3000–6000
Changchun Xi Hui Residential Aged Care Facilities	Changchun	6000	250	2013	yes	800–2000
Jilin Changchun Yee Lok Rehabilitation Centre	Changchun	54500	500	2015	no	1980–4800
Changchun Jingyueyikang Residential Aged Care Facilities	Changchun	28000	800	2017	no	2500–6000
Changchun Sunshine Home Residential Aged Care Facilities	Changchun	4900	290	2019	yes	2500–9500
Changchun Green Park Happy Care Home for the Elderly	Changchun	1500	110	1997	no	800–1500
Changchun Social Welfare Institute	Changchun	15000	300	2003	no	1000–3000

the spatial environment of care homes. Therefore, representative care home cases were selected for modeling and acoustic environment simulation. This section presents three cases of care homes situated in Beijing, Ma'anshan, and Guangzhou. In alignment with the (GB50176–2016) [6], they are located in cold areas, hot summer and cold winter areas, and hot summer and mild winter areas of China, respectively, exhibiting significant disparities in climatic conditions, which can to some extent mirror the differences in the architectural spatial environments of care homes across diverse regions of China. The specific conditions of each care home are delineated in Table 2.3.

2.1.2.1 Case 1-NH

Case 1-NH represents the inaugural urban comprehensive care-type elderly care facility demonstration project in China. This facility is a repurposing of an antiquated office building [7]. The original community was home to a substantial elderly population yet was devoid of corresponding care homes. Consequently, the building underwent renovation to fulfill the community's eldercare requirements. The primary service demographic of the care home comprises elderly individuals characterized by advanced age, disability, living alone, and empty nesters, offering them a spectrum of services, including care, assistance, and life support, encompassing accommodation, daytime care, and home nursing services [8].

The building boasts four floors housing 44 beds. The principal entrance is situated on the eastern facade of the building. The ground floor encompasses a lobby, reception area, nursing station, multipurpose activity hall, rehabilitation area,

Table 2.3 Basic information on care homes

Code	*Project name*	*Location*	*Opening time*	*Beds*	*Area*	*Service object*
Case 1-NH	Shoukai Cuncao Asian Sports Village home for the elderly	Beijing	2017	44	$2232.6m^2$	Disabled, semi-disabled, demented
Case 2-NH	Shabu Rong Yue Urban Elderly Care Center	Canton	2022	300	$4497m^2$	Self-care, semi-autonomous, disabled, bedridden intensive care, cognitive impairment
Case 3-NH	Zhongjiao Renyi Health and Elderly Care Center	Ma'anshan	–	254	$9235m^2$	Self-care, semi-autonomous, disabled, dementia, total care

Note: NH = Nursing Home.

dining hall, kitchen, and elderly living quarters (Figure 2.1). The second and third floors feature a common activity area, while the fourth floor houses a multipurpose hall and a rooftop platform. There are two traffic cores: one positioned centrally within the building near the common activity area and the other located at the southern terminus of the building, proximate to the elderly living quarters.

The care home implements a clustered layout, seamlessly integrating elderly living quarters with common activity areas. The common areas on each floor are strategically located in the central corner of the building and are equipped with nursing stations to facilitate timely access to elderly living quarters, thereby ensuring the provision of nursing services. All spaces within the building are meticulously designed to be age-friendly and barrier-free. Given that the original structure was a small-scale office building with a brick-concrete construction, the office dimensions of approximately $3300 * 6000mm$ generally align with the scale requirements of living spaces, necessitating no alterations to the span and depth. The elderly living quarters predominantly consist of single and double rooms, guaranteeing favorable living conditions and nursing quality.

Figure 2.1 additionally showcases photographs of the interior scenes of the corridors, communal activity areas, and elderly bedrooms within the nursing home. It is apparent that the public spaces of the care homes predominantly incorporate wooden materials, with the floors adorned with rubberized mats that possess certain sound-absorbing capabilities. The walls and ceilings of the activity areas are painted white, resulting in an interior environment that is appropriately scaled and comfortably minimalist, with the wooden tones infusing a warm and comforting atmosphere for the elderly residents. The arrangement of the elderly bedrooms is comparatively straightforward, with walls painted and not specifically treated for sound absorption. Considering that the primary clientele consists of physically and cognitively impaired seniors, the rooms are furnished with adjustable nursing beds,

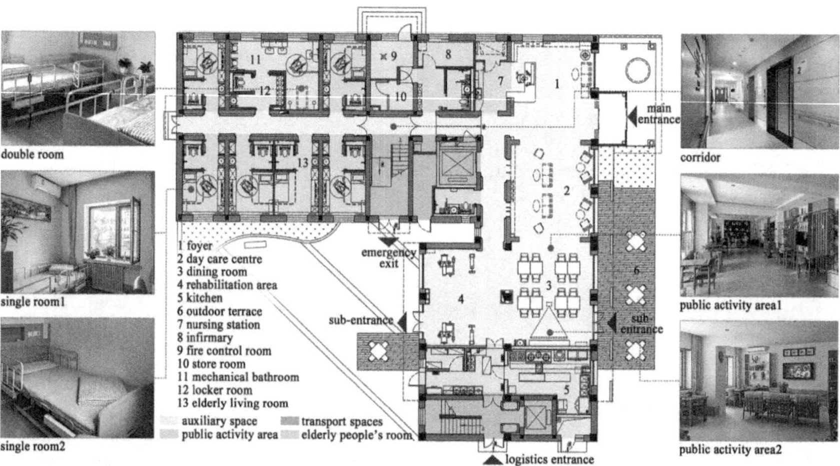

Figure 2.1 First floor plan and interior scene photograph

which, when juxtaposed with traditional beds, offer relatively less sound absorption. Overall, the acoustic environment within the bedroom spaces of the nursing home may necessitate further improvement and enhancement when contrasted with the public spaces.

2.1.2.2 Case 2-NH

Case 2-NH is situated in the Shaibu Urban Renewal Area of Huangpu district, Guangzhou. The land area is modest, measuring merely 2450 square meters. Consequently, in the design, the number of floors was augmented to expand the building scale and the number of beds. The building features a stepped design on each floor, allowing each level to encompass a landscaped terrace where elderly individuals can engage in communication and respite, which has a salutary effect on the physical and mental health and social interaction of the elderly.

The care home comprises five floors, with the first floor designated as the public area, equipped with a lobby, dining hall, rehabilitation room, medical room, conference room, kitchen, and equipment room, with traffic cores situated at both ends of the building (Figure 2.2). The second to fifth floors are residential and activity areas for the elderly. The second floor features a dining hall, unit living room, public entertainment area, nursing station, terrace, and elderly living quarters (Figure 2.3), all of which are double rooms. The layout of the third to fifth floors mirrors that of the second floor.

The image also presents the interior scenes of rooms frequently utilized by the elderly, encompassing the dining area, communal living room, and recreational zones. It is apparent that the care home's interior environment predominantly features warm color tones. Some walls and pillars are embellished with wooden veneer decorative panels, and the majority of the furniture is also wooden, offering a certain degree of

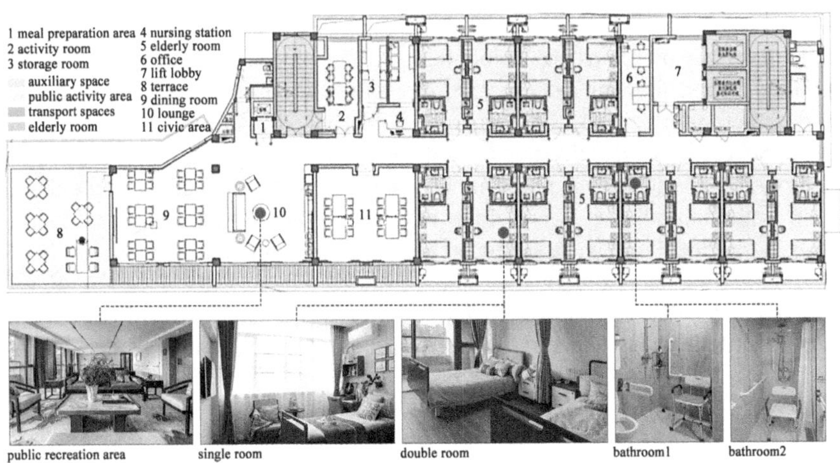

Figure 2.2 First floor plan and interior scene photograph

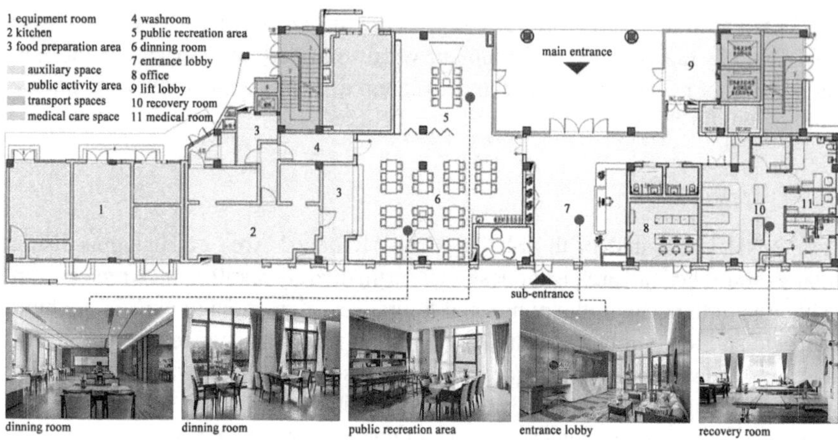

Figure 2.3 Second floor plan and interior scene photograph

sound absorption. The material combinations in the care home's public spaces are diverse; the dining and recreational areas boast wooden floors, with window-adjacent walls painted white, while the remaining walls are cloaked in wooden veneer. The material arrangement adjacent to the reading room mirrors that of the dining area. The communal living room features tiled floors with carpets spread out in seating areas and walls predominantly painted with minimal wooden veneer. The rehabilitation and care room has wooden floors, with all walls painted. Overall, the ceilings in public spaces are uniformly painted white without special sound-absorbing treatments, and while walls and furniture offer some sound absorption, the use of tiles in some rooms may result in suboptimal acoustic quality within those spaces.

Elderly living quarters can be categorized into single, double, and multi-person rooms, with double rooms being the most prevalent. Single and double rooms primarily cater to healthy seniors who can manage their daily lives independently, while multi-person rooms are mainly designed for physically and semi-physically impaired elders, allowing caregivers to attend to multiple residents simultaneously. As observed in Figure 2.3, the floors of the elderly bedrooms are all wooden, with walls and ceilings typically not treated for sound absorption. Therefore, sound absorption in the bedrooms relies mainly on the flooring and bedding. The design of the bathroom adheres to principles of aging-in-place, with the floor featuring anti-slip treatment and walls equipped with various safety grab bars according to the elderly's habits. Additionally, aging-in-place products that facilitate elderly bathing (such as mobile shower chairs) are provided, along with pull-cord alarms and call buttons that enhance safety during toileting and bathing for the residents.

2.1.2.3 Case 3-NH

Case 3-NH is situated in Ma'anshan City, Anhui Province. Its service targets are relatively comprehensive, encompassing self-care, nursing, and elderly individuals with cognitive impairment. The building integrates medical and care homes, offering services such as accommodation, medical treatment, eldercare, rehabilitation, and nursing. In terms of medical services, the center features a medical office and a rehabilitation hall equipped with departments such as general practice, rehabilitation, and traditional Chinese medicine, ensuring multi-level medical service needs for the elderly's daily diagnosis, rehabilitation, and other services.

The building comprises six floors, with the first floor being relatively compact, housing a lobby, negotiation room, and leisure reading area. The second floor is primarily dedicated to public activity spaces, including medical service areas, recreational activity areas, and dining areas (Figure 2.4a). These public areas provide leisure, entertainment, and social platforms for the elderly, fostering a pleasant living atmosphere. The third to sixth floors serve as residential and living activity areas for the elderly. Among them, the third floor caters to

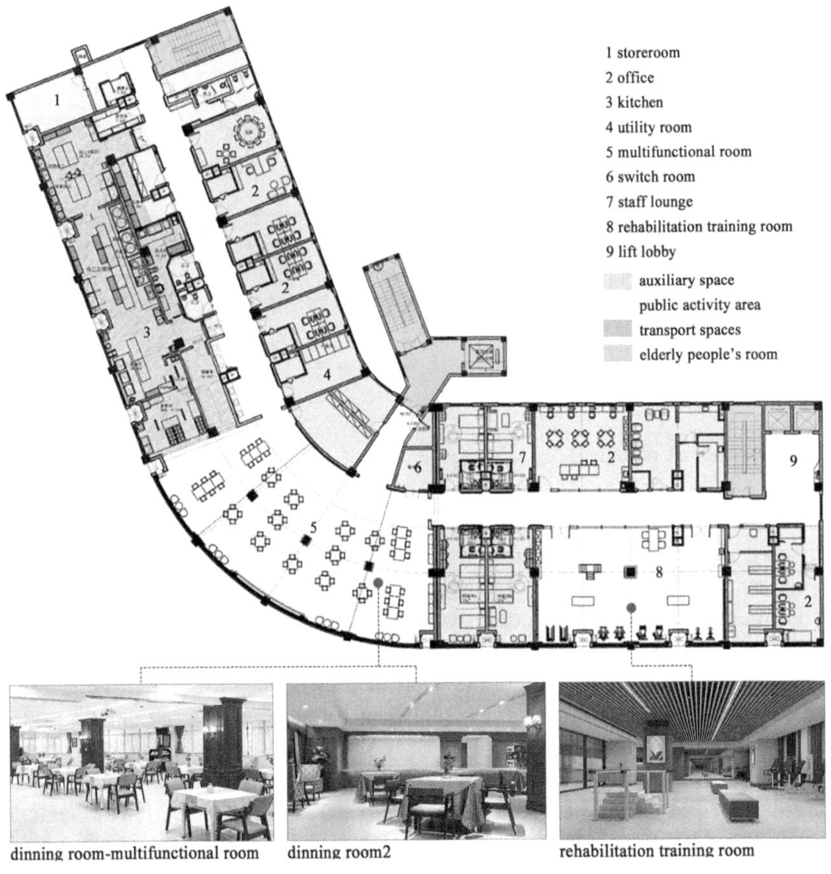

a) Second floor plan

Figure 2.4(a-b) Floor plan and interior scene photograph

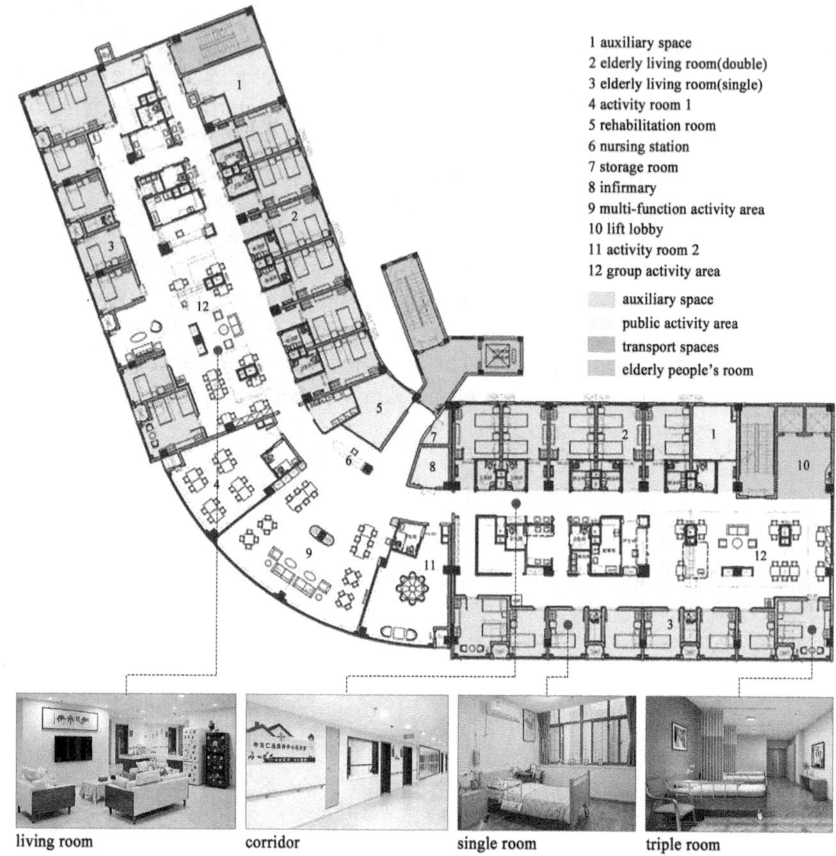

b) Sixth floor plan

Figure 2.4(a-b) (Continued)

self-care elderly living, the fourth and fifth floors accommodate disabled elderly living, and the sixth floor is designated for elderly individuals with cognitive impairment, equipped with a cognitive rehabilitation training area. The sixth floor implements a small-scale neighborhood-style clustered layout, with each cluster housing 10–20 elderly people. In the heart of each cluster, there are living rooms, activity halls, and memory spaces, realizing refined nursing services based on clusters (Figure 2.4b).

Figure 2.4 additionally showcases scenes of indoor spaces frequently utilized by the elderly in the care home. It can be discerned that, with the exception of the dining area and standard-level communal activity zones, the color scheme of other public spaces predominantly features white, with walls and ceilings painted white, and the floors covered with rubberized mats to prevent slipping and mitigate the risk of falls among the elderly. The indoor furniture is predominantly wooden, and some soft furnishings (such as sofas) possess certain sound-absorbing properties. However, due to the substantial volume of the building, the paucity of sound-absorbing materials may engender significant fluctuations in indoor sound pressure levels and protracted reverberation times, thereby diminishing the acoustic comfort for the elderly and potentially impacting their physical and mental well-being.

The standard-level elderly living quarters primarily consist of double and triple rooms, with a few VIP single rooms. The sixth-floor cognitive care specialty area mainly features single and double rooms. As depicted in Figure 2.4b, the floors of the elderly bedrooms are all wooden, with ceilings and walls predominantly white or light-colored, painted but not specifically treated for acoustics. Therefore, indoor sound absorption relies mainly on wooden floors and soft furnishings (such as beds and sofas). Given that the care home's bedrooms are predominantly double and triple rooms with larger areas, the quality of the indoor acoustic environment may be suboptimal, with potentially longer reverberation times, which could adversely affect the elderly's perception of the acoustic environment.

2.1.3 Method

Research indicates that critical indicators influencing indoor acoustic environments are sound pressure level and reverberation time [8]. Measurements of these parameters were carried out between 8:00 a.m. and 7:00 p.m. on weekdays from June 21, 2017, to May 15, 2018, and again from October 24, 2018, to March 10, 2019, in selected fixed rooms. The sound pressure level, recorded using an 801 Sound Level Meter, served as the key parameter for evaluating the acoustic environment. Each room was assessed once per season, with each assessment lasting two days. The background noise in the fixed rooms ranged from 30 to 35 dBA. Hourly data were averaged and plotted for analysis. During these measurements, sound level meters were set to a low-speed setting, and the distance from the measurement site to walls and other reflective surfaces was at least 0.999744 meters, while the height from the ground varied between 1.20091 and 1.49962 meters. If sudden noise occurred during testing, the acoustic environment tests were repeated.

In the simulation of acoustic environments, Odeon is acknowledged as the most comprehensive software for evaluating architectural acoustic performance, capable of simulating and measuring the indoor acoustic effects of care homes [9]. Consequently, the study utilized architectural drawings provided by architects to create three-dimensional models of various nursing facilities using Sketchup 2018. These models were then imported into Odeon 16 to simulate the building's acoustic environment. The analysis primarily focused on reverberation time and sound pressure level. Based on the simulation results, the study identified existing issues in the acoustic environment of care homes and proposed strategies for improvement by adjusting indoor materials and furniture arrangements. Additionally, a database of the acoustic environment of care homes was constructed using SPSS 27, and Pearson correlation and regression analyses were conducted to explore the influence of factors such as the scale, type, functional spaces, and seasons of care homes on the measured values.

2.2 Sound pressure level of care homes

Through field investigations, it was discovered that the primary activity areas for the elderly are the activity room and the bedroom. Consequently, the acoustic environment data of these two types of rooms were the main focus of the measurements, with some care homes' test data illustrated in Figure 2.5.

2.2.1 Sound pressure levels in different functional rooms

The sound pressure level measurement results for different functional spaces are presented in Figure 2.6. It is observed that the sound pressure level in bedrooms and activity rooms shows regular variations throughout the day. Between 7:00 a.m. and 9:00 a.m. and from 12:30 p.m. to 2:00 p.m., the sound pressure levels in both rooms are relatively low, fluctuating around 46 dBA. This can be attributed to the reduced occupancy in the bedrooms and activity rooms during these times, as the elderly typically dine in the cafeteria. In contrast, from 9:30 a.m. to 12:00 p.m. and between 3:00 p.m. and 7:00 p.m., the sound pressure levels in these rooms are higher, with levels fluctuating around 53 dBA in the morning and around 56 dBA in the afternoon. Compared to summer and autumn, there is a relatively greater fluctuation in sound pressure levels during winter, though no significant differences were noted in other aspects.

Figure 2.7 presents boxplots of the sound pressure levels in different functional rooms, revealing that the average sound pressure level in bedrooms is higher than in activity rooms. Additionally, across all seasons, the average sound pressure level in activity rooms is lowest during autumn, while at other times, both bedrooms and activity rooms exhibit sound pressure levels fluctuating around 51.8 dBA.

2.2.2 Influence of season on indoor sound pressure level

The measurement results of indoor sound pressure levels in care homes across different seasons are illustrated in Figure 2.8. It is observed that, regardless of the season, the fluctuation patterns of sound pressure levels in both bedrooms and activity rooms are generally similar. Indoor sound pressure levels are lower between 7:00 a.m. and 9:00 a.m. and between 12:30 p.m. and 2:00 p.m., while they are higher during other times of the day. Additionally, unlike in winter and transitional seasons, the sound pressure levels in care homes during summer are more stable, gradually increasing between 9:00 a.m. and 12:00 p.m. and declining noticeably around 12:30 p.m. In other seasons, sound pressure levels exhibit fluctuating decreases between 9:00 a.m. and 12:00 p.m., which could be related to summer activity patterns.

2.2.3 Indoor sound pressure levels of care homes of different scales

Figures 2.9 and 2.10 display the indoor sound pressure levels in care homes of different scales, indicating significant fluctuations across various time periods but consistent overall patterns. The sound pressure levels in both bedrooms and

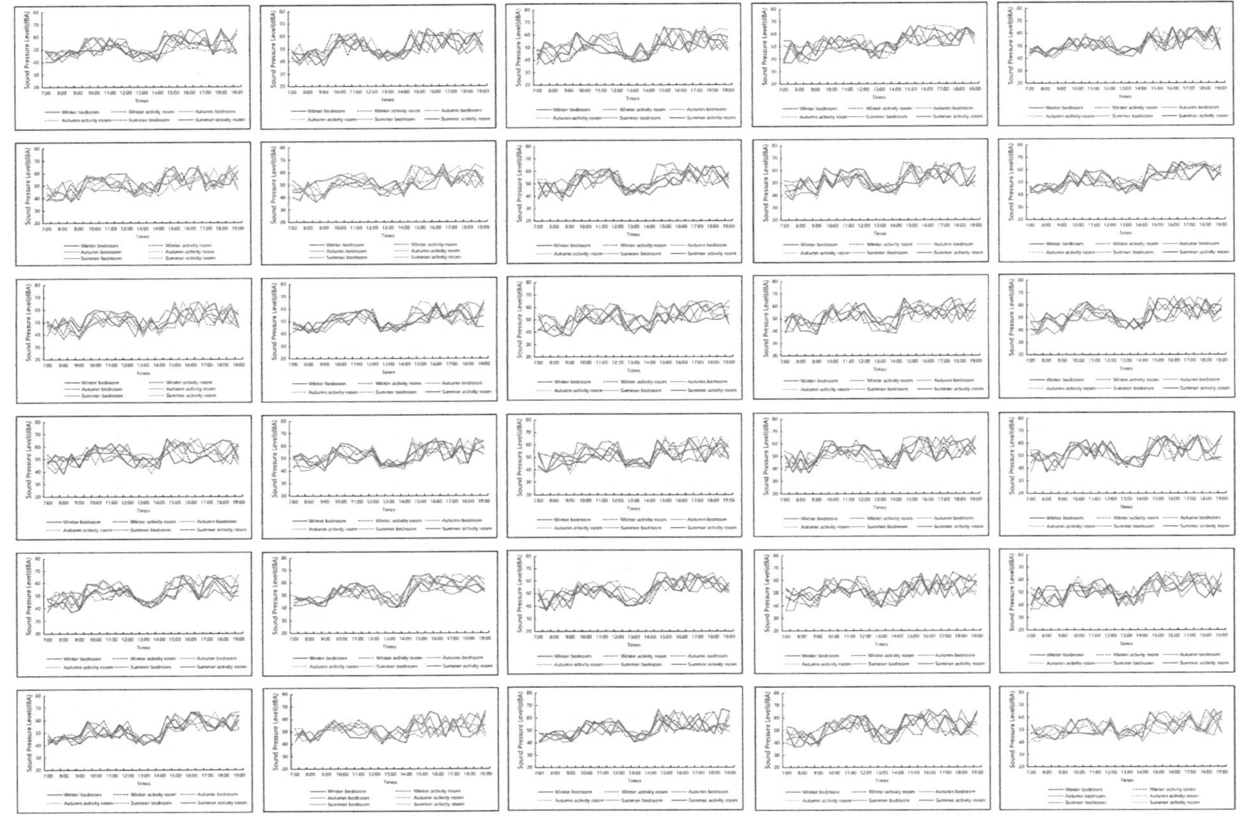

Figure 2.5 Indoor sound pressure levels in some researched care homes

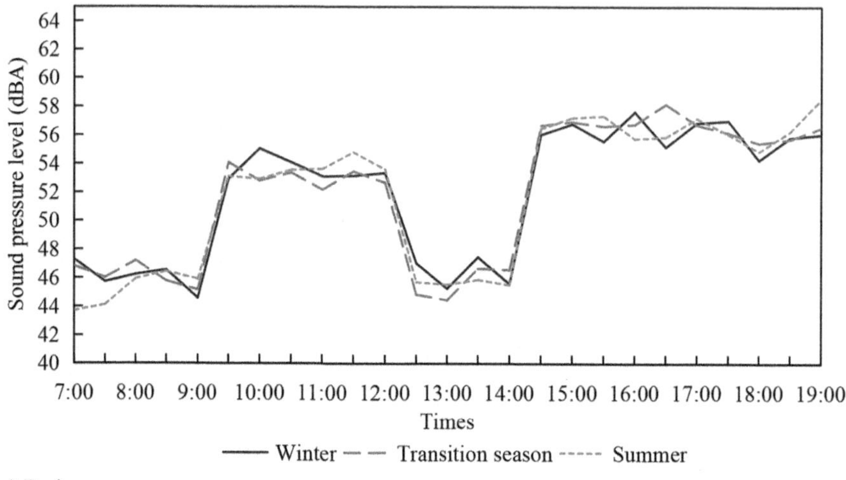

a) Bedroom

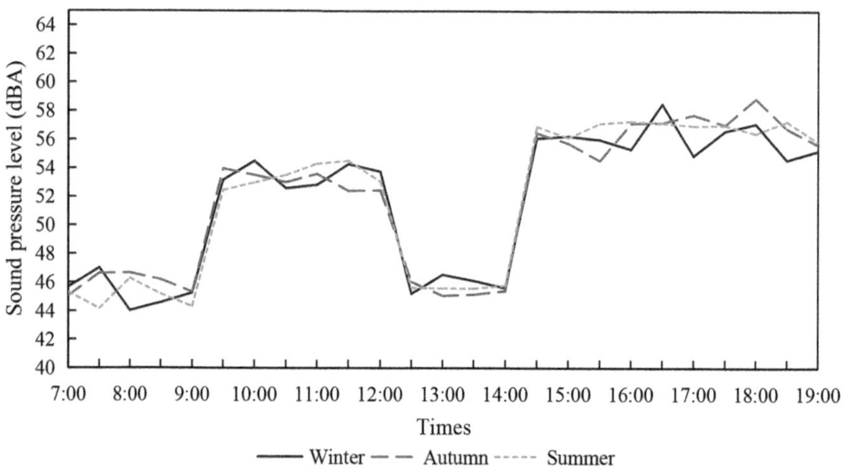

b) Activity room

Figure 2.6(a-b) Sound pressure level in bedroom and activity room

activity rooms peak between 9:30 a.m. and 12:00 p.m. and between 2:30 p.m. and 7:00 p.m., with lower levels observed at other times.

Figure 2.10 presents boxplots of sound pressure levels in care homes of different scales, revealing that as the scale of the care home increases, the average sound pressure level gradually decreases, stabilizing when the scale reaches large or extra-large. Additionally, compared to large-scale care homes, those of other

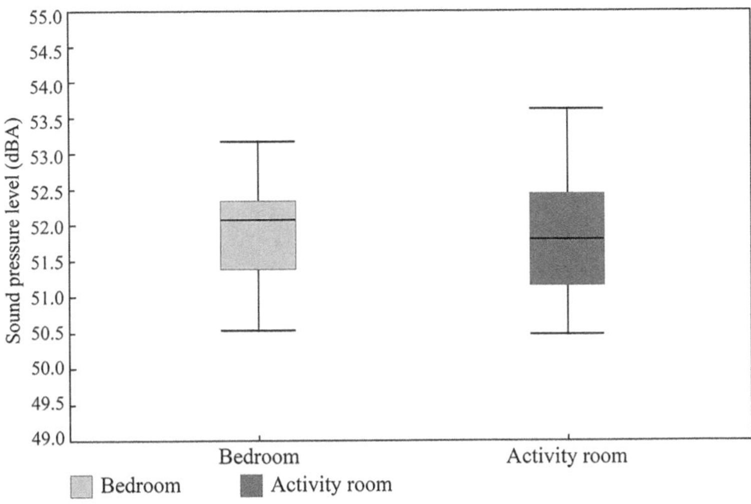

a) Function room sound pressure level

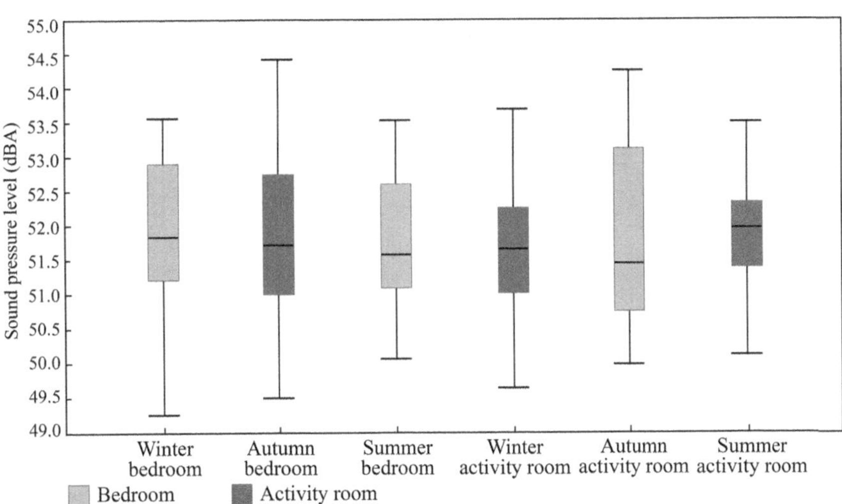

b) Function room sound pressure levels in different seasons

Figure 2.7(a-b) Boxplots of sound pressure level in different functional rooms

scales exhibit greater fluctuations in indoor sound pressure levels. Notably, unlike in large and extra-large care homes, the average sound pressure level in activity rooms of small and medium-sized facilities is generally higher than that in bedrooms (Figure 2.10b). Moreover, except for activity rooms in large care homes, indoor sound pressure levels in other care homes are distributed around 52 dBA.

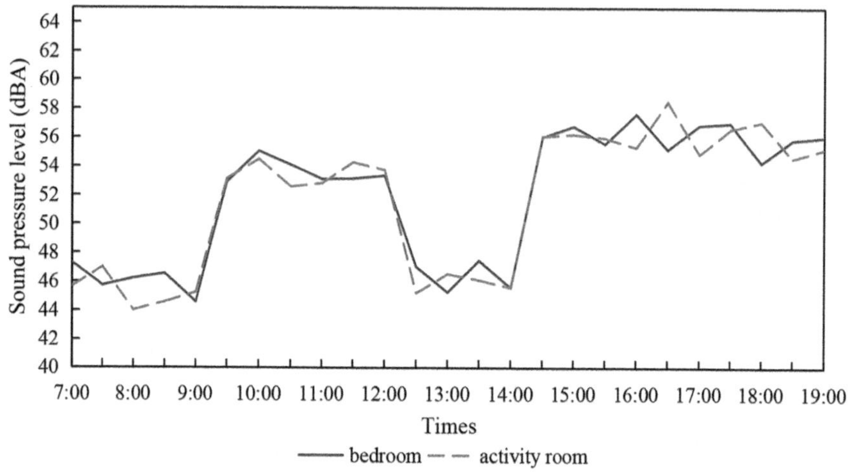

a) Winter

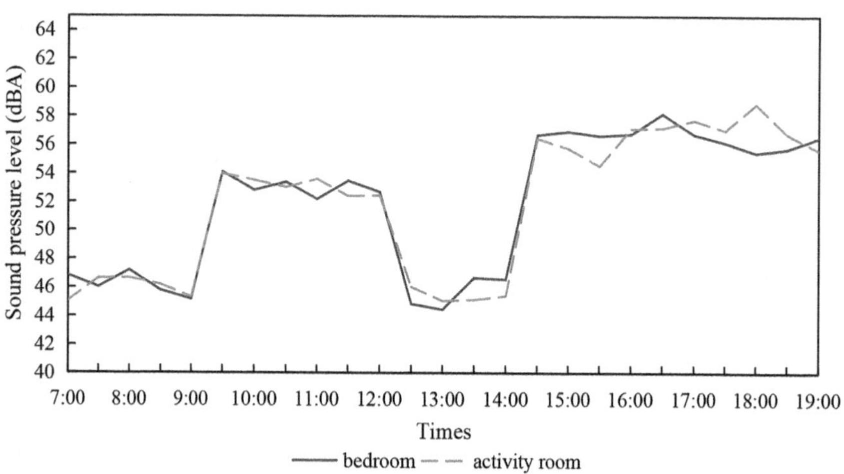

b) Transition season

Figure 2.8(a-c) Indoor sound pressure levels of care homes in different seasons

Figure 2.11 illustrates the distribution of sound pressure levels in bedrooms and activity rooms of care homes of different scales across seasons, indicating significant differences among these facilities. The data for medium-sized care homes are more stable, with sound pressure levels generally distributed around 51.5 dBA, while those for small-sized care homes are primarily distributed around 52 dBA. Large and extra-large care homes exhibit more pronounced fluctuations, with the average sound pressure levels in bedrooms generally higher than those in activity rooms.

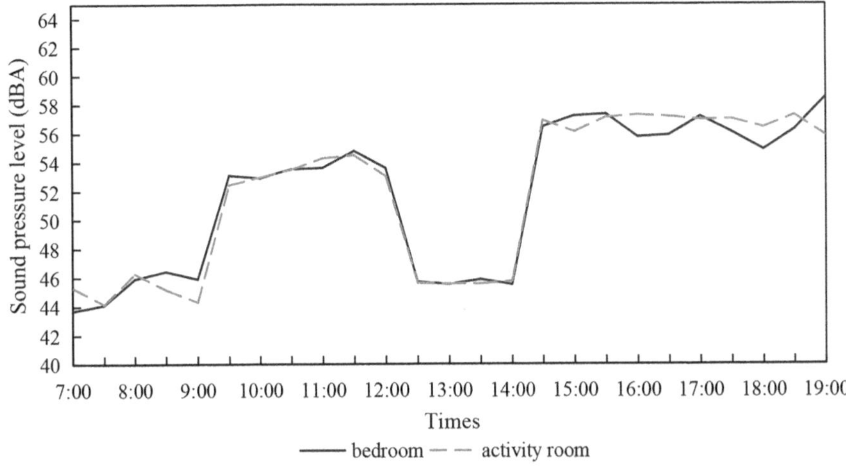

c) Summer

Figure 2.8(a-c) (Continued)

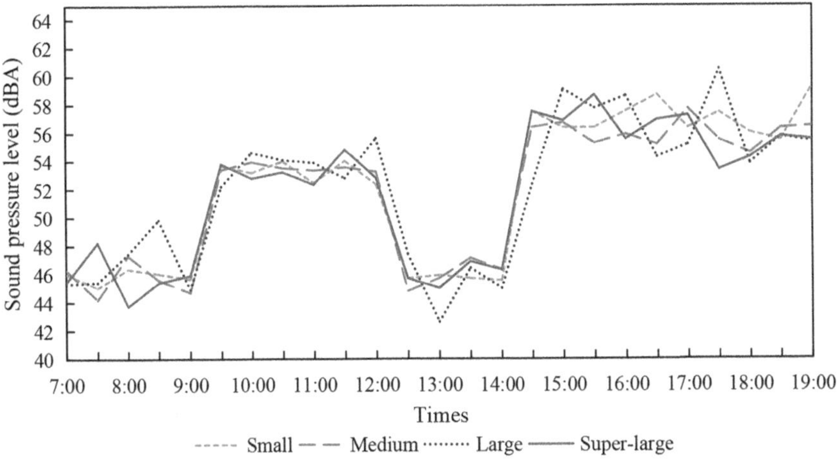

a) Bedroom

Figure 2.9(a-b) Indoor sound pressure levels of care homes of different sizes

2.2.4 Indoor acoustic environments for different types of care homes

Figures 2.12 and 2.13 depict the indoor sound pressure levels in different types of care homes. The data reveals that unreconstructed care homes have a lower sound pressure level, fluctuating around 51.5 dBA, whereas reconstructed care homes exhibit sound pressure levels around 52 dBA, with greater fluctuations.

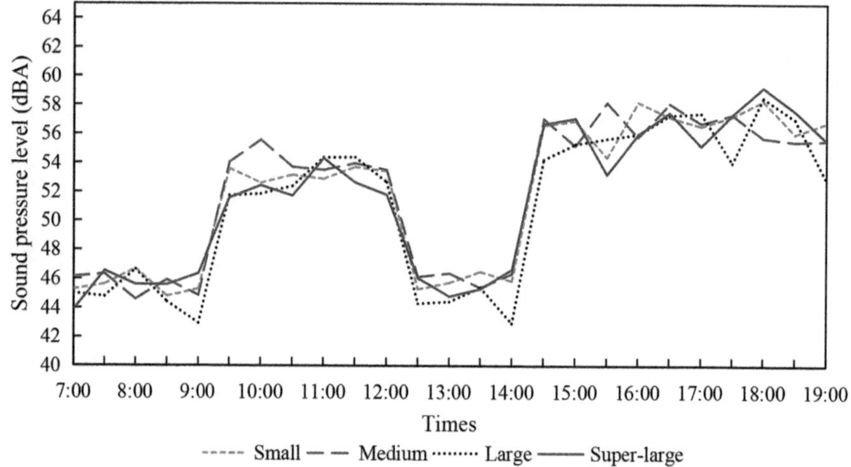

b) Activity room

Figure 2.9(a-b) (Continued)

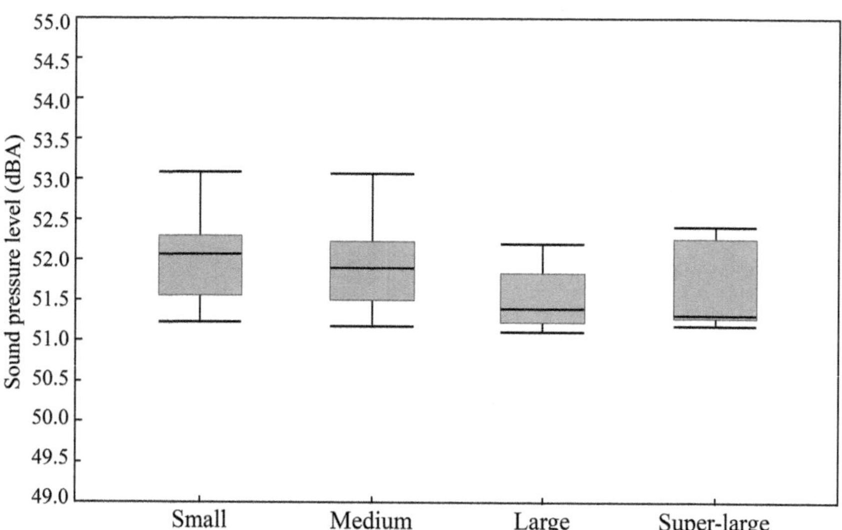

a) Indoor sound pressure levels for different scales of care homes

Figure 2.10(a-b) Indoor sound pressure levels for different scales of care homes

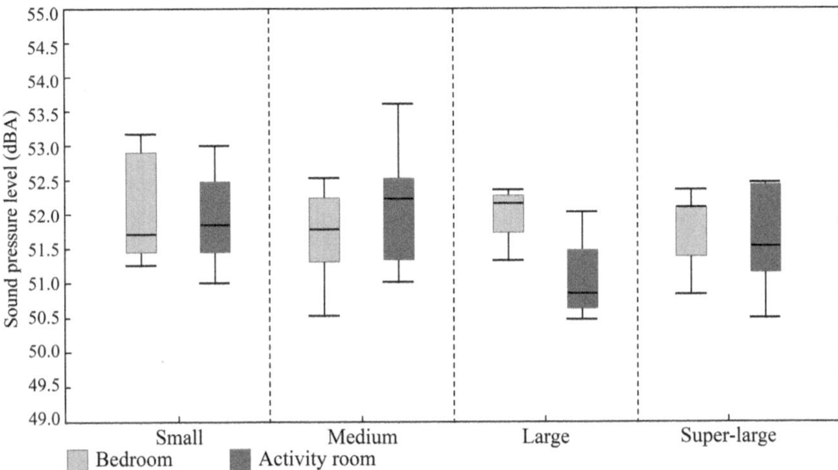

b) Functional room sound pressure level in care homes of different sizes

Figure 2.10(a-b) (Continued)

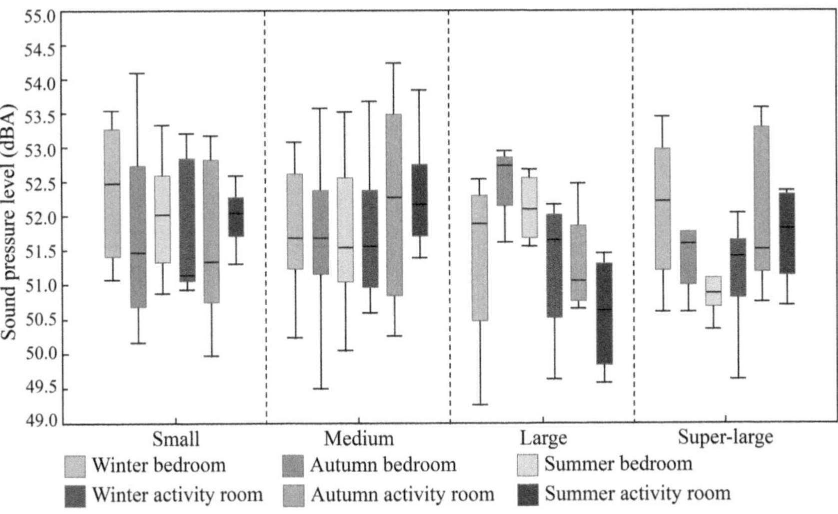

Figure 2.11 Sound pressure level distribution of bedrooms and activity rooms in care homes of different sizes in different seasons

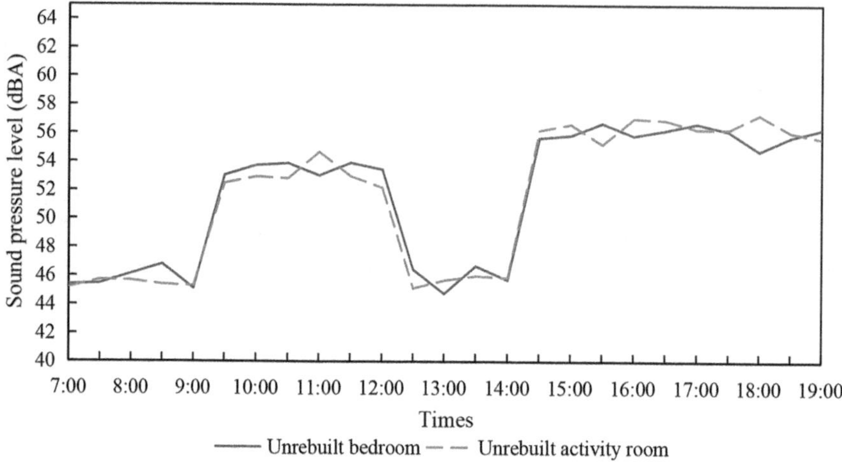

a) Sound pressure levels in bedrooms and activity rooms of non-reconstructed care homes

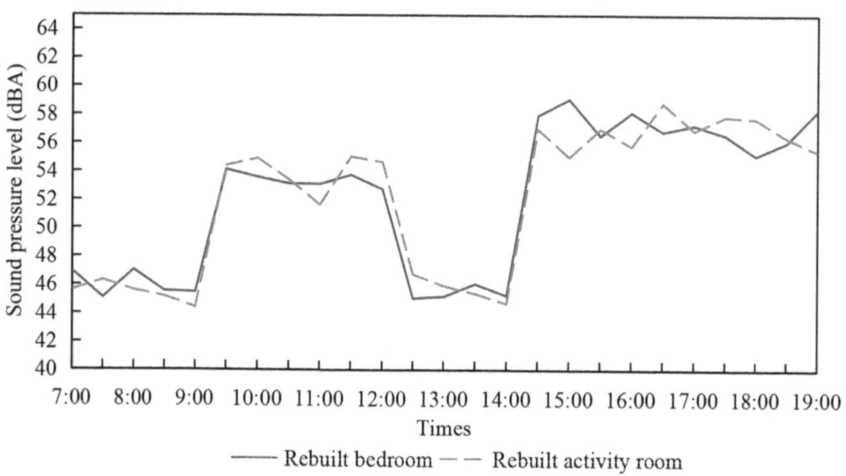

b) Sound pressure levels in bedrooms and activity rooms of reconstructed care homes

Figure 2.12(a-b) Indoor acoustic environment for different types of care homes

Additionally, the average sound pressure levels in bedrooms and activity rooms in both types of facilities are relatively similar, though activity rooms demonstrate greater fluctuations than bedrooms.

Figure 2.14 illustrates the sound pressure levels in different types of care homes across various seasons. It can be observed that in unreconstructed care homes, aside from the bedrooms in winter and the activity rooms in summer, the indoor

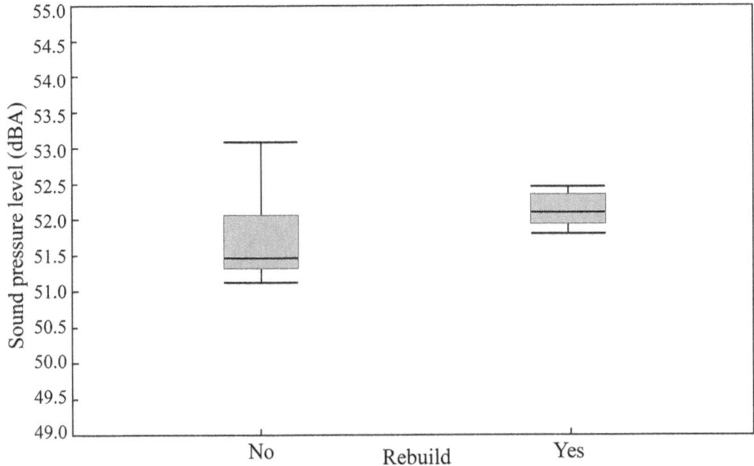

a) Indoor sound pressure levels for different types of care homes

Figure 2.13(a-b) Indoor acoustic environment boxplots for different types of care homes

average sound pressure level hovers around 51.4 dBA at other times. There are significant fluctuations in sound pressure levels for both bedrooms and activity rooms during autumn. In reconstructed care homes, apart from bedrooms in winter, which have an average sound pressure level of 51.8 dBA, the sound pressure level at other times exceeds 52 dBA. This graph substantiates the earlier findings that reconstructed care facilities generally have higher sound pressure levels than unreconstructed ones.

2.2.5 *Indoor acoustic environments for care home in different geographical regions*

The study selected three cities located in distinct climatic zones: Beijing, Ma'anshan, and Guangzhou, with one care home from each city chosen for analysis. Preliminary field research revealed that the bedroom environments of these care homes were quite similar, featuring wooden floors, solid wood furniture, and ceilings and walls typically painted without sound-absorbing treatments. In contrast, the public spaces of these care homes varied significantly; thus, this section primarily focuses on simulating the public spaces within the care homes.

Public spaces in care homes are generally open, with strong connectivity between different functional areas, often interconnected with corridors and other circulation spaces. Therefore, the simulation process integrated these spaces, including corridors, for analysis. The study utilized the acoustic software Odeon to simulate

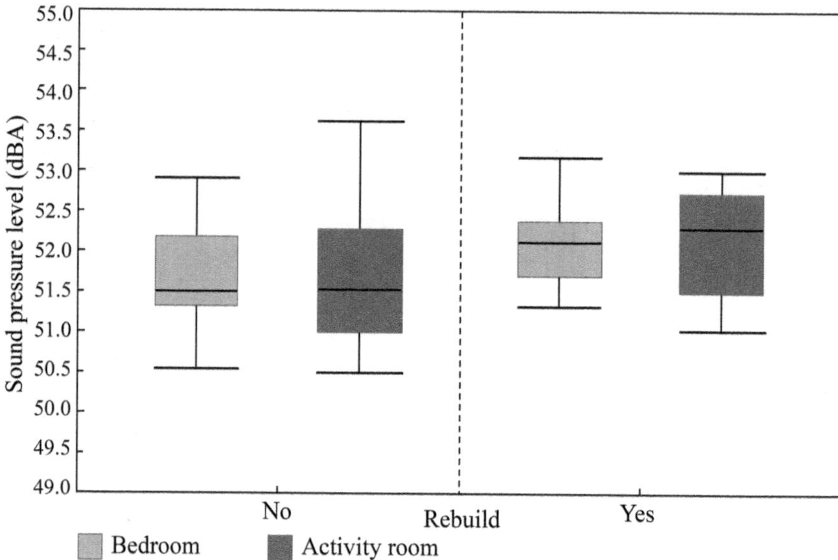

b) Indoor sound pressure levels of functional rooms in different types of care homes

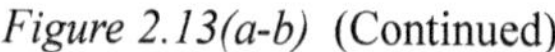

Figure 2.13(a-b) (Continued)

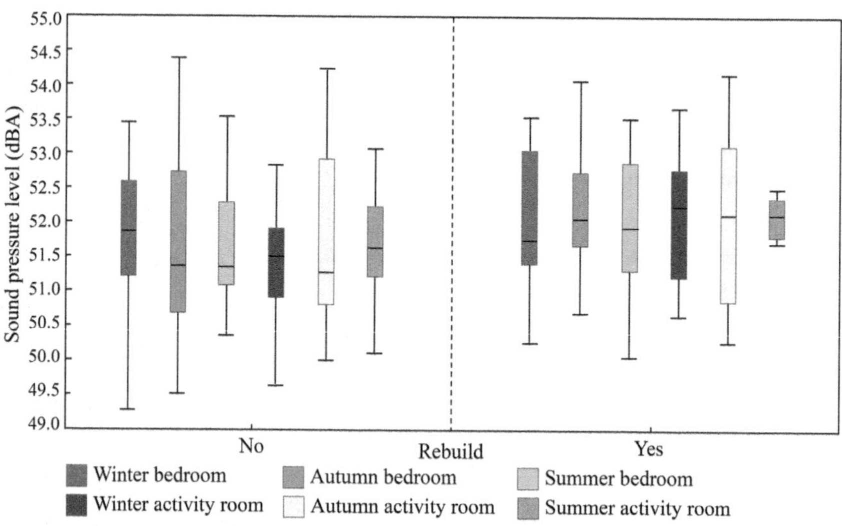

Figure 2.14 Sound pressure level of functional rooms in different types of care homes in different seasons

the indoor sound pressure levels of the three care homes. Since the material types of the public spaces in these care homes were relatively similar, a uniform setting was applied to the indoor materials of all three facilities, with the material sound absorption coefficients shown in Table 2.4.

Table 2.4 List of sound absorption coefficients for indoor materials in public spaces of care homes

Area	*Odeon material type*	*63Hz*	*125Hz*	*250Hz*	*500Hz*	*1000Hz*	*2000Hz*	*4000Hz*	*8000Hz*
Floor	linoleum or vinyl stuck to concrete	0.02	0.02	0.02	0.03	0.04	0.04	0.05	0.05
Glass	glass, ordinary window	0.35	0.35	0.25	0.18	0.12	0.07	0.04	0.04
Walls/Ceiling	painted plaster surface	0.02	0.02	0.02	0.02	0.02	0.02	0.02	0.02
Seats	moderately upholstered chairs	0.44	0.44	0.56	0.67	0.74	0.83	0.87	0.87
Wooden furniture	solid wooden furniture	0.48	0.48	0.77	0.38	0.27	0.65	0.35	0.35
Wooden veneer	Plywood paneling, 1 cm thick	0.28	0.28	0.22	0.17	0.09	0.1	0.11	0.11
Wooden flooring	Thin plywood paneling	0.44	0.44	0.56	0.67	0.74	0.83	0.87	0.87

The simulation results of sound pressure levels in the three care homes, illustrated in Figure 2.15, reveal significant spatial variations in indoor sound pressure levels across the facilities. The sound pressure levels in the activity areas are generally high, often exceeding 52 dBA, while those in the corridor spaces are relatively lower. Additionally, the degree of openness in a space can influence sound propagation to some extent. Overall, the magnitude of indoor sound pressure levels in care homes is closely related to the number of occupants and the scale of the building. Areas with a higher concentration of the elderly, such as activity and recreational zones, typically have higher sound pressure levels. Corridors, primarily used for circulation, see less occupancy and, therefore, have lower sound pressure levels. As a result, sound pressure levels in the public spaces of care homes generally decrease from activity areas along the corridors.

Significant climatic differences across geographical regions lead to substantial variations in architectural design. For example, buildings in the north are often more enclosed due to cold climates (Figure 2.15a), whereas those in the south, with its warm and humid climate, tend to have more open and diverse architectural styles (Figure 2.15c). The differences in architectural styles and materials due to

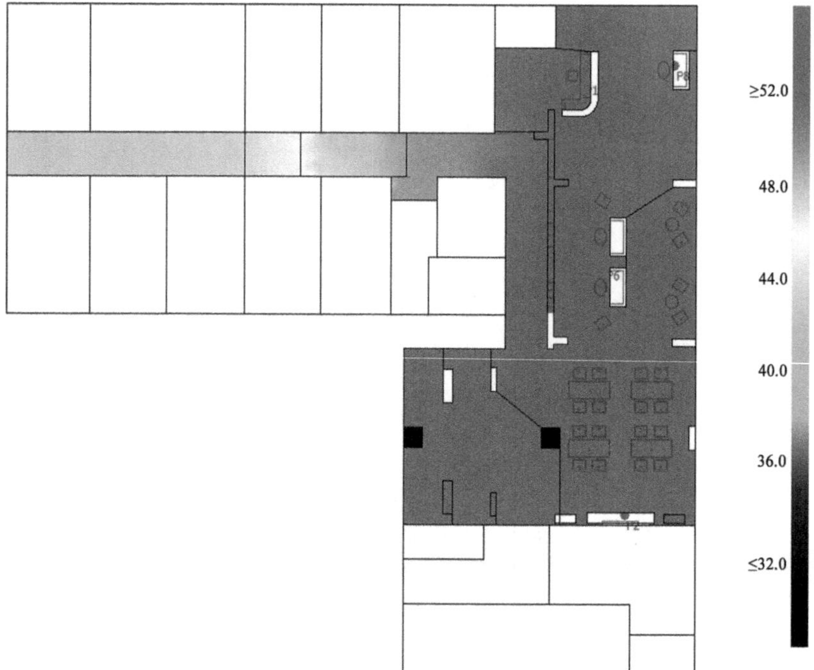

a) Case 1-NH

Figure 2.15(a-c) Sound pressure level(dB)

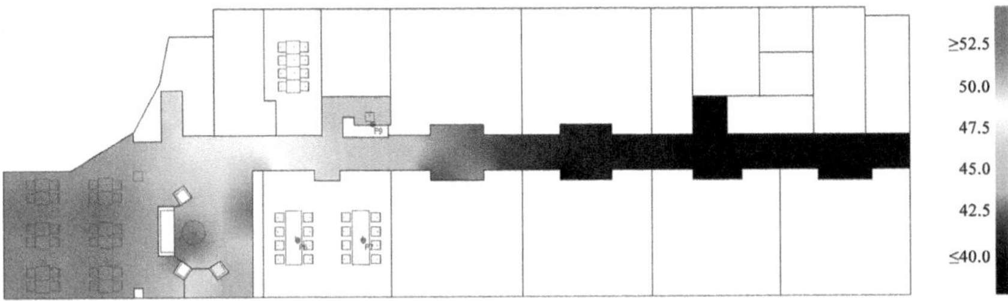

b) Case 2-NH

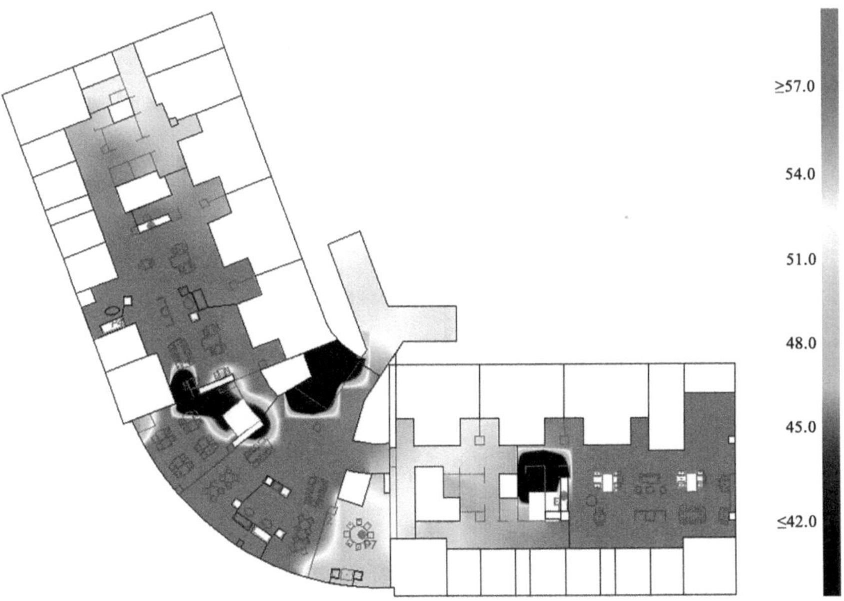

c) Case 3-NH

Figure 2.15(a-c) (Continued)

climate can also result in variations in indoor acoustic environments. Compared to northern facilities, the indoor acoustic environments of southern care homes may be more complex and variable.

2.3 Reverberation time of care homes

2.3.1 Reverberation time in different functional rooms

The study measured the reverberation time in the activity rooms and bedrooms of care homes, as depicted in Figure 2.16. Figure 2.17 reveals that while the

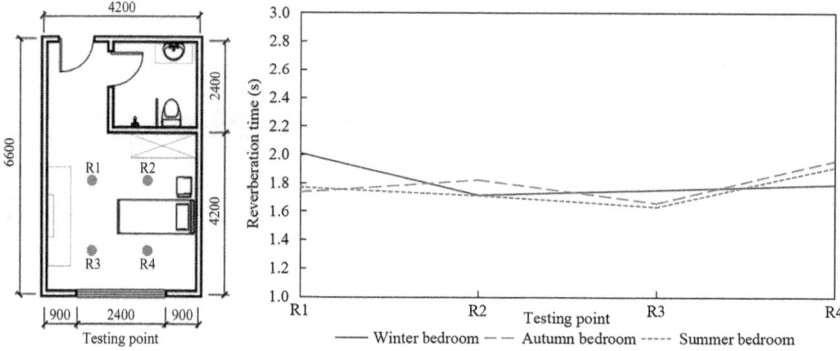

a) Reverberation time in bedroom

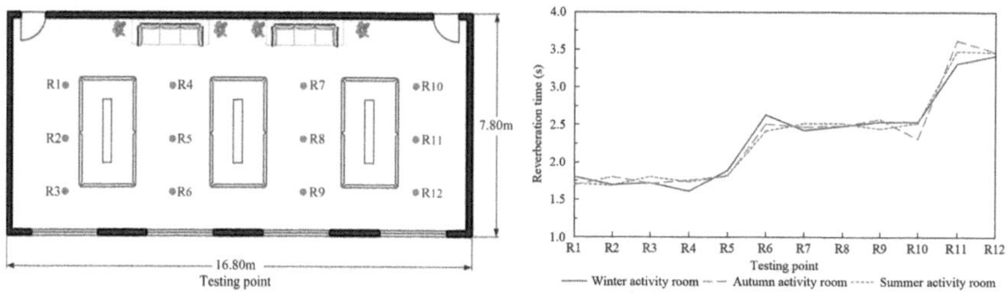

b) Reverberation time in activity room

Figure 2.16(a-b) Reverberation time in functional rooms

reverberation time in activity rooms fluctuates considerably, it is generally shorter than that in bedrooms, averaging around 3.52 seconds. This indicates a relatively longer reverberation time in bedrooms. Research suggests that when the reverberation time is around 3.5 seconds, elderly individuals rate their acoustic environment most favorably. However, when the reverberation time exceeds 4 seconds, background noise increases, interfering with daily communication among the elderly and reducing their perception of acoustic comfort [10]. This suggests that the current indoor reverberation time in the surveyed care homes is generally suitable for the elderly.

2.3.2 *Reverberation time of care homes of different scales*

Figures 2.18 and 2.19 illustrate the reverberation time in care homes of different scales. Large care homes have the longest average reverberation time, at

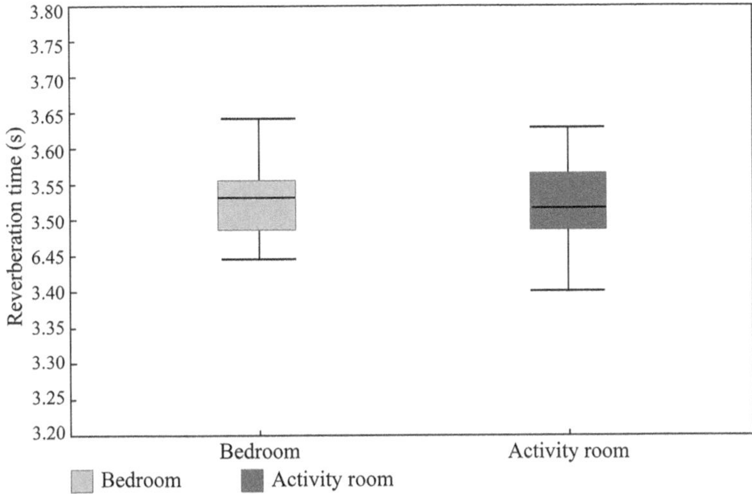

a) Reverberation time of different function rooms

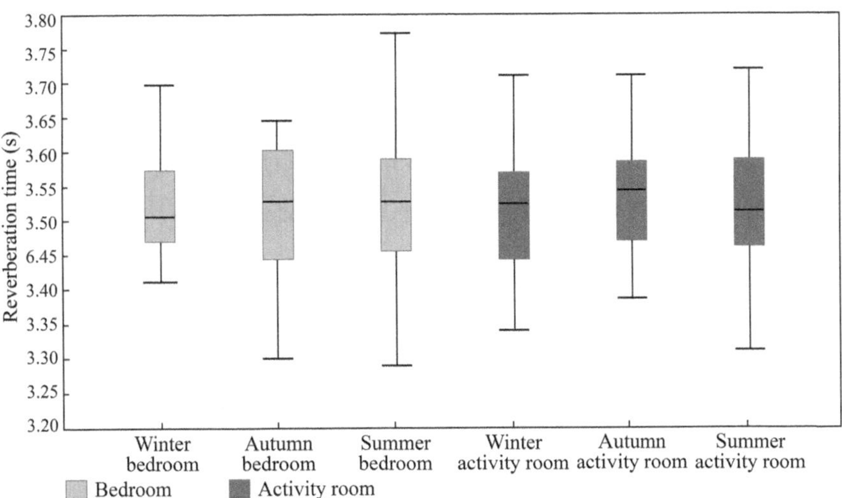

b) Reverberation time of different functional rooms in different seasons

Figure 2.17(a-b) Reverberation time in activity room and bedroom

3.54 seconds, followed by medium and small facilities, while extra-large care homes have the shortest average reverberation time, at 3.48 seconds. Additionally, in the distribution of reverberation time across different functional spaces, the reverberation time in the bedrooms of large care homes is significantly lower

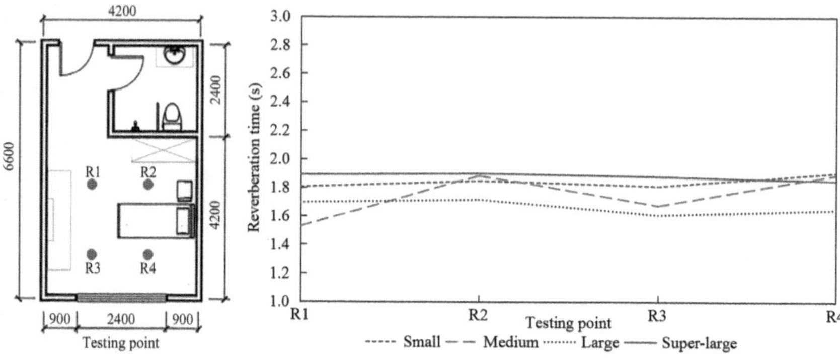

a) Reverberation time of bedroom in care homes of different sizes

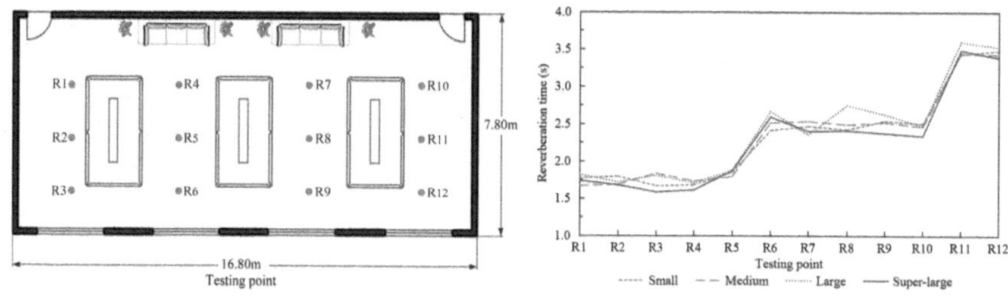

b) Reverberation time of activity rooms in care homes of different sizes

Figure 2.18(a-b) Reverberation times for different scales of care homes

than that in activity rooms. In contrast, in other scales of care homes, the reverberation time in bedrooms equals or exceeds that in activity rooms.

Figure 2.20 illustrates the distribution of reverberation time in functional rooms of care homes across seasons, revealing significant fluctuations in data among different-sized care homes. Medium and large care homes exhibit relatively stable indoor average reverberation times, fluctuating around 3.54 seconds, with bedroom reverberation times generally lower than those in activity rooms. Small and extra-large care homes show greater fluctuations, with the average reverberation time in bedrooms generally higher than that in activity rooms.

2.3.3 Reverberation time for different types of care homes

The study analyzed the reverberation time of reconstructed and unreconstructed care homes, revealing that unreconstructed facilities have significantly higher and more variable reverberation times. In contrast, the reverberation time in reconstructed facilities is more stable, fluctuating around 3.52 seconds (Figure 2.21).

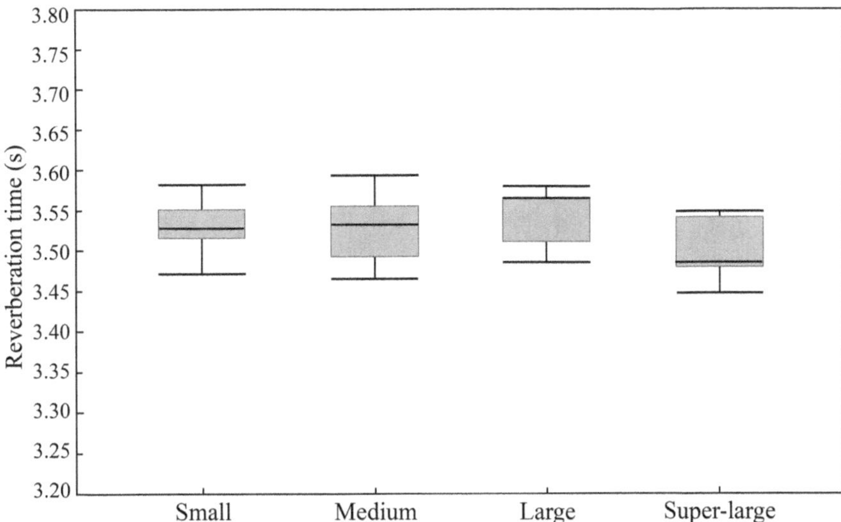

a) Reverberation time for different scales of care homes

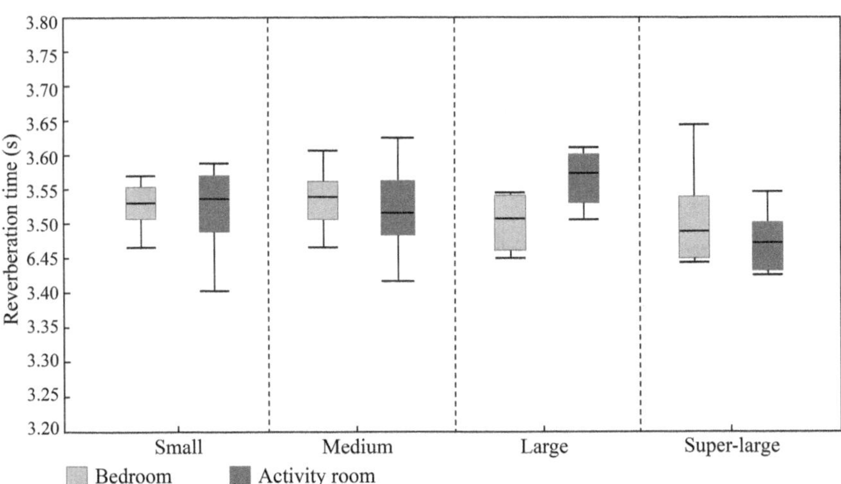

b) Reverberation time of various functional rooms in different scales of care homes

Figure 2.19(a-b) Reverberation time in different scales of care homes

In unreconstructed care homes, the reverberation times for bedrooms and activity rooms are similar. However, in reconstructed facilities, the reverberation time in activity rooms is significantly lower than in bedrooms. Overall, the reverberation times in both types of care homes generally meet the daily needs of the elderly.

Figure 2.22 illustrates the variation of reverberation time in different functional rooms of care homes across seasons, showing that in unreconstructed facilities,

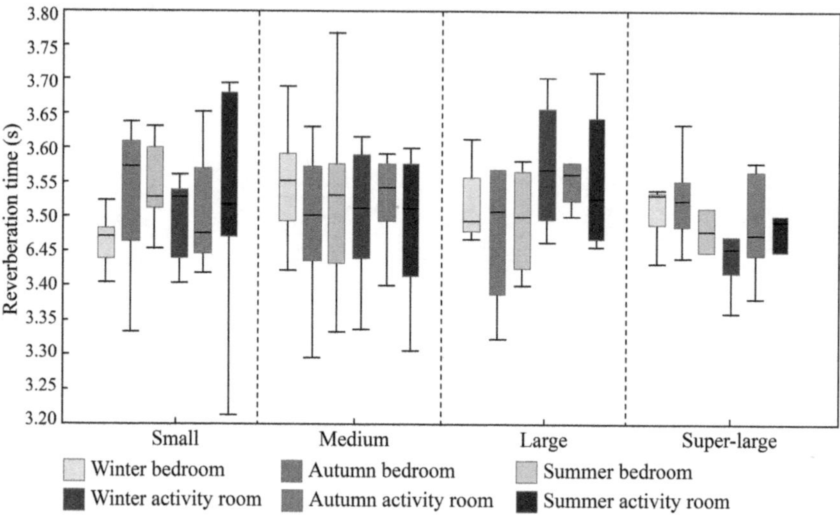

Figure 2.20 Reverberation time in care homes of different sizes

the reverberation time is relatively consistent, fluctuating around 3.52 seconds. In contrast, reconstructed facilities exhibit more variation, with bedroom reverberation times being higher than those in activity rooms. Seasonally, the shortest reverberation times are observed in winter bedrooms and summer activity rooms, both at 3.5 seconds.

2.3.4 *Reverberation time for care homes in different geographical regions*

Based on simulations using Odeon 16, the reverberation times for the public spaces of these three care homes were analyzed (Figure 2.23), revealing significant differences among the care homes. Case 2-NH exhibited the shortest reverberation time, with a maximum value of approximately 1.8 seconds, while the reverberation times for Case 1-NH and Case 3-NH were relatively longer, with maximum values around 2.4 seconds. These two nursing homes showed similar patterns in the variation of reverberation times across different sound frequencies: higher reverberation times in the 63 to 1000 Hz range, which decreased as the frequency increased. Conversely, Case 2-NH exhibited higher reverberation times between 500 and 2000 Hz, with lower times at other frequencies.

Figure 2.24 shows the spatial distribution of reverberation time in a nursing home, revealing a significant correlation between the length of indoor reverberation and the scale of the space. Activity areas, which are more open, result in shorter reverberation times. In contrast, corridors, being mostly narrow and long, cause sound to reflect multiple times during transmission, leading to longer reverberation times. Therefore, the indoor reverberation time in nursing homes

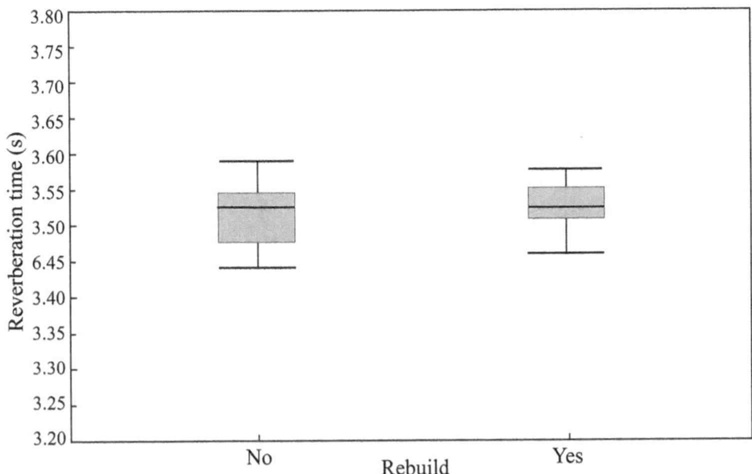

a) Indoor reverberation time for different types of care homes

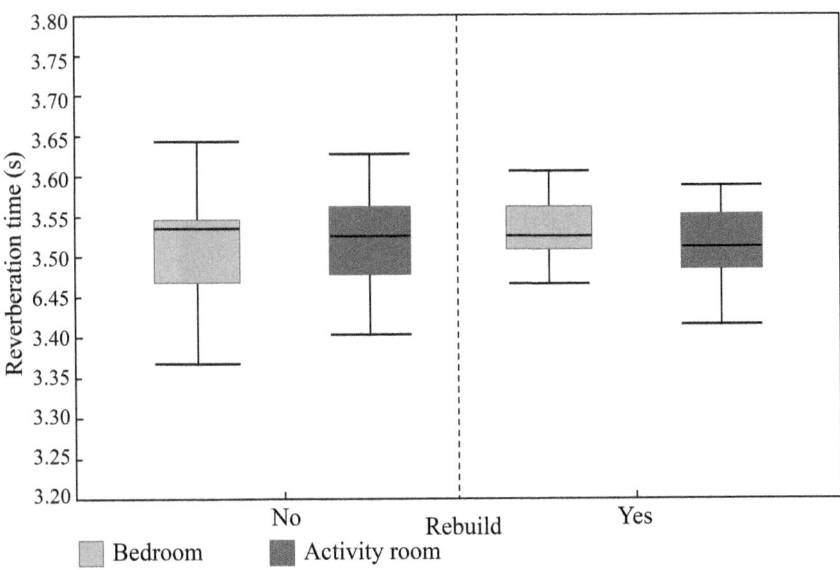

b) Reverberation time of different functional rooms in different types of care homes

Figure 2.21(a-b) Reverberation time of different types of care homes

generally increases from open activity spaces to corridors, with longer corridors experiencing increased reverberation times. This indicates that reverberation time is influenced by the spatial form of the nursing facility. Architectural styles in the north and south of China are greatly influenced by regional and climatic factors.

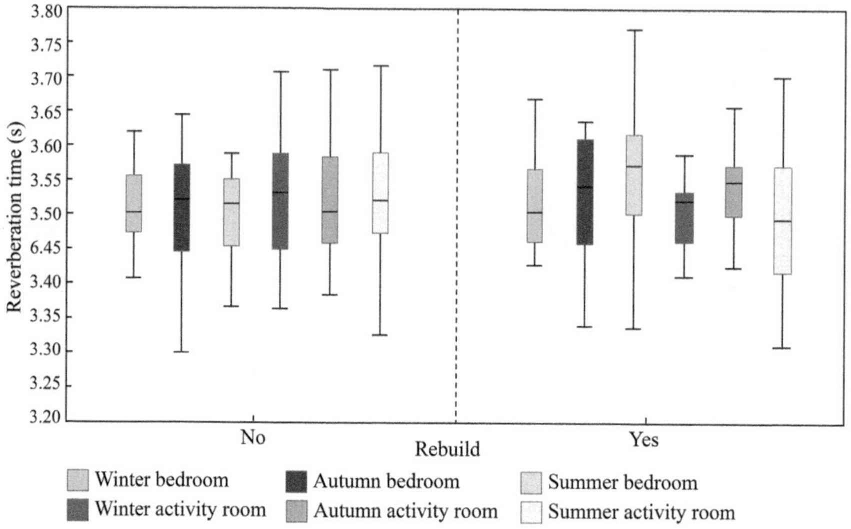

Figure 2.22 Reverberation time in functional rooms of different types of care homes in different seasons

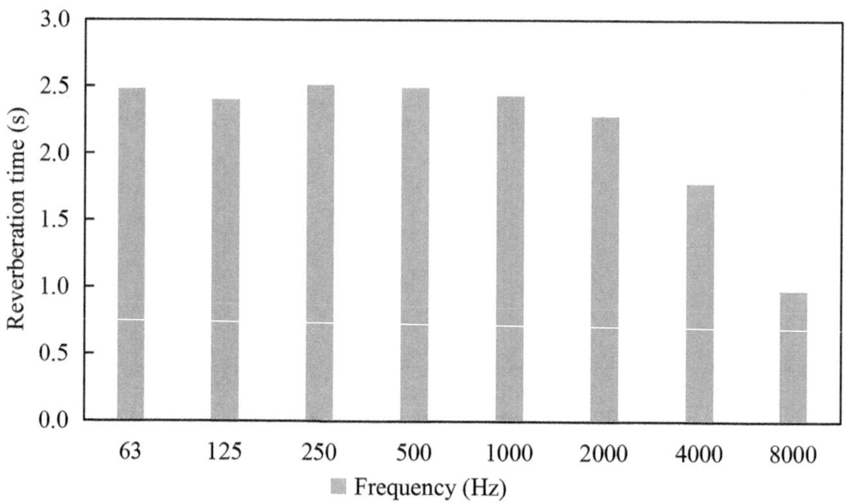

a) Case 1-NH

Figure 2.23(a-c) Reverberation time in care homes

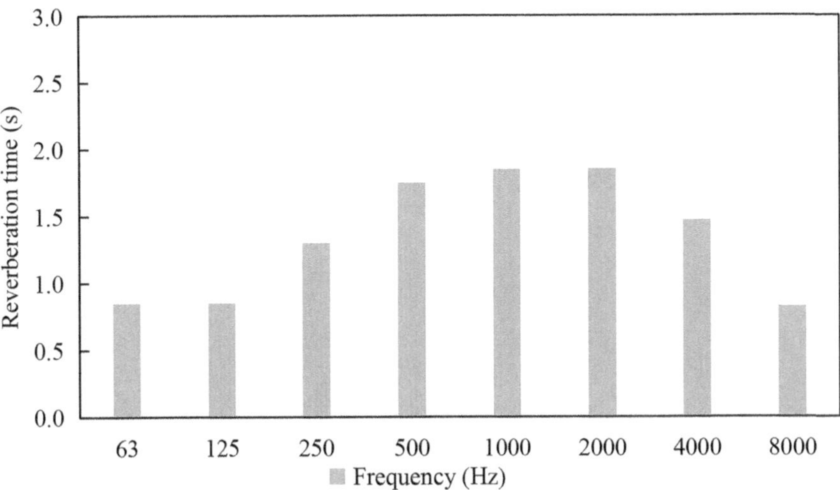

b) Case 2-NH

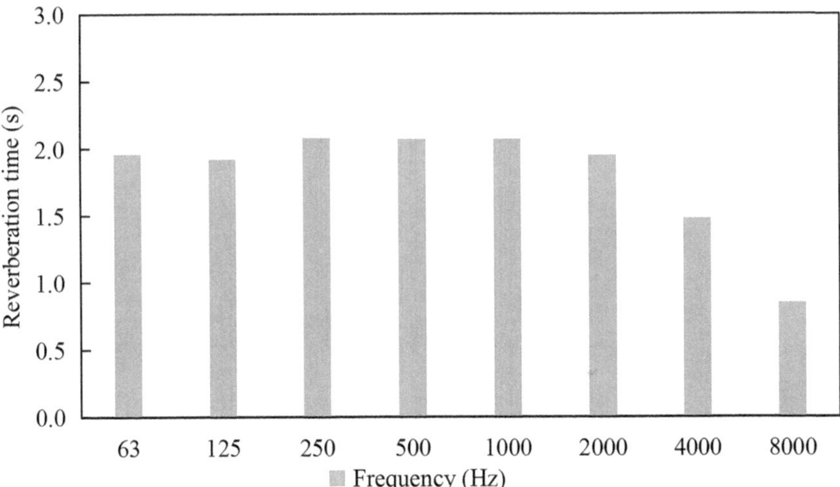

c) Case 3-NH

Figure 2.23(a-c) (Continued)

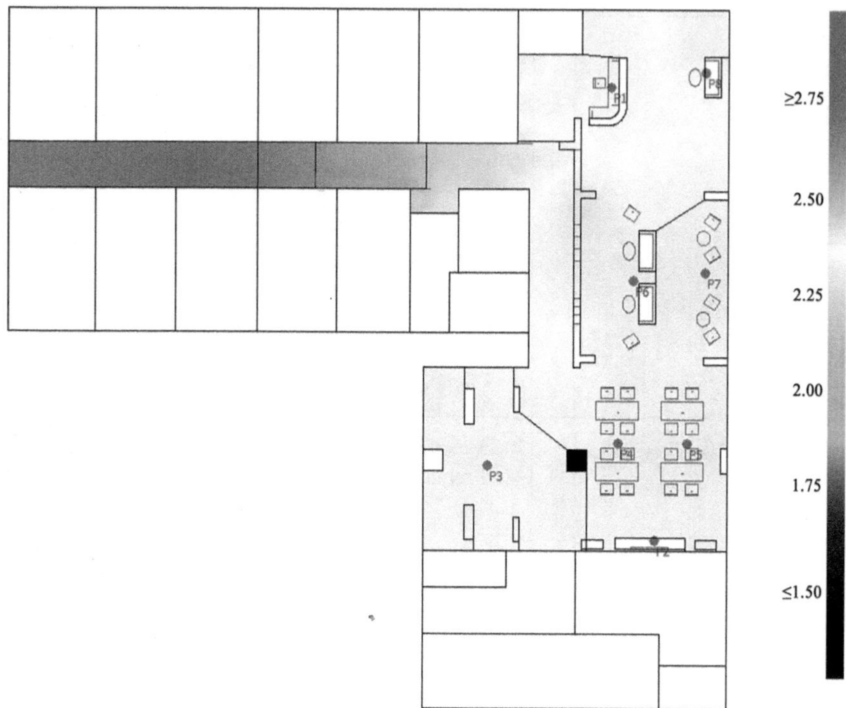

a) Case 1-NH

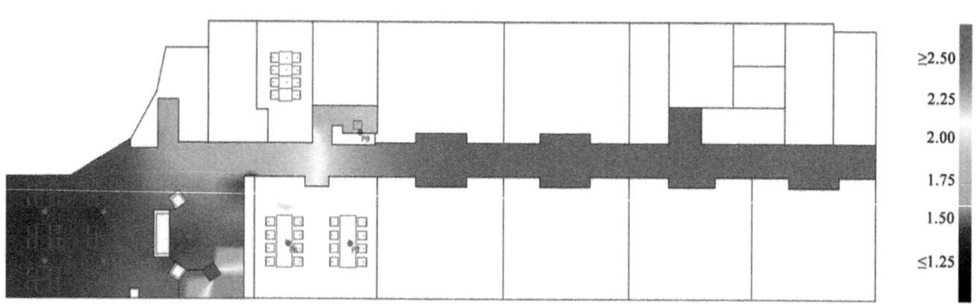

b) Case 2-NH

Figure 2.24(a-c) Spatial distribution of reverberation time in care homes

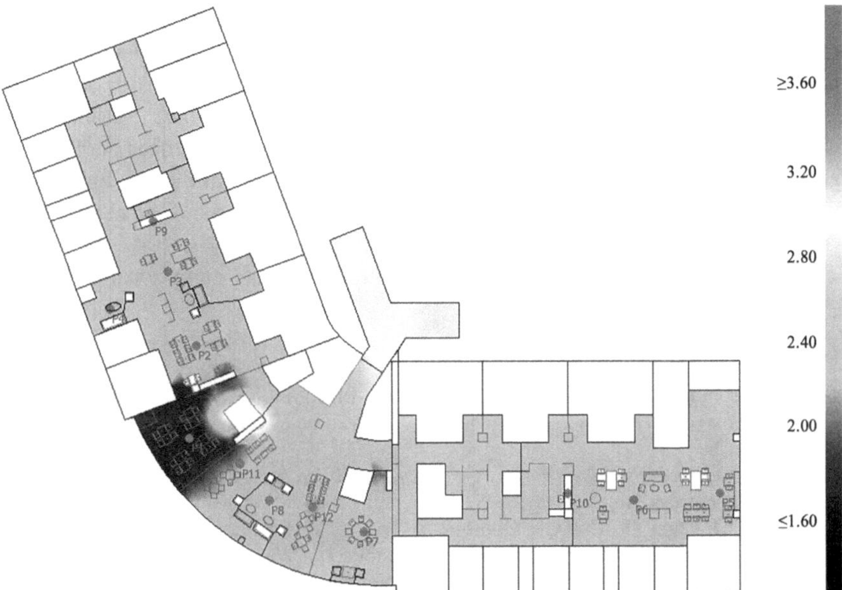

c) Case 3-NH

Figure 2.24(a-c) (Continued)

Consequently, the architectural styles and spatial forms under different regional influences vary significantly, impacting the indoor acoustic environment of buildings.

2.4 Conclusion

This chapter conducted a comprehensive one-year survey on the acoustic environment of 34 care homes located in four provincial capital cities in Northeast China. The objective was to gain insights into the current indoor acoustic conditions of care homes in this region. The study found that the fluctuation patterns of sound pressure levels in bedrooms and activity rooms were generally consistent across all seasons. Moreover, the results indicated that as the scale of the care homes increased, the average sound pressure level gradually decreased, stabilizing once the care homes reached large and extra-large sizes. Additionally, it was observed that the indoor sound pressure levels in unreconstructed care homes were lower compared to those in reconstructed ones.

The survey also examined the reverberation time in these care homes, revealing that activity rooms exhibited more fluctuation and had shorter reverberation times than bedrooms. Differences were noted in the reverberation times among care homes of varying scales. Large care homes had the longest average reverberation time, followed by medium and small ones, while extra-large cares homes had the shortest average reverberation time.

The study also utilized the acoustic software Odeon to simulate the sound environments in care homes in other regions. The analysis highlighted that the magnitude of indoor sound pressure levels is closely related to the number of occupants and the scale of the building, while reverberation time is significantly influenced by the architectural form. Moreover, significant climatic differences across various geographical regions lead to substantial variations in building design. These differences in architectural style and materials, driven by climate, can also result in variations in the indoor acoustic environment. Compared to the north, the indoor acoustic environment in southern care homes may be more complex and varied.

References

[1] Scheepmans K, de Casterlé BD, Paquay L, Milisen K. Restraint use in older adults in home care: A systematic review[J]. *International Journal of Nursing Studies*, 2018, 79.

[2] JGJ450–2018. *Standard for design of care facilities for the aged*[S]. Beijing: China Architecture & Building Press, 2018.

[3] Zhen M, Chen ZL, Zou QS. Combined effects of thermal and acoustic environments on outdoor human comfort in university campus[J]. *Urban Climate*, 2023, 49:101566.

[4] Chen J, Ma H. An impact study of acoustic environment on users in large interior spaces[J]. *Building Acoustics*, 2019, 26(6):1351010X1984811.

[5] Mu JY, Kang J, Zheng S. Evaluating the objective and subjective physical environments of residential care facilities[J]. *Indoor and Built Environment*, 2023, 32(5):1033–1050.

[6] GB50176–2016. *Code for thermal design of civil building*[S]. Beijing: China Architecture & Building Press, 2017.

[7] Liu DW, Liu XG. Shokai Cuncao Asian sports village home for the elderly, Beijing, China[J]. *Contemporary Architecture*, 2023, (03):60–65. (In Chinese)

[8] Liu DW, Qin S, Pan JW, et al. A study on composite care facilities for the elderly based on urban renewal of residential areas[J]. *Architectural Journal*, 2017, (10):23–30. (In Chinese)

[9] Nannariello J, Fricke FR. The use of neural network analysis to predict the acoustic performance of large rooms Part I.: Predictions of the parameter *G* utilizing numerical simulations[J]. *Applied Acoustics*, 2001, 62(8):917–950.

[10] Mu J, Kang J, Wu Y. Acoustic environment of comprehensive activity spaces in nursing homes: A case study in Harbin, China[J]. *Applied Acoustics*, 2021, 177(24):107932.

3 The acoustic perception of the elderly in care homes

3.1 Acoustic environment and sound perception

3.1.1 Introduction

The global population is rapidly aging, posing significant challenges to local healthcare and elderly care services [1]. Care homes, as essential components of the elderly care system, primarily provide accommodation, leisure activities, and medical rehabilitation services for the elderly [2]. Research indicates that the indoor environmental quality of care homes profoundly impacts the comfort and mental well-being of the elderly [3]. Therefore, creating a comfortable living environment for the elderly is crucial to promote their overall health.

As a key element of the physical environment, the acoustic environment significantly influences the elderly. Studies have shown that prolonged exposure to sound levels exceeding 65 dB(A) can lead to severe health issues, such as sleep disorders, hearing loss, tinnitus, hypertension, and cardiovascular diseases [4, 5]. Although older adults may have a higher tolerance for sound, they are also more sensitive to it [6]. Background noise can disrupt sleep for many elderly individuals, leading to a lack of concentration and physical fatigue, thereby affecting daily communication. Hence, providing a healthy and comfortable acoustic environment for the elderly is crucial.

Acoustic comfort reflects people's subjective evaluations of the acoustic environment [7]. Relevant studies have shown that when the reverberation time in the activity hall of care homes exceeds 4 seconds, or the sound pressure level exceeds 65 dB(A), the subjective evaluation of acoustic comfort for the elderly decreases [8]. Additionally, compared to fast-paced music, slow-paced music is more effective in improving the emotional state of the elderly. Under natural sound backgrounds, individual activities bring more happiness than collective activities [9]. Music not only has positive effects on emotions and arousal but also significantly influences human behavior [10].

While there is a foundation for research on the acoustic environment of care homes, studies specific to the Northeast region are relatively scarce, and specific standards for the acoustic performance of care homes are lacking [11–13]. Furthermore, individuals' evaluations of acoustic comfort are influenced not only

DOI: 10.1201/9781003407232-3

by the objective acoustic environment but also by their physiological conditions (age, health status) and social backgrounds (education level, marital status). Other physical environmental factors may also affect the subjective evaluations of the elderly.

Therefore, this study explores the acoustic environment in the Northeast region from four perspectives [9, 14]: (1) investigating the satisfaction of the elderly with the indoor acoustic environment; (2) analyzing the impact of demographic and social backgrounds on the assessment of the acoustic environment by the elderly; (3) investigating the influence of the acoustic environment on the activities of the elderly; and (4) analyzing the relationship between the acoustic environment and other indoor physical environmental factors. To achieve these objectives, five representative care homes were selected, and an in-depth study of their indoor acoustic environments was conducted. The behavior of the elderly was recorded, followed by surveys to study the impact of acoustic environmental factors on their perception and activities.

3.1.2 Case study

In this study, 30 care homes were randomly selected from the officially registered care homes' database in Changchun City, Jilin Province. Following initial communications, 21 care homes agreed to participate in the research. After conducting preliminary investigations of these 21 facilities, five nursing homes with similar layouts and internal designs were chosen for in-depth study. The specific details are shown in Table 3.1.

These five care homes offer a range of services for the elderly, including accommodation, meals, leisure activities, medical rehabilitation, and more. In terms of spatial layout, they all feature single and double rooms equipped with essential facilities such as televisions, private bathrooms, emergency call systems, and internal telephones. The public areas include recreation rooms, dining halls, cultural corners, indoor gyms, and public activity areas. Based on their scale and number of beds, the surveyed care homes were categorized into small-scale (≤150 beds), medium-scale (151–300 beds), large-scale (301–500 beds), and extra-large-scale (>500 beds). The selected care homes are representative of the functional layout and spatial environment typically found in care homes in Northeast China [15].

In China, care homes can be classified by their nature into public and private institutions. Public care homes, organized by the government, primarily serve vulnerable groups such as impoverished and disabled elderly individuals, emphasizing a strong welfare orientation. Conversely, private care homes are primarily established through entrepreneurial investments and feature more comprehensive infrastructure and eldercare services, albeit with higher fees. Among the five care homes examined, only one is public, while the rest are private. To provide a more comprehensive and clear understanding of the differences between public and private care homes in China, this section also includes two highly representative public care homes from the south as case supplements. The specific information about these care homes is detailed in Table 3.2.

Table 3.1 Demographic statistics of the participants

RCFs	*Location (district)*	*Beds*	*Funding*	*Flooring*	*Walls*	*Furniture*	*Heating system*	*Ventilation system*
RCF 1	Kuancheng	4730	Public	Private area: wooden; public area: tiles	Plaster, white paint	Wooden	HVAC	HVAC
RCF 2	Kuancheng	68	Private	Wooden	Plaster, white paint	Wooden	Water radiators	Natural ventilation
RCF 3	Chaoyang	30	Private	Vinyl	Plaster, white paint	Wooden	Water radiators	Natural ventilation
RCF 4	Nanguan	50	Private	Vinyl	Plaster, white paint	Wooden	Water radiators	Natural ventilation
RCF 5	Nanguan	50	Private	Vinyl	Plaster, white paint	Wooden	Water radiators	Natural ventilation

Note: RCF = Residential care facility.

Table 3.2 Basic information on public care homes

Code	*Project name*	*Location*	*Completion time*	*Beds*	*Area*	*Service recipient*
Case 1-G/WH	Suzhou Yangshan Nursing Home	Suzhou	2014	290	29843.13m^2	Self-care, semi-self-care/semi-disabled/assisted elders
Case 2-G/WH	Shuanglian Xinzhuang Social Welfare Center	Taiwan	2015	0	2092.41m^2	Self-care, semi-self-care/semi-disabled/assisted elders

Note: G/WH = Geracomium/Welfare Home.

3.1.2.1 Case 1-G/WH

Case 1-G/WH is situated at the eastern foot of Mount Yangshan in the Dapeng Mountain National Forest Park, Gaoxin district, Suzhou city. The terrain gently slopes from west to east, with an approximate height difference of eight meters. In its design, three courtyard clusters are strategically positioned along this elevation variation, covering a total above-ground building area of 26,500square meters. This area encompasses 216 residential units and accommodates 324 beds [16].

To enhance connectivity between these courtyard clusters, several "streets" have been incorporated in both east-west and north-south directions, fostering the involvement of the elderly in various activities and social engagements (Figure 3.1). The central east-west public space within the courtyard holds a prominent position in terms of scale and design, functioning as the bustling "main street." [17] This thoroughfare plays a vital role in linking the three courtyards. Public amenities such as lobbies, supermarkets, game rooms, fitness centers, exhibitions, and dining establishments line the "main street," enriching the activity zones for the elderly and fostering interaction among residents from different courtyards.

Additionally, interior scene photographs of the care home depicted in Figure 3.1 showcase various functional areas predominantly furnished with anti-slip rubber flooring and walls adorned with warm-toned paints, some sections featuring wooden veneer accents to evoke a cozy ambiance. The indoor furniture, predominantly crafted from solid wood, includes plush sofas for added comfort. Certain areas, such as activity rooms, reading spaces, and corridors, boast expansive high-ceiling spaces; however, the walls and ceilings lack acoustic treatments, potentially causing excessive sound reflections and prolonged reverberation times. Moreover, with "alleyways" connecting most public spaces, significant acoustic interference between different functional zones may compromise the clarity of the sound environment and hinder daily communication among the elderly.

As for the living quarters, the care home comprises a total of 216 residential units, comprising 63 standard rooms ($38\mathrm{m}^2$), 99 compact suites ($47\mathrm{m}^2$), and 54 family suites ($78\mathrm{m}^2$). Figure 3.1 showcases the interior scenes of the elderly living quarters, revealing bedrooms adorned with warm hues and solid wood furnishings. The majority of bedroom floors feature wooden finishes, complemented by painted walls and ceilings lacking specialized acoustic treatments. Most beds are standard double beds, which inherently possess better sound absorption properties compared to nursing beds. The bathrooms feature tiled surfaces and have been thoughtfully designed for aging-in-place. Overall, neither the public spaces nor the elderly living quarters in the care home have undergone specific acoustic enhancements. Given the expansive spatial scale, the absence of sound-absorbing materials may potentially compromise the indoor sound environment's quality, impacting the comfort and daily interactions of the elderly residents.

3.1.2.2 Case 2-G/WH

Case 2-G/WH, nestled in New Taipei City, Taiwan, was established by the Shuanglian Social Welfare Charity Foundation, serving as a vital welfare institution.

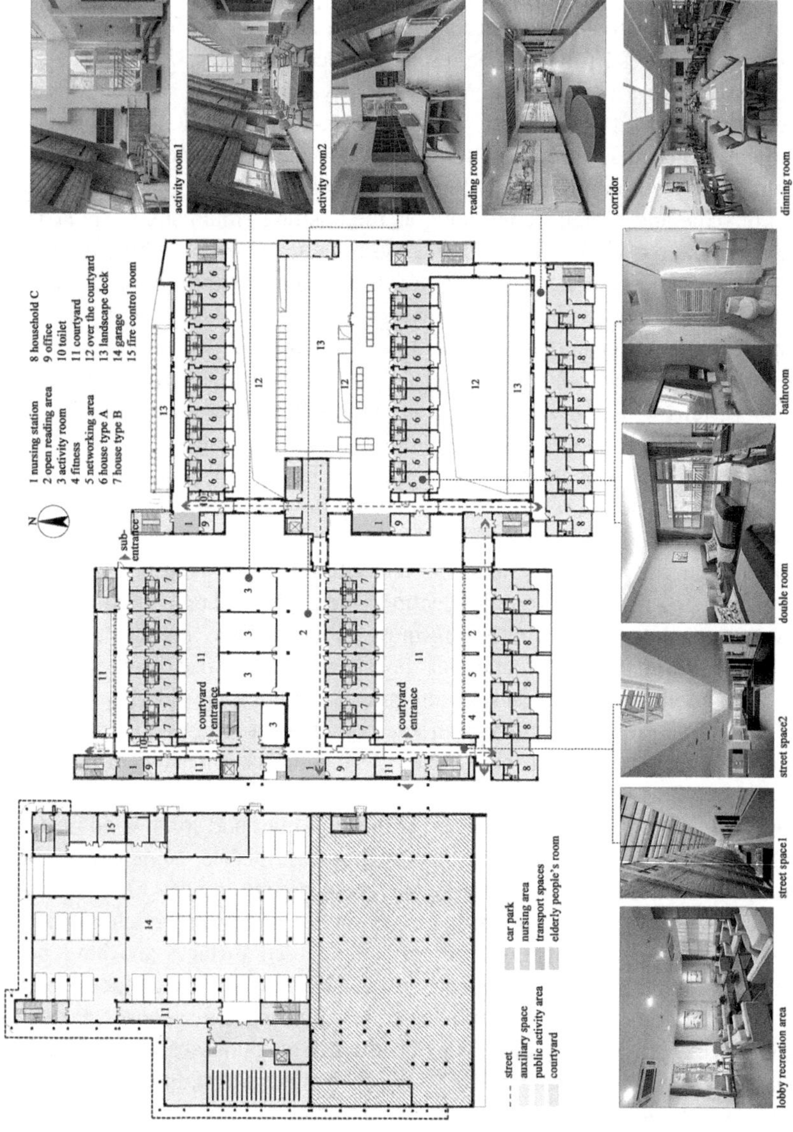

Figure 3.1 Floor plan of basement level of block C, 1st floor of block B, and 2nd floor of block A

Positioned in a densely populated urban enclave grappling with increasingly pressing aging challenges, the charity foundation's initiative to establish a welfare center aims to champion the health and well-being of the elderly.

Strategically nestled within the city's bustling heart, the building occupies a modest site area with a relatively compact building volume. Anchored in the ethos of "care normalization" and "service community," the center prioritizes home care and community services tailored to the elderly [18]. Its repertoire encompasses home care, day care, nutritional, and medical rehabilitation services, with no provision for beds due to the limited building volume. Spanning four floors, the center's ground level hosts the lobby and the rehabilitation clinic alongside ancillary spaces like offices, recycling rooms, and distribution hubs (Figure 3.2). The subsequent levels cater to day care services, boasting activity rooms, terraces, and day care centers, while the top floor is predominantly dedicated to dining services, featuring kitchens, cafes, versatile dining areas, and rooftop gardens, fulfilling the dietary and recreational requisites of the elderly.

Illustrations in Figures 3.2 and 3.3 offer glimpses into the public spaces within the welfare center. Notably, the medical zone on the ground floor exudes a predominant purple hue, while other areas boast warm color palettes, accentuating environmental recognition and imbuing primary activity zones for the elderly with a welcoming, snug ambiance. Upon scrutinizing the indoor materials adorning various functional quarters, it becomes apparent that most indoor flooring boasts a wooden finish. While walls and ceilings are painted sans acoustic treatments, some sections feature wooden veneer, offering modest sound absorption capabilities, albeit limited in distribution. Overall, the indoor milieu of the welfare center remains bereft of acoustic enhancements, with sound absorption predominantly reliant on soft furnishings and wooden embellishments. Given the center's more

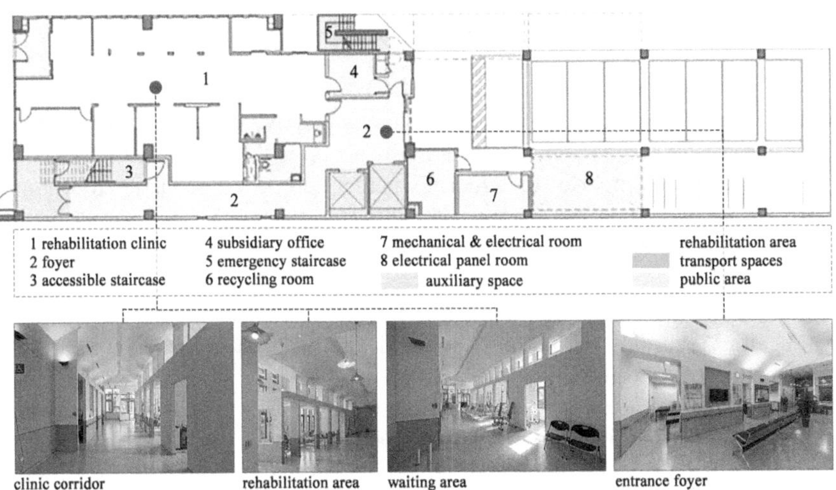

Figure 3.2 First floor plan and interior scene photograph

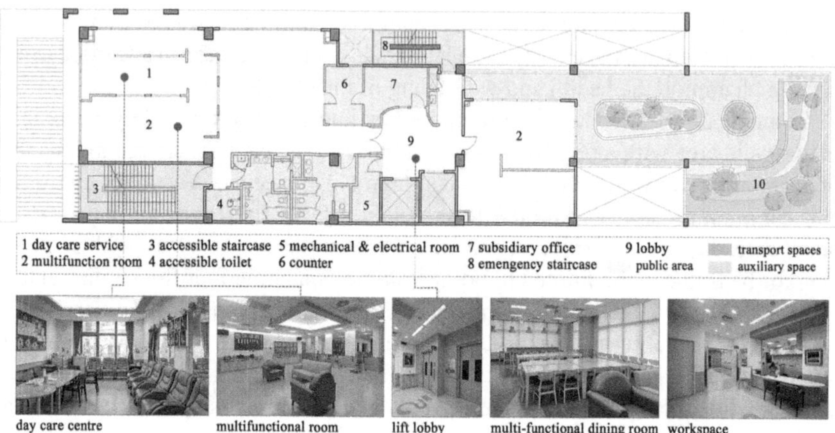

Figure 3.3 Second floor plan and interior scene photograph

modest spatial scale, limited occupancy, and the inherent challenge in generating prolonged reverberation times, it's conjectured that the indoor sound environment may be conducive for the elderly.

In comparison to their private counterparts, public care homes tend to exhibit simpler indoor furnishings, often constrained by budgetary considerations. Moreover, these facilities typically forego sound absorption treatments, potentially fostering a tighter nexus between acoustic environment quality and variables such as spatial scale and population density. The dearth of sound-absorbing materials renders these care homes more susceptible to instances of elevated sound pressure levels or protracted reverberation times, underscoring the imperative for substantial enhancements in their indoor acoustic environments.

3.1.3 Method

In the acoustic environment perception study, objective data regarding the physical environment of care homes were initially acquired through measurements, followed by an assessment of the elderly's perception of the acoustic environment via questionnaire surveys. Approval for this study was obtained from the ethics review committees of the University of Sheffield and the School of Architecture, Harbin Institute of Technology. The survey participants were elderly individuals who had resided in care homes for more than three months and were in good physical health. According to the frailty scales developed by Rockwood et al., participants scoring between 1 and 4 were deemed suitable for inclusion in the survey, indicating their sufficient physiological and psychological well-being to partake in the study [19]. The selected elderly participants were thus relatively healthy, totaling 618 individuals who met the aforementioned criteria, with 500 consenting to participate in the survey and providing informed consent. Participants retained

Table 3.3 Demographic statistics of the participants

Statistical indicators	*Number of samples*	*Proportion (%)*
Gender		
Female	210	43.8
Male	270	56.2
Age distribution		
Under 60 years old	122	25.4
60–70 years old	107	22.3
70–80 years old	175	36.5
80–90 years old	55	11.5
Over 90 years old	21	4.3
Room type		
Single room	153	31.9
Double room	218	45.4
Triple room	109	22.7
Membership structure		
Single person	168	35
Couple	312	65

the freedom to withdraw from the study at any point, and the confidentiality of their data was rigorously upheld. The demographic details of the participants are outlined in Table 3.3.

The questionnaire comprised two sections: the first section aimed to gather background information about the elderly, including age, gender, education level, marital status, and more. The second section solicited the elderly's assessments of the indoor acoustic environment. Validated by both experts and participants, the questionnaire underwent necessary adjustments following pilot studies with select participants. Its reliability was assessed by Cronbach's α coefficient, yielding a value of .784, indicative of acceptable internal consistency. To minimize ambiguity among the elderly, the survey was conducted through one-on-one interviews, requiring only 15 minutes for completion by each participant. The acoustic environment questionnaire predominantly utilized a 7-point Likert-type scale, enabling participants to evaluate the acoustic environment based on their genuine sentiments, ranging from 'very dissatisfied' to 'very satisfied.' A total of 500 questionnaires were collected, comprising 480 valid responses and 20 invalid ones (e.g., incomplete due to participant dropout).

Measurements of the acoustic environment were conducted in bedrooms and public areas, such as dining rooms and activity rooms. Selecting the most typical bedrooms and public spaces in each care homes, measurements were undertaken from 8:00 a.m. to 6:00 p.m. Continuous measurements were conducted in each area, employing a BSAB 801 sound level meter. The average values of the measurement results were then computed for subsequent analysis.

All subjective and objective measurement data were input into the SPSS 20.0 database to calculate the average and median scores of environmental measurements and questionnaire responses. Given the study's implementation across five distinct care homes, which varied in geographical location, scale, and furniture arrangement, one-way analyses of variance (ANOVAs) were employed to assess potential differences among the measurement results of these facilities. Subsequently, Pearson correlation analysis and linear regression analysis were conducted to explore the elderly's assessment of indoor acoustic environment comfort, while mean differences were analyzed to examine the influence of season and region on variations in indoor acoustic environments within care homes. The statistical significance threshold was set at $p < 0.05$.

3.1.4 Results

3.1.4.1 Acoustic environment perception of care homes in different functional rooms

Figure 3.4 portrays the acoustic comfort ratings of elderly individuals across different functional spaces, revealing that the elderly rank the acoustic quality of serene areas the highest, garnering a score of 4.5. Following closely are the corridors, resting zones, and compact activity areas, with the activity zones receiving the lowest evaluation in terms of acoustic ambiance. This finding indirectly supports a prior study suggesting the elderly's preference for relatively tranquil surroundings [8].

3.1.4.2 Acoustic environment perception of care homes in different seasons

Sound characteristics evaluation indicators primarily encompass acoustic comfort, loudness, noise level, and preference level. The analysis predominantly centered on the activity rooms and bedrooms of the five care homes, as depicted in Figures 3.5–3.8. Substantial discrepancies in acoustic comfort were noted among

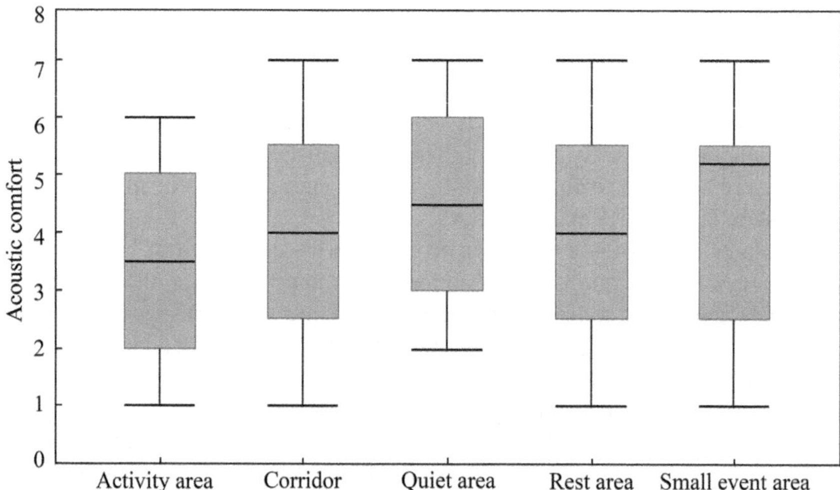

Figure 3.4 Acoustic comfort in different functional rooms

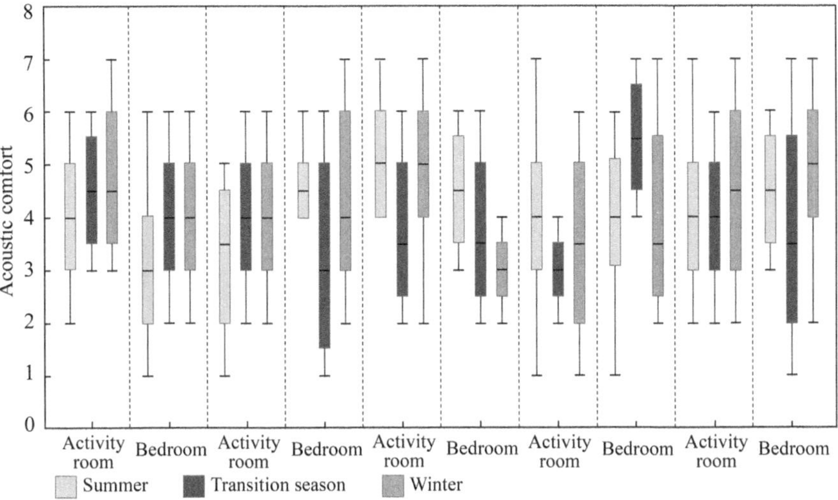

Figure 3.5 Acoustic comfort in care homes in different seasons

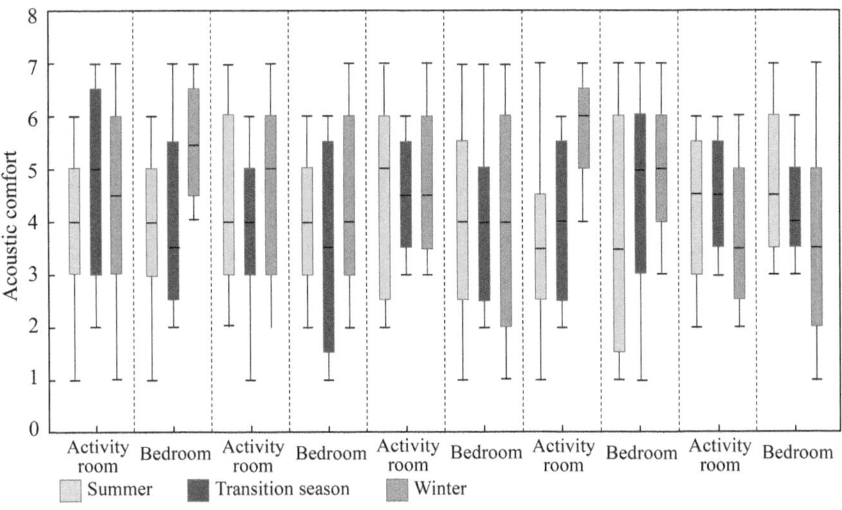

Figure 3.6 Sound loudness in care homes in different seasons

the care homes. Relative to summer and transitional seasons, acoustic comfort in activity spaces was higher during winter, whereas during the transitional season, bedrooms experienced diminished acoustic comfort, exhibiting significant deviations in analysis outcomes for the other two seasons.

Concerning sound intensity, activity rooms generally registered higher volumes in winter, trailed by the transitional season, with summer exhibiting the lowest sound intensity. Bedrooms tended to have relatively elevated sound volumes during winter, whereas values fluctuated widely across care homes in the other seasons (Figure 3.6).

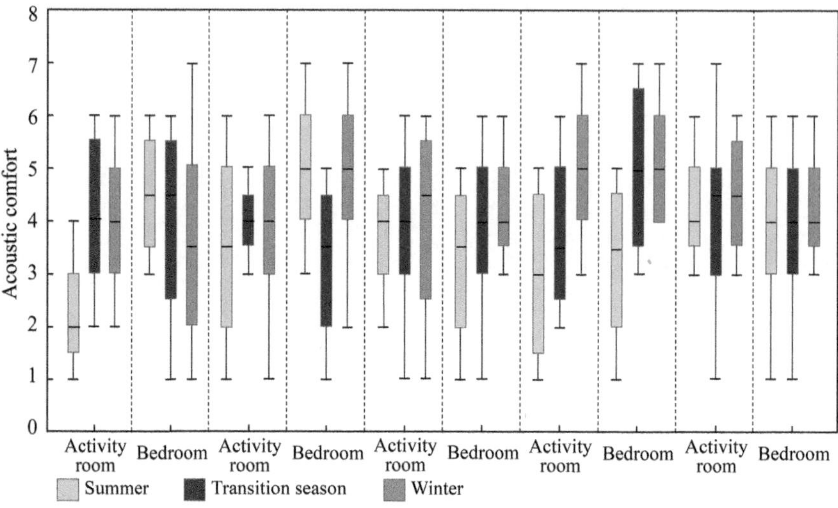

Figure 3.7 Noise levels in care homes in different seasons

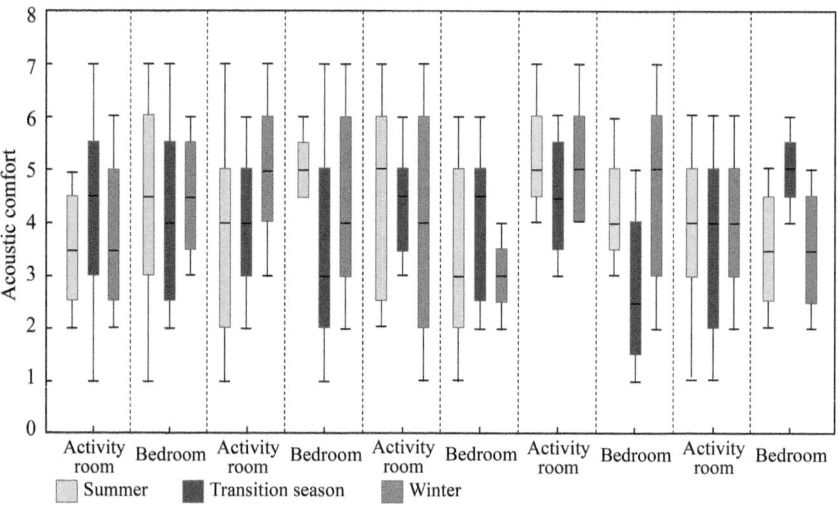

Figure 3.8 Sound preference levels in care homes in different seasons

As for noise levels, activity spaces in care homes recorded their peak noise levels in winter, followed by the transitional season, and the least noise in summer (Figure 3.7), aligning with the sound level distribution in activity zones across varying seasons. Significant variances in noise levels were observed among the bedrooms of different care homes, with heightened noise levels during winter compared to the other two seasons.

In terms of sound preferences, the elderly expressed a greater preference for sound during the transitional season, with comparatively lower preferences for sound in winter and summer. Conversely, the sound preference outcomes for bedrooms were contrary to those in activity areas, with diminished preferences for sound during the transitional season and heightened preferences during winter and summer (Figure 3.8).

The sound preferences of A, B, and C increased with the seasonal variation in a year. The sound preference of E was higher in summer. The sound preference of D is higher than that of others.

3.1.4.3 Acoustic environment perception of care homes in different scales

Figure 3.9 presents the indoor sound pressure levels across care homes of varying sizes, illustrating a direct relationship between sound pressure levels and the dimensions of care homes. As the area of these facilities increases, so do the sound pressure level values. The average sound pressure level in medium-sized care homes was measured at 52.5 *dBA*, whereas in large and extra-large facilities, it reached 57.5 *dBA*, with an observed maximum sound pressure level of 65 *dBA* in extra-large care homes. Concerning satisfaction, seniors express the lowest contentment with medium-sized care homes, whereas their satisfaction with the other three types of care homes is notably higher.

3.1.4.4 Acoustic environment perception for different types of care homes

Upon comparing the satisfaction levels of the elderly residing in renovated and non-renovated care homes, it was observed that the average sound pressure

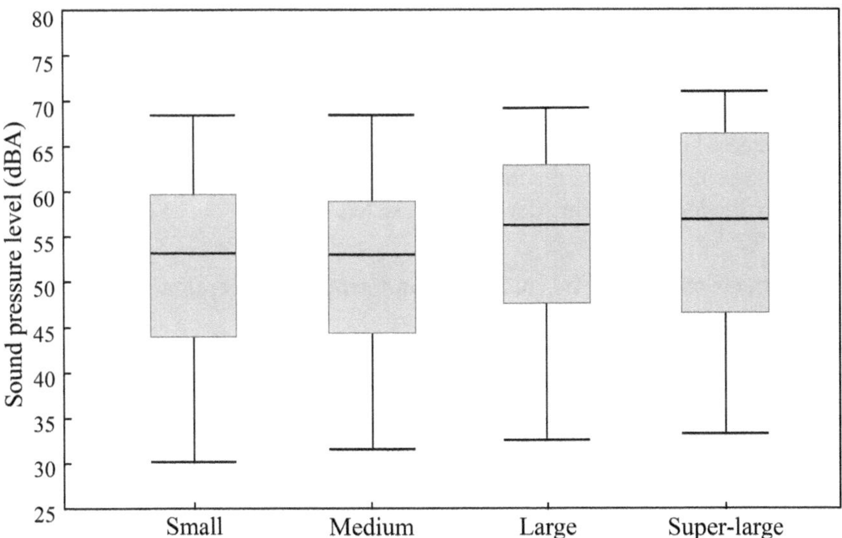

a) Indoor sound pressure levels in different scales of care homes

Figure 3.9(a-b) Acoustic environment perception of care homes at different scales

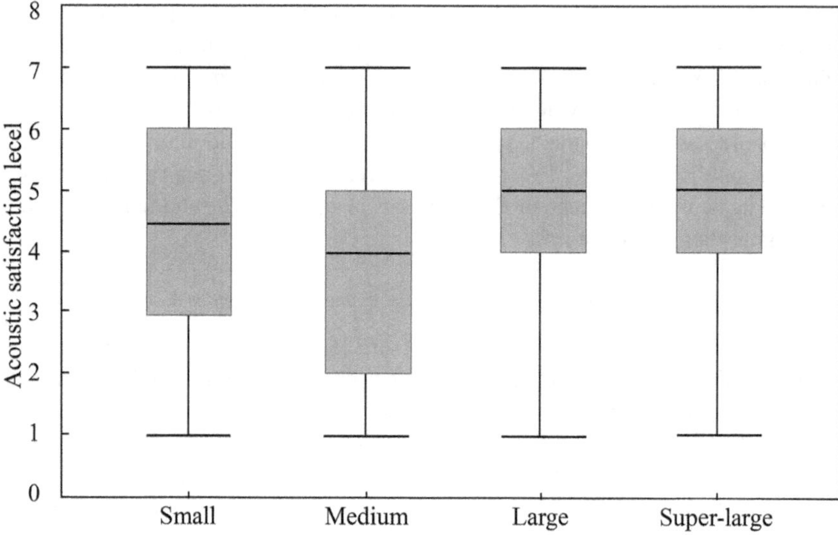

b) Acoustic environment satisfaction in different scales of care homes

Figure 3.9(a-b) (Continued)

level recorded in care homes converted from other structures surpassed that of non-renovated care homes ($p < 0.05$). Following reconstruction, the elderly's satisfaction with the acoustic environment declined (Figure 3.10).

3.1.4.5 *Acoustic environment perception for care homes in different geographical regions*

Figure 3.11 showcases the perception data of the elderly regarding the acoustic environment in care homes across diverse geographical regions. The satisfaction levels of care homes in urban settings ranked the highest, trailed by suburban areas, while those in rural areas recorded the lowest satisfaction levels, possibly influenced by the local economic development status.

3.2 Effects of the elderly's behaviors and acoustic perception in care homes

To delve deeper into the impact of the acoustic environment on the behavior of the elderly, we chose a representative extra-large care home for our investigation [9]. Its expansive indoor public space was segmented into three distinct sections: a grand, sunlit hall shaped like a fan (occupying 1560 m^2 with a height of 14m), corridors (covering 720 m^2, with a length of 72*m*, width of 10m, and height of 4.5*m*), and smaller activity rooms (comprising art studios and lecture halls). Preliminary examinations revealed that the elderly's activities could be categorized into three types: tranquil activities (such as resting, reading, and internet browsing), moderate-decibel activities (like chatting, strolling, and playing chess), and

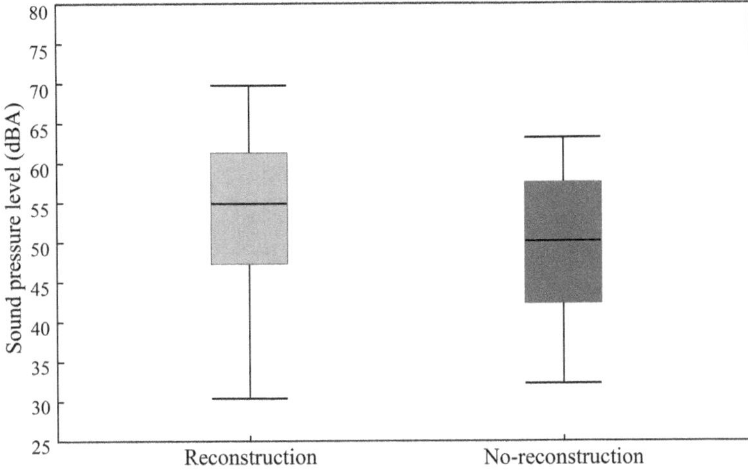

a) Average sound pressure levels in different types of care homes

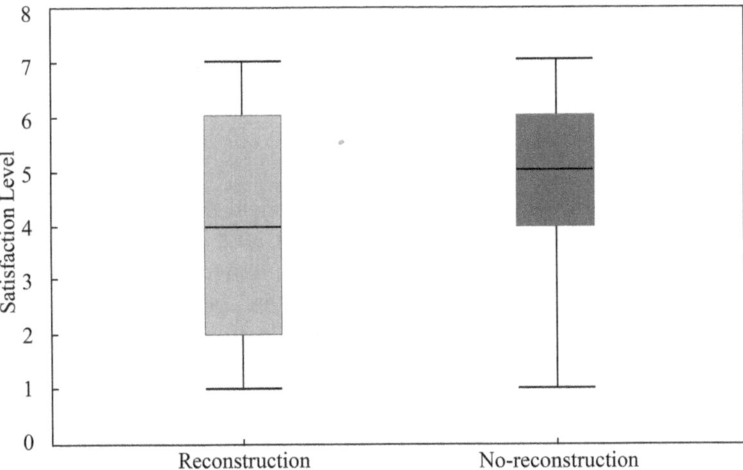

b) Satisfaction level in different types of care homes

Figure 3.10(a-b) Perception of acoustic environment for different types of care homes

high-decibel activities (such as dancing, among others). Video cameras were strategically placed to record crowd density and elderly behavior while different types of music were played in the activity hall. To avoid disrupting the seniors' activities, the cameras were positioned around the sunlit hall and corridors on the second floor, capturing the entirety of the hall from above. Photos were taken every 30 seconds, with continuous shooting lasting for five minutes each time [20]. Following this, individual interviews were conducted with the elderly to gather their assessments of various acoustic environments.

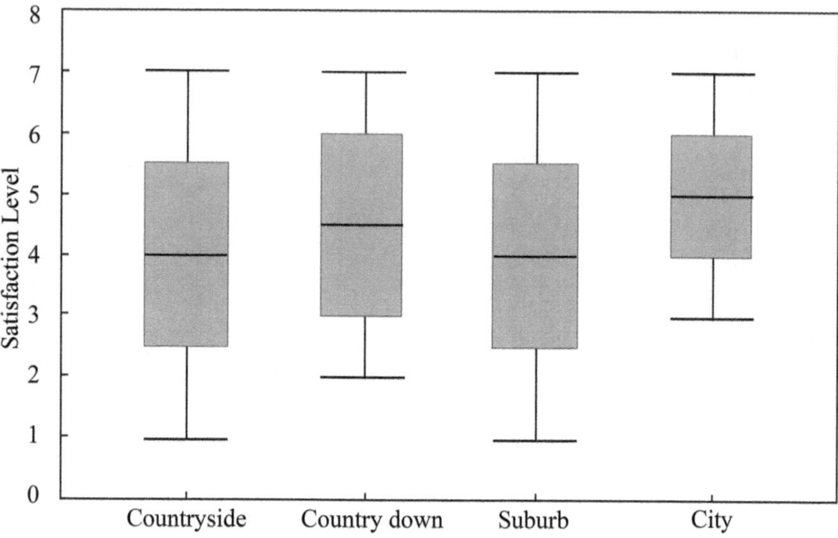

Figure 3.11 Satisfaction with the acoustic environment of care homes in different geographical areas

3.2.1 Activity types

Figure 3.12 visualizes the effects of different music environments on the three activity types (high-decibel, moderate-decibel, and tranquil) across various activity areas (the fan-shaped hall, the corridor promenade, and the small activity rooms). The outcomes demonstrate that as natural sounds increased, most elderly individuals engaged in moderate-decibel activities across all three activity areas, with statistically significant differences $\left(p < 0.001\right)$. Introducing instrumental music with lyrics resulted in a noticeable increase in the proportion of elderly individuals participating in high-decibel activities in the fan-shaped hall and small activity room compared to those engaged in moderate-decibel activities in the promenade area. Moreover, when exposed to music with language, lyrics, and slow tempos, no one engaged in high-decibel activities in the promenade area.

In the natural soundscape, there was a notable 15% rise in high-decibel music activities across the entire activity space, with a slight 5% dip in the corridor and a significant 18% surge in the activity room. While the differences were not strikingly pronounced in the experimental groups with or without lyrics, a subtle uptick was observed overall. These results imply that music has the potential to

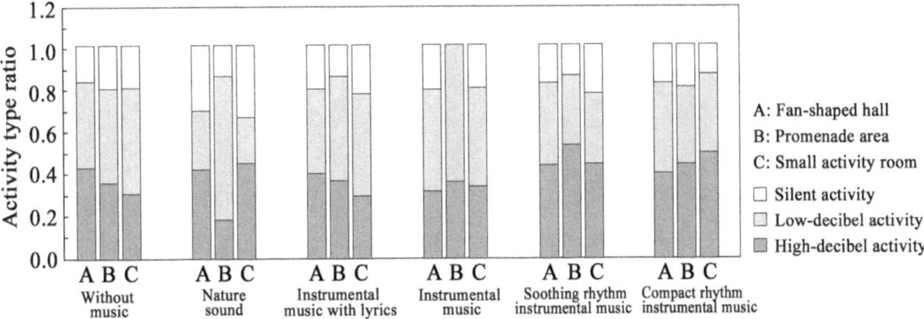

Figure 3.12 Proportion of various types of activities in the activity space under different acoustic environments

encourage elderly individuals to partake in physical activities willingly. Moreover, compared to other musical genres, slow-paced instrumental music was linked to heightened activity levels, attributed to its ability to trigger the release of endorphins [21]. Conversely, in the presence of natural sounds, activity levels saw a decrease, possibly due to increased introspection and planning, as noted in earlier studies [22]. By promoting physical activities and integrating music, the irritation stemming from noise can be alleviated, and gentle, slow-paced music can positively impact the mood of elderly individuals [23]. Previous research has shown that concerts with low arousal potential can have a beneficial effect on human activities [24].

3.2.2 Participation degree

The impact of the acoustic environment on the level of activity involvement among the elderly is substantial. Illustrated in Figure 3.13 is the assessment of specific music types by three distinct groups of elderly individuals: active participants (engaged in dancing, chess, and Tai Chi), spectators (observing and watching), and those engaged in miscellaneous activities. This figure delineates five key indicators: satisfaction, behavior, pleasure, arousal, and dominance. Among the elderly individuals immersed in dancing, there was a marked preference for fast-paced instrumental music, which elicited high satisfaction levels. Conversely, chess enthusiasts leaned towards slow-paced instrumental melodies. This discovery corresponds with previous comprehensive analyses on the correlation between active engagement in music and dance, highlighting the elderly's inclination towards dancing to music owing to its potential benefits for overall well-being, health, and life quality. Additionally, chess aficionados tend to favor slow-paced music for its conducive effect on clear thinking within a serene ambiance [25].

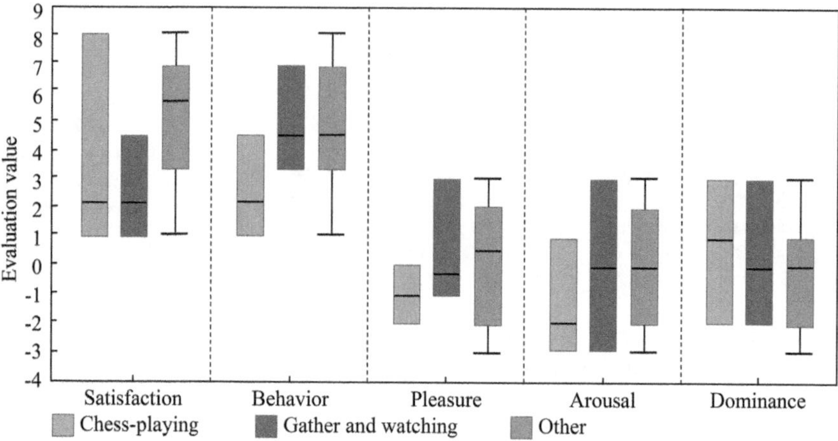

a) Chess-playing activity under fast-rhythm instrumental music

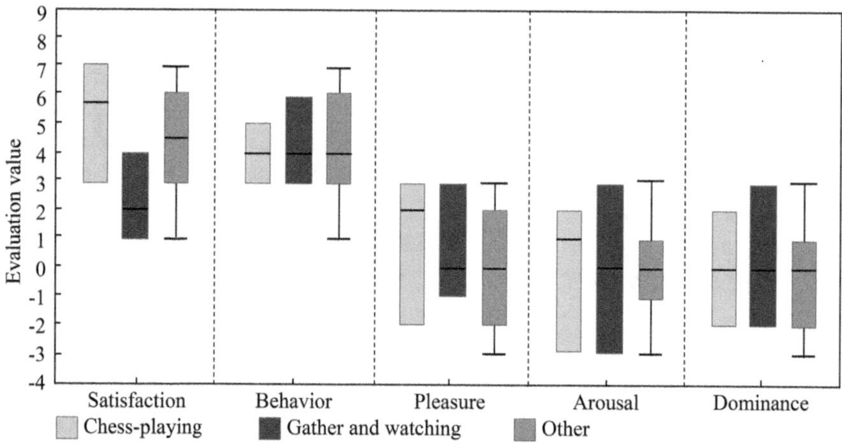

b) Dancing activity under fast-rhythm instrumental music

Figure 3.13(a-j) Impact of different acoustic environments on different activities performed by the participants

The average pleasure ratings (ranging from -1 to 0) for elderly participants in Tai Chi and dancing were comparable. As depicted in Figure 3.13, chess, Tai Chi, and dancing showcased more individual involvement than collective engagement in terms of approach-avoidance behavior and satisfaction ($p < 0.01$). This suggests a preference among the elderly for active participation in these activities over mere observation or engaging in other pursuits while music plays. Overall, the average satisfaction ratings for elderly individuals actively involved in activities and others were notably higher than those for mere observers. Furthermore, the findings

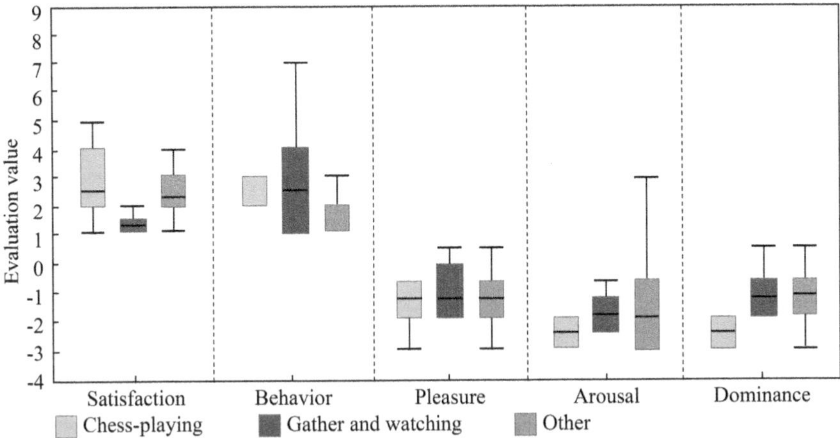

c) Chess-playing activity under slow-rhythm instrumental music

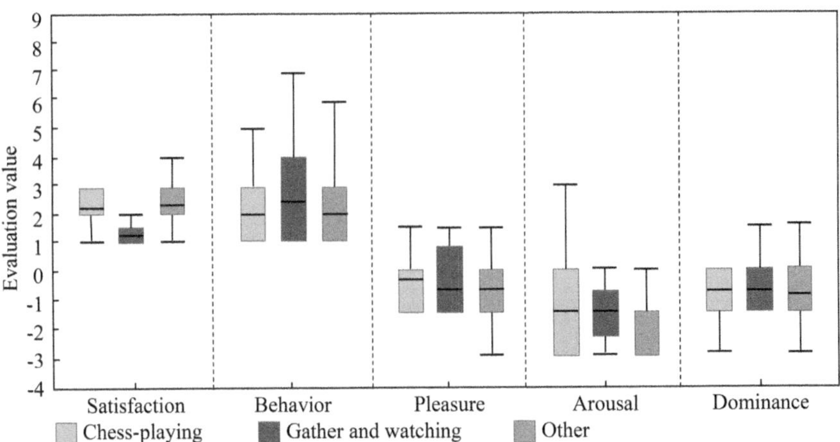

d) Tai Chi under slow-rhythm instrumental music

Figure 3.13(a-j) (Continued)

indicate a preference for natural sounds among elderly individuals during simple activities like playing chess, as these sounds are perceived as invigorating or calming by the majority [26].

3.2.3 Crowd density

The correlation between crowd density and the perception of the acoustic environment, along with satisfaction in various acoustic settings (with or without music),

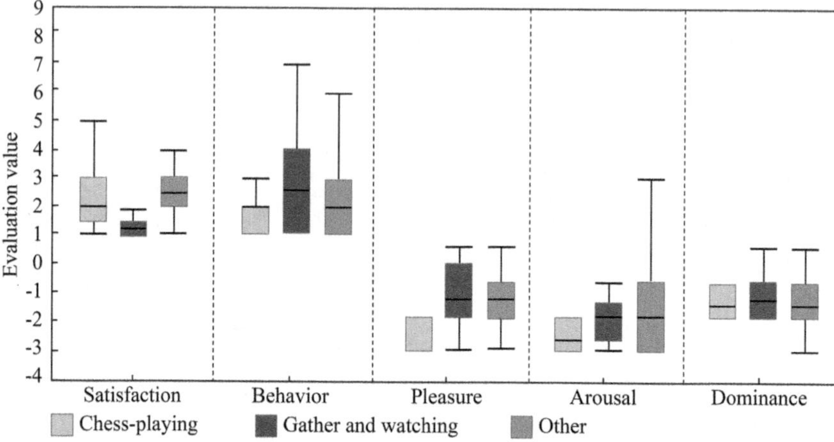

e) Dancing activity under slow-rhythm instrumental music

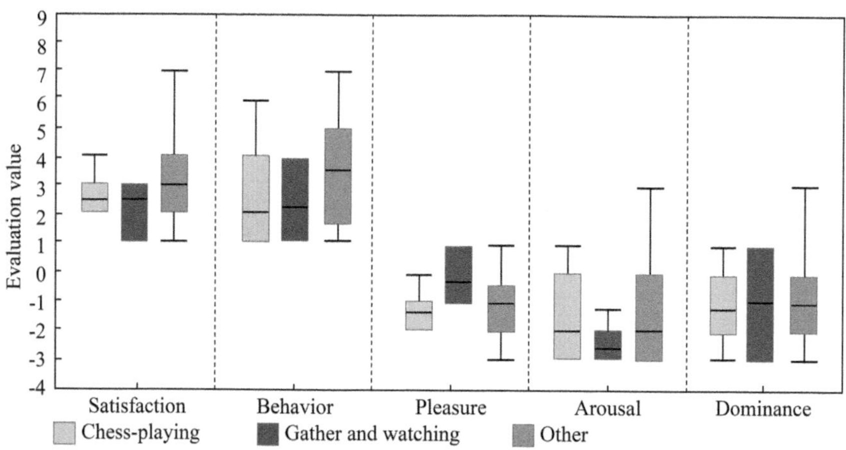

f) Chess-playing activity under instrumental music

Figure 3.13(a-j) (Continued)

is illustrated through linear regressions and their coefficients of determination (R2) in Figures 3.14 and 3.15. As crowd density increases during low-decibel activities, the impact of music diminishes. The association between crowd density and satisfaction perception during low-decibel activities in environments with music was moderate ($R2 = 0.36$). However, in the absence of music in activity spaces, the R2 value rose to 0.65. Conversely, the correlation between crowd density and satisfaction perception during high-decibel activities in environments without

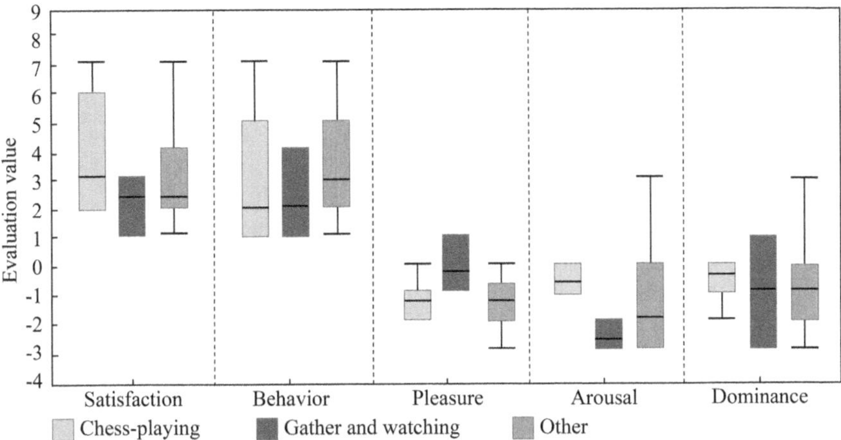

g) Tai Chi exercise under instrumental music

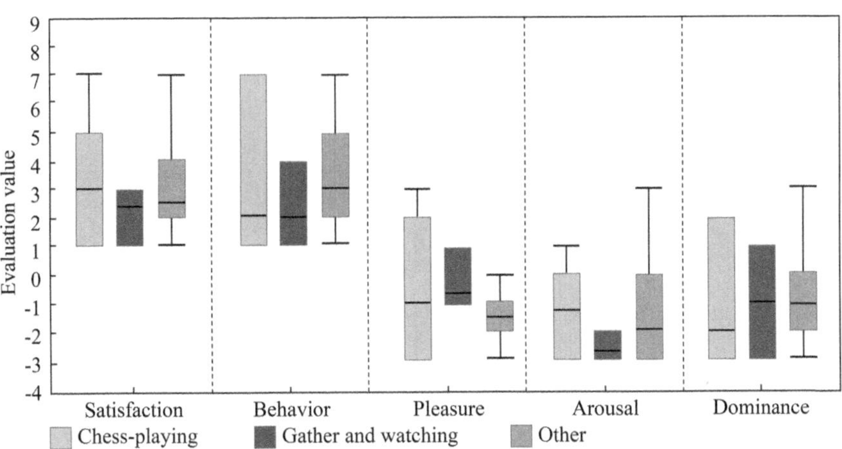

h) Dancing activity under instrumental music

Figure 3.13(a-j) (Continued)

music was relatively robust ($R2 = 0.74$), surpassing that in environments with music ($R2 = 0.68$).

Nevertheless, irrespective of the presence of music, the overall trend declined with an uptick in crowd density, as depicted in Figure 3.14. If music accompanies low- or high-decibel activities, the correlation of satisfaction continues to rise with a decrease in crowd density. In the fan-shaped sunshine hall, satisfaction and boredom increased, while the correlation with pleasure decreased (Figure 3.15).

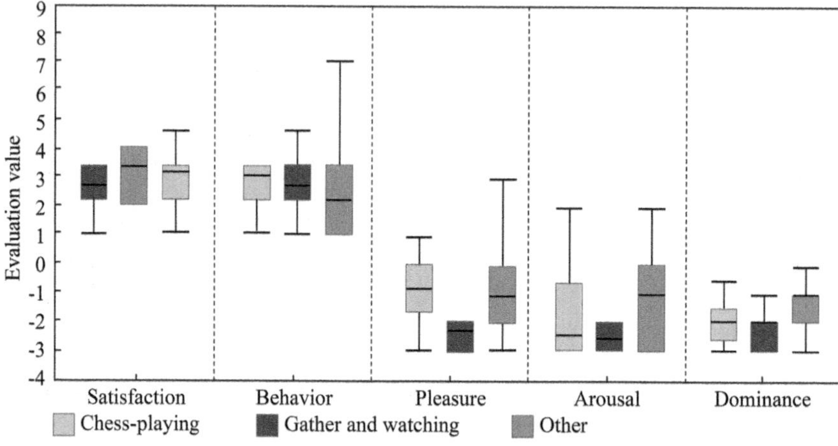

i) Chess-playing activity under natural sounds

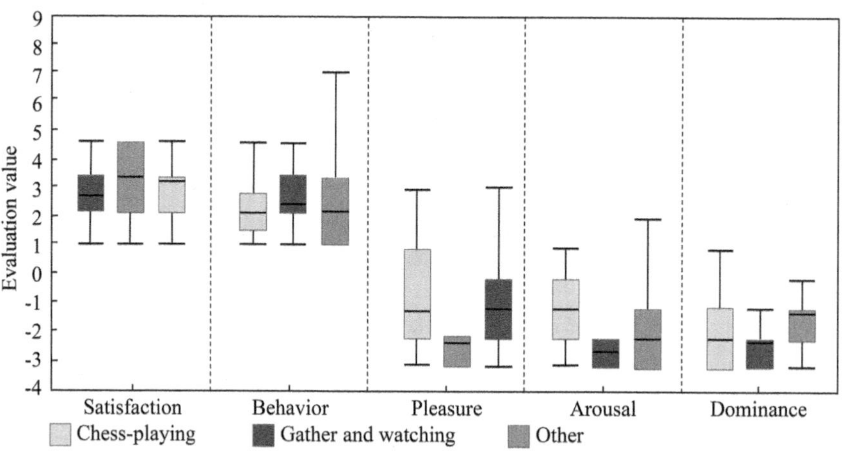

j) Tai Chi exercise under natural sounds

Figure 3.13(a-j) (Continued)

A similar decline in pleasure has been documented in prior studies [27]. However, Lawton and Fujiwara [28] emphasized the disparities in satisfaction and arousal levels across varying decibel levels; satisfaction was higher in quieter external environments and lower in louder ones, suggesting that sound pressure levels significantly influence the elderly's acoustic environment experience.

Figure 3.16 illustrates that in the absence of music, the R^2 value of 0.31 indicates a weak correlation between crowd density and satisfaction. Similarly, settings with natural sounds, music with lyrics, and instrumental music also exhibited weak correlations, with R^2 values of 0.40, 0.36, and 0.48, respectively. However, the R^2 values for

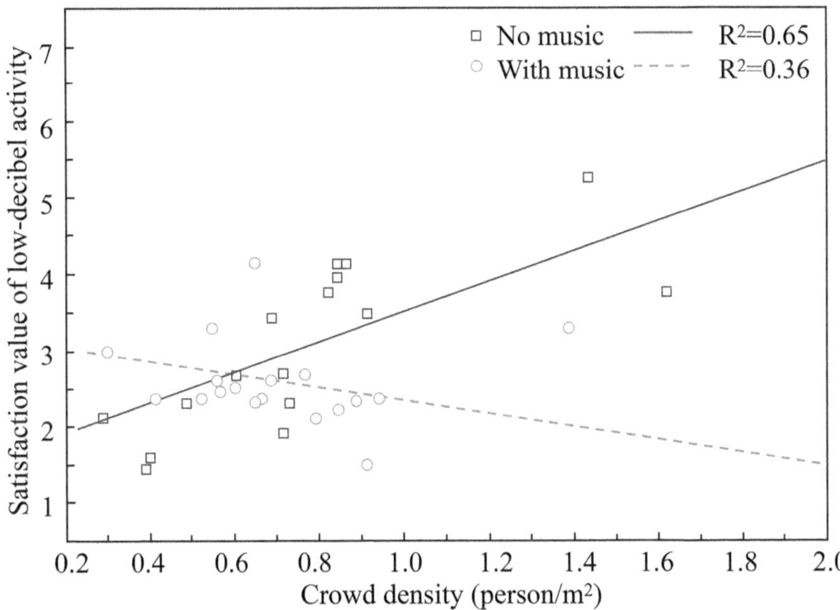

a) Relationship between crowd density and acoustic environment satisfaction with low-decibel activity

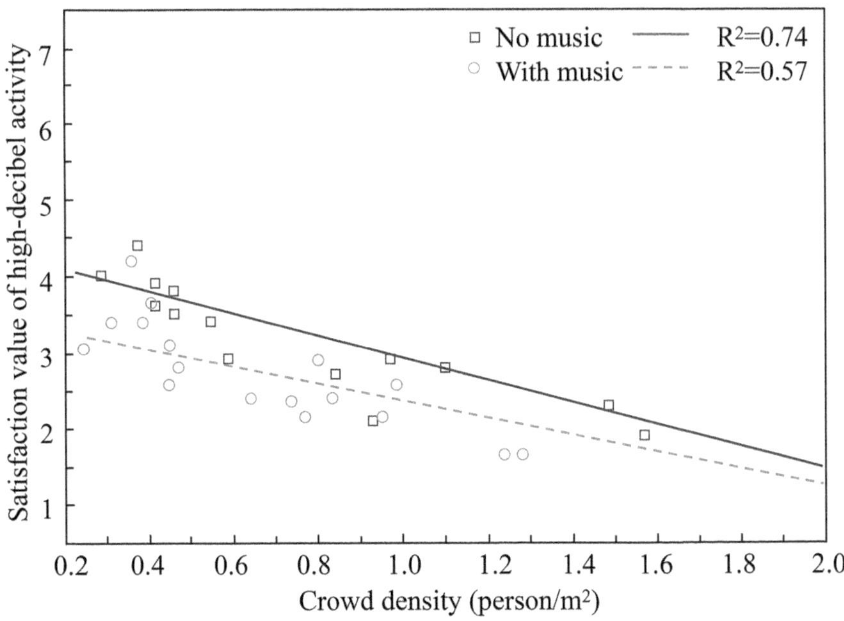

b) Relationship between crowd density and acoustic environment satisfaction with high-decibel activity

Figure 3.14(a-b) Impact of music on different types of activities

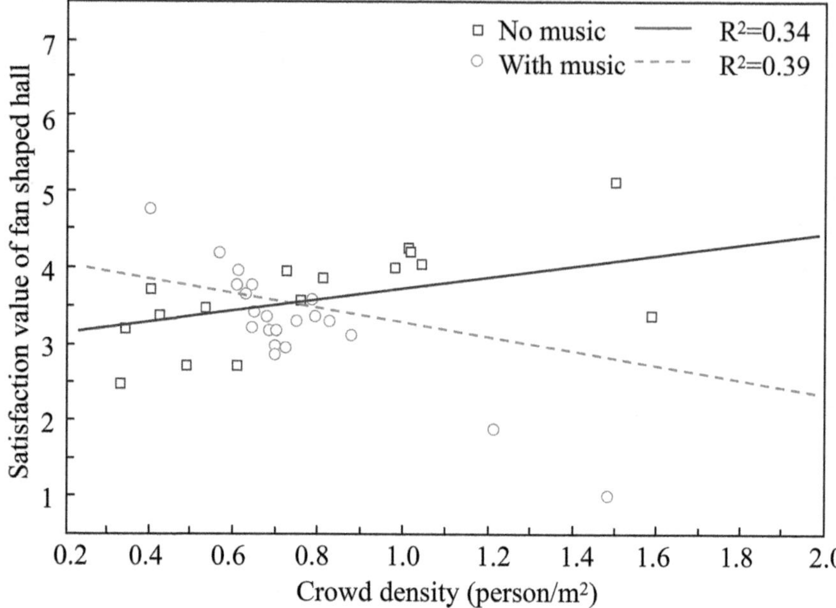

a) Relationship between crowd density and acoustic environment satisfaction in the fan-shaped hall.

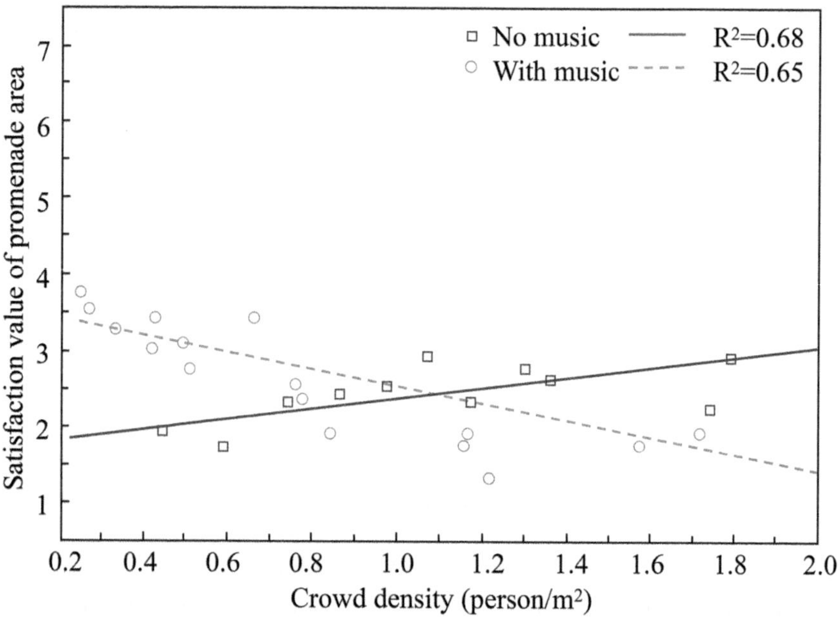

b) Relationship between crowd density and acoustic environment satisfaction in the promenade area.

Figure 3.15(a-b) Impact of music in different areas on crowd density

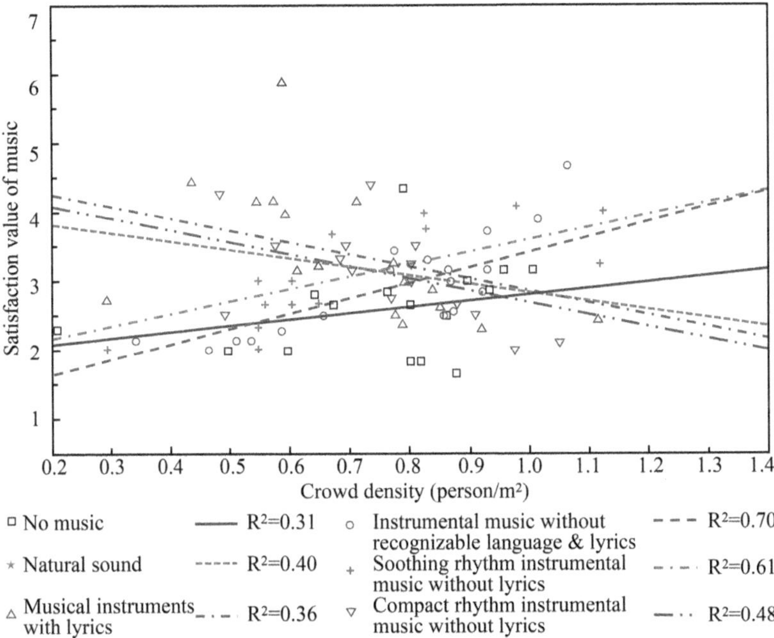

a) Relationship between sound evaluation and crowd density

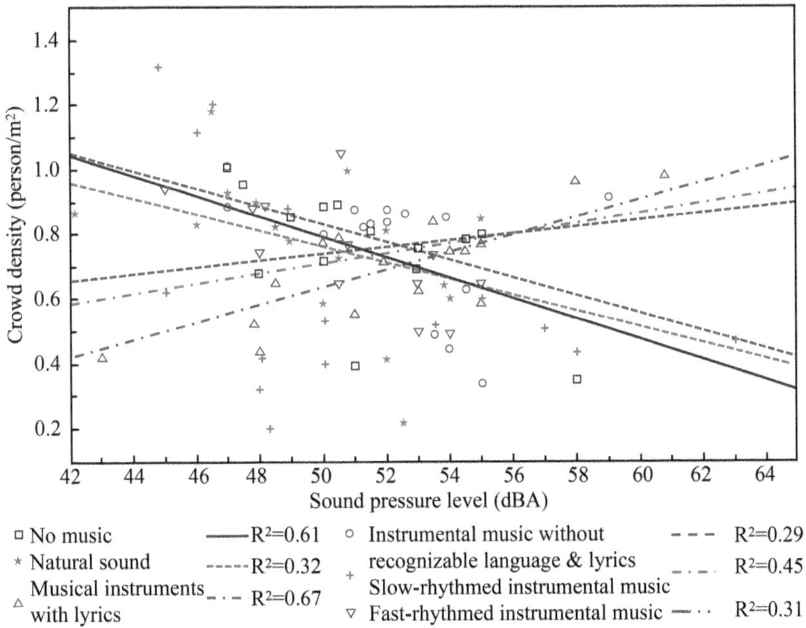

b) Relationship between crowd density and sound pressure level

Figure 3.16(a-b) Relationship between various music situations and sound evaluation in large activity spaces

slow-paced instrumental music and instrumental music were 0.70 and 0.61, respectively. These findings suggest that elderly individuals prefer slow-paced instrumental melodies in expansive environments. Additionally, the sound pressure level demonstrated a trend of initially increasing and then decreasing. With heightened crowd density, a positive correlation was noted between instrumental music and lyrics and crowd density. Moreover, under fast-paced instrumental music, satisfaction levels for these two behaviors decreased more rapidly. Previous research has indicated that in locales with high crowd density, slow-paced instrumental music can enhance the mental state of elderly individuals and alleviate physical discomfort and mental stress [29].

3.3 The satisfaction threshold range of sound pressure level in care homes

3.3.1 *Functional rooms*

The linear correlation between acoustic assessment and sound pressure levels illustrates a decrease in acoustic evaluation with rising sound pressure levels (Figure 3.17). Various room types exhibit linear relationships with acoustic evaluations [30], albeit the correlation between bedroom and restaurant sound pressure levels and acoustic evaluations is relatively weak.

An evaluation score surpassing four points signifies contentment with the surrounding physical environment. For bedrooms and activity rooms, satisfactory

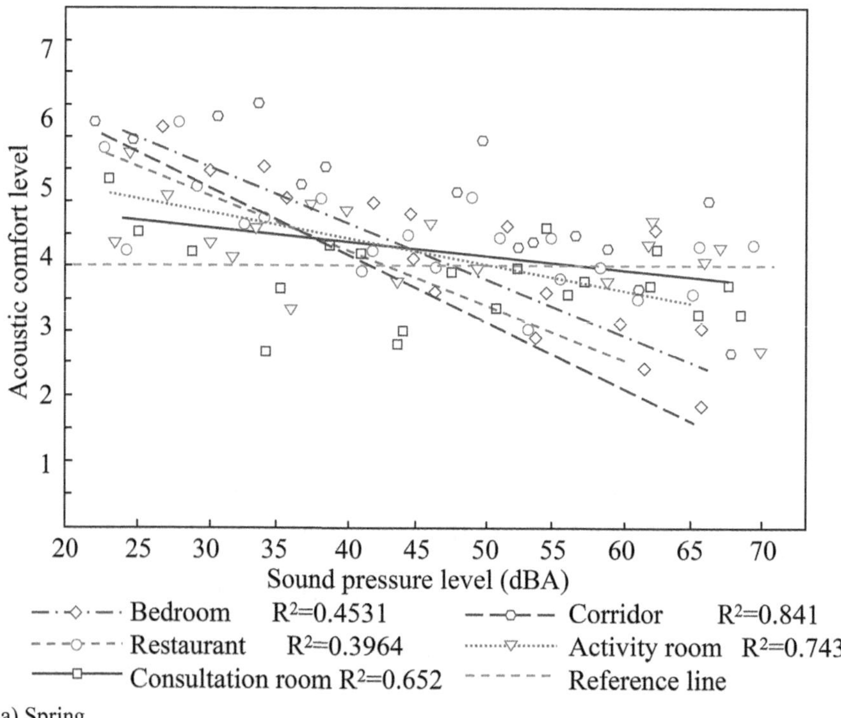

a) Spring

Figure 3.17(a-d) Fitting between sound pressure level and acoustic evaluation based on seasonal differences

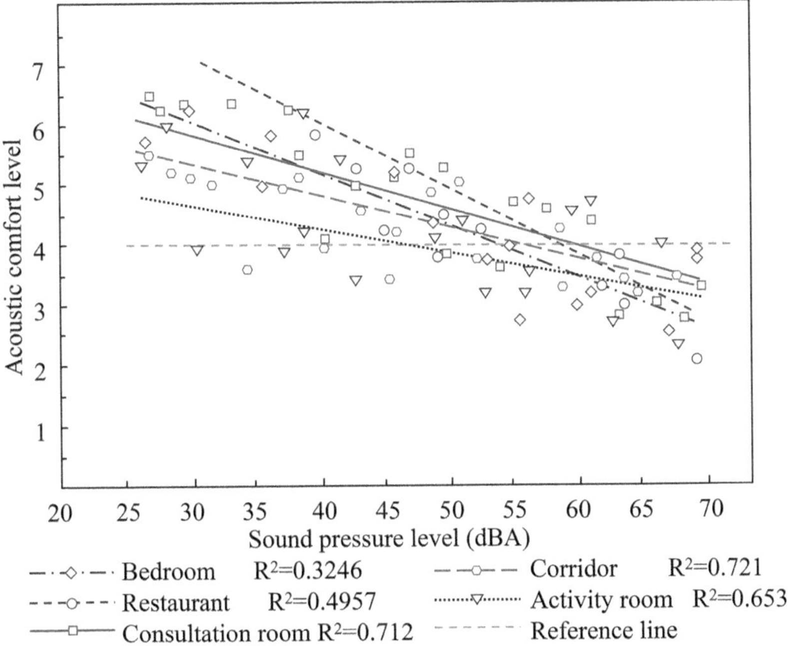

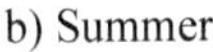
b) Summer

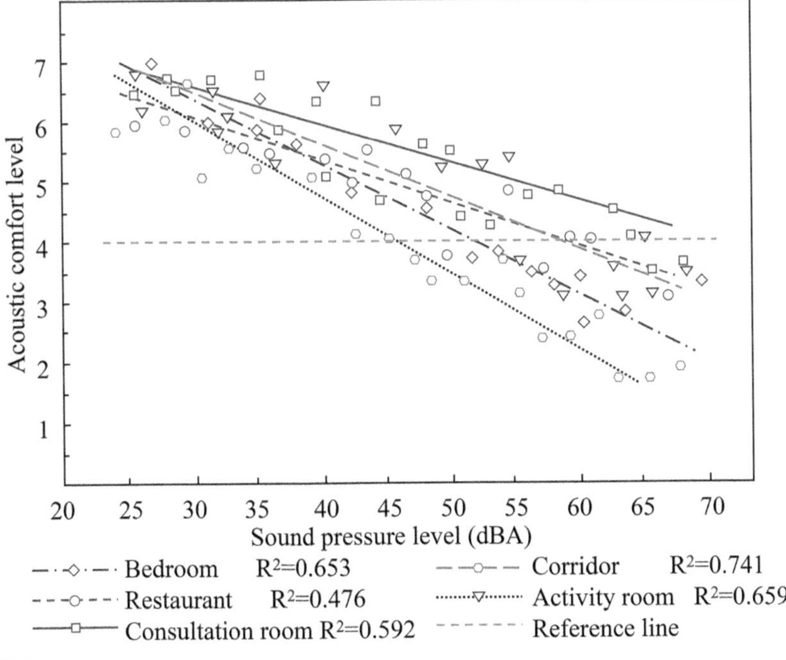

c) Autumn

Figure 3.17(a-d) (Continued)

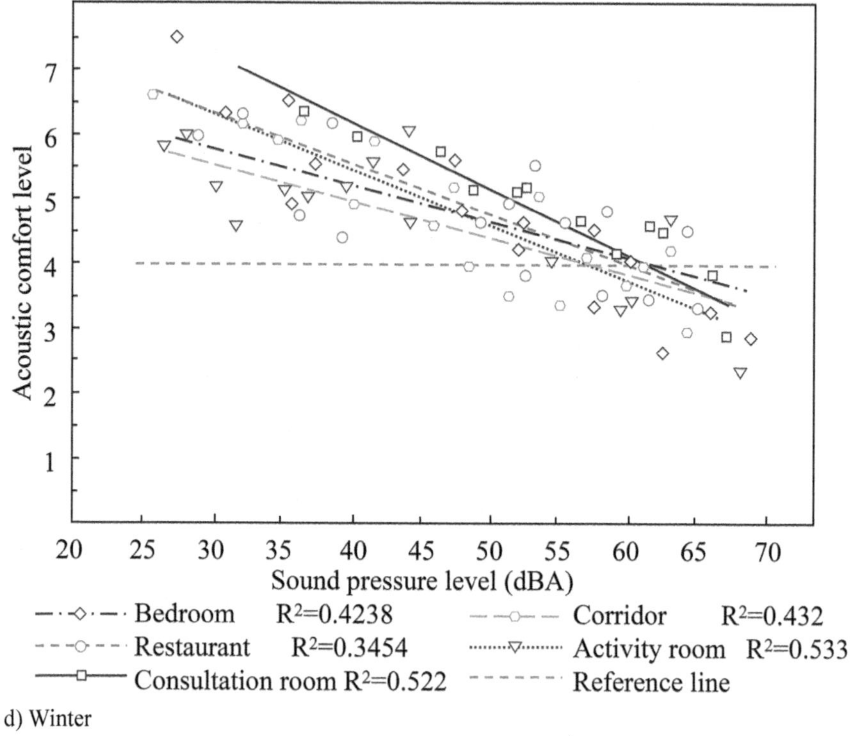

d) Winter

Figure 3.17(a-d) (Continued)

levels ranged between 60 dBA and 65 dBA. However, once noise levels exceed 70 dBA, dissatisfaction among elderly individuals significantly escalates [31].

In this investigation, acoustic levels in both bedrooms and activity rooms surpassed recommended values, likely attributed to floor contact noise [32]. Additionally, sporadic movements by staff members contributed to noise levels. However, when the majority of elderly individuals were engaged in activities or outdoors, bedroom noise levels decreased. The correlation between sound pressure level in bedrooms and dining areas and acoustic evaluation was deemed inadequate (R-squared < 0.653, $p < 0.01$). Hence, further exploration of the relationship between sound pressure levels in bedrooms and dining areas and satisfaction with the acoustic environment is imperative to effectively cater to the needs of the elderly residents.

3.3.2 Seasons

Regarding seasonal variations, Figure 3.17 depicts distinctive trends in the linear relationship between sound pressure levels and acoustic evaluations across different room types. The correlation between corridor sound pressure levels and acoustic evaluation was more robust during spring, summer, and autumn $(R - square > 0.7, p < 0.01)$ but weaker during winter $(R - square = 0.432, p < 0.01)$. Conversely, the relationship between consultation room sound pressure levels and acoustic evaluation displayed minimal seasonal variation (R-square between 0.522 and 0.712, $p < 0.01$). Generally, during summer, dissatisfaction with the acoustic environment surfaced when sound pressure levels exceeded 65 dBA. In autumn and winter, discontent was evident when sound pressure levels reached 60 dBA. This might be attributed to the colder weather during autumn and winter, causing the elderly to spend more time indoors, thereby significantly increasing their requirements for the acoustic environment in elderly care facilities compared to summer.

3.4 Effects of the elderly's demographic factors and acoustic perception in care homes

Satisfaction with the acoustic environment in care homes is significantly intertwined with individuals' backgrounds [33]. These background factors encompass physiological aspects like gender and age; age-related factors such as education, retirement income, and marital status; and lifestyle factors including length of residency and birthplace. Based on preliminary investigations, this section delineates seven potential individual and social factors that may influence satisfaction with the acoustic environment (Table 3.4). Gender differences, overall, do not exert

Table 3.4 Relationship between acoustic evaluations and residents' background

Variable	*Classification*	*Data*
Gender	Male	4.71
	Female	4.34
	F	4.945
	P	0.345
	η_p^2	3.661
Age	<65	5.12
	65–75	4.13
	75–85	4.24
	>85	5.31
	F	9.848
	P	0
	η_p^2	3.554
Education	Basic-Edu	3.56
	Secondary-Edu	4.55
	Higher-Edu	4.61
	F	28.965
	P	0
	η_p^2	3.443
Residence time	<1 year	3.92
	1–3 years	4.22
	3–5 years	4.86
	>5 years	5.31
	F	13.398
	P	0
	η_p^2	3.513

(*Continued*)

Table 3.4 (Continued)

Variable	*Classification*	*Data*
Former residence	Countryside	4.23
	Country town	4.05
	Suburb	3.94
	City	4.63
	F	1.942
	P	0.164
	η_p^2	3.593
Marital status	Single	5.52
	Married	4.83
	Widowed	3.04
	Divorced	4.53
	F	12.106
	P	0.001
	η_p^2	3

significant impacts on acoustic environment assessment, whereas marital status does. Age, education level, and length of residency all markedly influence the evaluation of acoustic environment satisfaction ($p < 0.01$).

3.4.1 *Physiological factors*

This study delves into the influence of different age groups on acoustic environment evaluation. Groups under 65 and over 85 years old rate the indoor acoustic environment higher (Figure 3.18). Additionally, some studies have showcased that as individuals age, their evaluation of acoustic environment comfort increases, suggesting that elderly individuals exhibit higher tolerance to acoustic environments compared to younger counterparts [34].

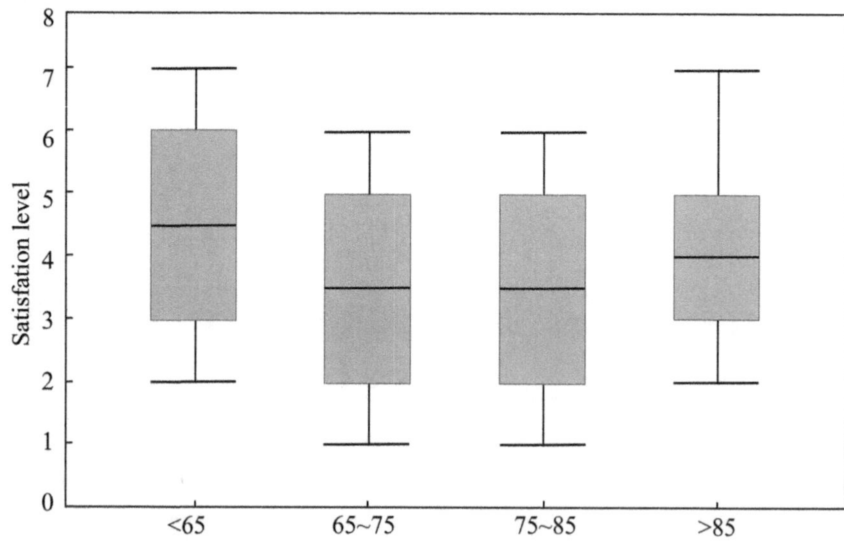

Figure 3.18 Acoustic evaluation based on age difference

3.4.2 Social factors

Regarding educational attainment, primary education or below constitutes basic education, middle education encompasses junior high or high school, and tertiary education refers to college or above. Analysis of satisfaction with the acoustic environment across different groups is illustrated in Figure 3.19. It's evident that in tranquil environments, individuals with higher education levels express the highest satisfaction with the care home's acoustic environment, followed by those with lower education levels, while individuals with intermediate education exhibit the lowest satisfaction. Conversely, in noisy environments, acoustic comfort diminishes with higher levels of education. The boundary between quiet and noisy environments is a sound pressure level of 60 dBA [35]. When sound exceeds 60 dBA, elderly individuals with higher cultural backgrounds significantly reduce their satisfaction with the acoustic environment.

Marital status significantly influences elderly individuals' satisfaction with the acoustic environment. As depicted in Figure 3.20, single individuals express the highest satisfaction with the acoustic environment, followed by divorced individuals. Married and widowed individuals rate the acoustic environment of care homes the lowest, with scores below 4. Research results suggest that single and divorced older adults are more satisfied with the acoustic environment compared to married individuals, possibly because the former may experience loneliness more easily, and the care homes' environment enhances their social skills, compensating for the lack of intimate relationships, thereby positively affecting their physical and mental health.

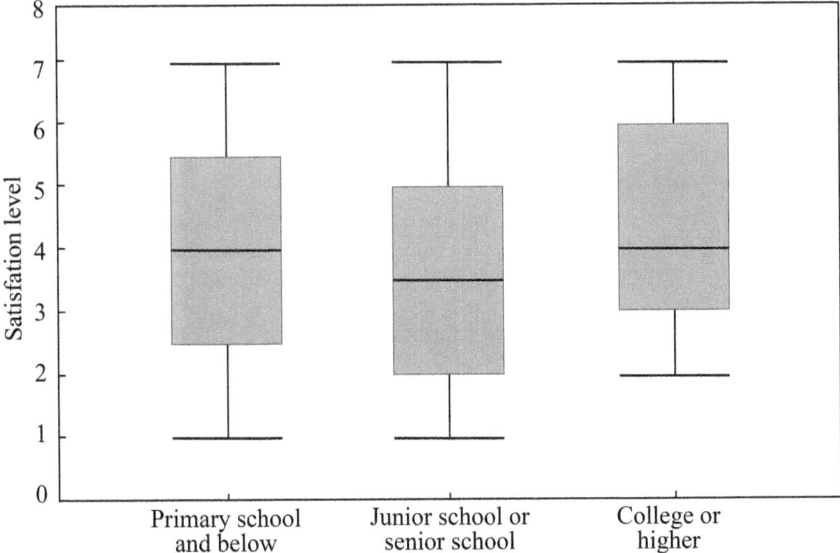

Figure 3.19 Acoustic evaluation based on the difference in education level

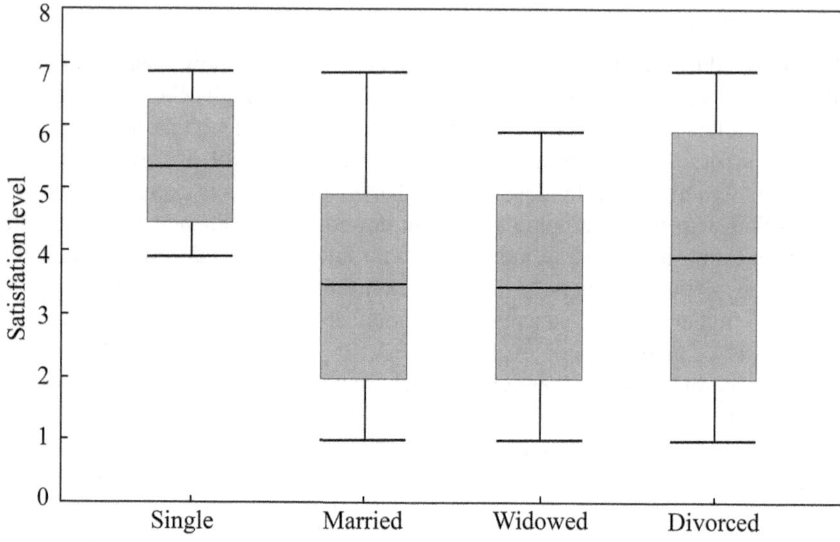

Figure 3.20 Acoustic evaluation based on marital status

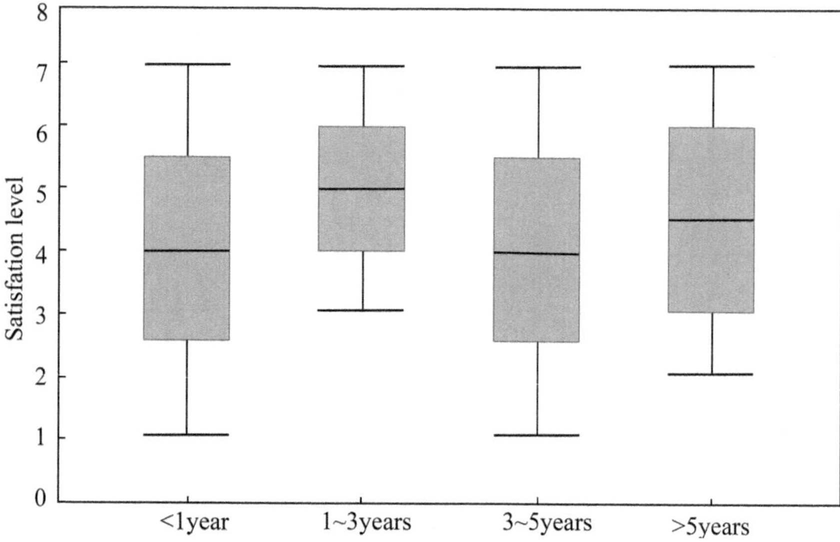

Figure 3.21 Acoustic evaluation based on residence time

3.4.3 Lifestyle factors

The duration of residence in care homes significantly impacts individuals' evaluation of the acoustic environment. As evident in Figure 3.21, elderly individuals who have resided for less than a year rate the indoor acoustic environment relatively low, whereas those who have resided for 1–3 years and over 5 years offer higher evaluations, scoring 5 points. This phenomenon might be attributed to the

Table 3.5 Instruments for measurements of the environment

Test	*Instrument*	*Test range/Accuracy*
Sound pressure level	BSAB801 sound level meter	19–37 dBA (±0.1 dBA)
Illumination	T-10A illuminance meters	0.01–299,000 lx (±5%)
Brightness	GPH-1001 brightness meters	20 cd/m2x–2,000 kcd/m2
Temperature	K-type thermocouple (Centre 314 temperature/humidity data logger)	−40–80 °C (± 0.1 °C); 40–76 °F (± 32.18 °F)
Relative humidity (RH)	RH sensors (Center 314 data logger)	0–99% (± 3%)

fact that longer-term residents have adapted to the indoor acoustic environment of the care homes. Overall, different groups express satisfaction with the care homes' acoustic environment, with average satisfaction scores of ≥4.

3.5 Relationship between acoustic environment and other indoor physical environment factors

Research suggests that the overall physical environment of care homes plays a crucial role in the physical and mental well-being and comfort of the elderly. Additionally, the subjective evaluation of the acoustic environment by the elderly may be influenced by other physical environmental factors, such as thermal and lighting conditions. Therefore, investigating the interaction between these factors in care homes is essential to better promote the health and happiness of the elderly [36].

In this study, comprehensive on-site measurements were conducted to assess the indoor physical environment of the aforementioned five care homes. These measurements encompassed sound pressure levels, lighting conditions, brightness, temperature, and relative humidity. Data collection occurred from December 2018 to February 2019, spanning from 8:00 a.m. to 6:00 p.m., with continuous measurements taken in each area for two days. The instruments utilized for measurement are detailed in Table 3.5.

Following data collection, elderly residents participated in surveys. Consistent with the aforementioned methods, the questionnaire comprised two sections. The first part aimed to gather background information on the elderly, including gender, age, length of residency, and so forth. The second part focused on the comprehensive physical environmental assessment of care homes by the elderly, covering aspects such as sound, light, and thermal environments. Questions in the questionnaire were based on a 7-point Likert-type scale, and the survey was conducted through one-on-one interviews, taking approximately 15 minutes for each participant to complete. A total of 480 valid questionnaires were collected. Key questions from the second part of the questionnaire are outlined in Table 3.6.

Data analysis utilized SPSS 20.0, employing the t-test, Pearson's correlation coefficient, and regression analysis to explore the relationships between light, thermal, and acoustic environments and the respective questionnaire results. The significance of the results was evaluated based on the p-value of each index, with $p < 05$considered significant, $p < 01$highly significant, and $p < 001$extremely significant [37].

Table 3.6 Definition of environmental evaluation in questionnaire

Question category	*Questions*	*Scale (1–7)*
Light environment	1. What is your general impression of the light environment in the care home?	1 = *very uncomfortable*; 7 = *very comfortable*
	2. Do you think the lighting condition in your current facility has a significant impact on your life?	1 = *not at all*; 7 = *very much*
	3. How do you rate the lighting in your room?	1 = *very bad*; 7 = *very good*
	4. Do you think there is enough light in your place?	1 = *not at all*; 7 = *very much*
	5. Will the light environment in your current facility affect your daily life?	1 = *not at all*; 7 = *very much*
Acoustic environment	1. What is your general impression of the acoustic environment in the care home?	1 = *very uncomfortable*; 7 = *very comfortable*
	2. Do you think the acoustic environment in your current facility has a significant impact on your life?	1 = *not at all*; 7 = *very much*
	3. How do you rate the acoustic environment in your room?	1 = *very bad*; 7 = *very good*
	4. Do you think your place is noisy?	1 = *not at all*; 7 = *very much*
	5. Does the acoustic environment in your current facility affect your mood?	1 = *not at all*; 7 = *very much*
	6. Do you think there is an echo in the place where you live?	1 = *not at all*; 7 = *very much*
	7. Can you hear what others say in the facility?	1 = *not at all*; 7 = *very much*
Thermal environment	1. What is your general impression of the thermal environment in the care home?	1 = *very uncomfortable*; 7 = *very comfortable*
	2. Do you think the temperature in the current facility has a significant impact on your daily life?	1 = *not at all*; 7 = *very much*
	3. Do you think the temperature in the facility is suitable?	1 = *not at all*; 7 = *very much*
	4. Do you think the indoor temperature during winter meets your needs?	1 = *not at all*; 7 = *very much*
	5. Do you think the humidity meets the demand when the indoor temperature is high?	1 = *not at all*; 7 = *very much*

Table 3.7 Comfort evaluation statistics, ratings on a 7-point likert-type scale

Statistical measure	*Light environment*	*Air temperature*	*Humidity*	*Wind speed*
Mean value	3.41	2.69	3.31	0.43
Standard deviation	1.018	1.211	0.996	0.031
Standard error of the mean	0.097	0.117	0.095	0.086
Kurtosis	−0.411	0.933	−0.215	0.697
Skewness	−0.218	0.202	−0.015	−.517

Table 3.8 The adaptability relationship among the light, thermal, and acoustic environments

Variable	*Correlation coefficient*	*Progressive standard error*	*Approximate t value*	*Approximate significance value*
Light environment	0.418	0.144	2.511	0.01
Thermal environment				
Temperature	0.435	0.119	2.143	0.025
Humidity	0.265	0.116	3.611	0
Wind speed	0.311	0.155	1.796	0.058
Overall evaluation	0.3573	0.142	2.5152	0.001

3.5.1 Interactions among physical environment influencing factors

Research results indicate that the physical environment – including sound, light, and thermal conditions – significantly influences the comfort and satisfaction of older adults in care homes [38]. When analyzing the correlation between sound, light, and thermal environments, we conducted statistical analyses based on sensory comfort parameters [36], as detailed in Table 3.7.

As shown in Table 3.6, older adults perceive the light environment in care homes as the most comfortable, with a score of 3.41, followed by the acoustic environment and humidity. With the exception of wind speed, the values for other factors were relatively high. Based on this data, we analyzed the correlation between the acoustic comfort of older adults and the comfort of other physical environments, as presented in Table 3.8.

The findings in Table 3.8 reveal that the acoustic environment has a stronger correlation with temperature than with humidity. A multiple regression analysis was conducted to predict the overall level of environmental comfort – represented by the mean value of questionnaire results – based on measurements of lighting, acoustic, and thermal parameters. The results, shown in Table 3.9, demonstrate significant correlations between the lighting, acoustic, and thermal environments and overall environmental comfort. Notably, the coefficients for lighting and acoustic evaluation were the highest, at 0.0208and 0.0547, respectively. While both parameters were statistically significant, only the coefficient for lighting evaluation was highly significant ($p < .001$).

To further examine the relationships among the three variables – lighting, acoustic, and thermal environments – Pearson's correlation coefficients were computed using the objective measurement results. As depicted in Table 3.10, the objective

Table 3.9 Multiple regression analysis

Overall environmental comfort	*Unstandardized coefficients*		*t*	*Significance*	*95% Confidence interval*
	B	*Std. Error*			
Constant	23.47	3.081	7.617	$p < .001$*	13.413
Illuminance level	0.0208	0.0033	6.296	$p < .001$*	0.042
Sound pressure level	0.0547	0.0352	1.551	$p = .02$*	
Temperature	−0.1607	0.0871	−1.8444	$p = .05$*	13.261

* Significant results.

Table 3.10 Pearson's correlation analysis of the three environmental variables

Variable	*Acoustic*	*Lightning*	*Thermal*	*p Value*
Acoustic	–	$r = -.22$		0.058
Lightning		–	$r = .27$	.024*
Thermal	$r = -.04$		–	0.764

* Statistically significant.

parameter of the acoustic environment exhibited a negative association with the objective parameters of both lighting and thermal environments. The sole significant association was observed between the objective parameters of the thermal and lighting environments (r = .27).

The study results indicate significant correlations between the acoustic, lighting, and thermal environments and the overall comfort of elderly residents. Our analysis revealed that the acoustic environment is more closely associated with temperature than humidity. Illumination, indoor temperature, and humidity collectively influence the comfort within the indoor acoustic environment. Both the acoustic and lighting environments significantly impact the physical environment of care homes, thereby affecting elderly residents' evaluations of their surroundings. Consequently, managing the acoustic environment in care homes could potentially affect residents' perceptions of the thermal environment. Additionally, the lighting environment influences the comfort of the indoor acoustic environment. Ultimately, our findings underscore the interdependence of these three factors and suggest that achieving a balance among them could enhance the indoor comfort of the elderly [39].

3.5.2 *Correlation between indoor environmental quality indicators rating and physical environment*

To investigate the influence of the physical environment on the overall indoor environmental quality evaluation [30], we initially examined the correlation between different physical environments and the overall indoor environmental quality, as shown in Table 3.11. Elderly residents provided favorable overall indoor environmental quality evaluations for the four physical environmental parameters, each

Table 3.11 Correlations between indoor environmental quality and four environmental parameters

Overall IEQ	*Acoustic*	*Lighting*	*Thermal-Env*	*IAQ*
Evaluation	4.64	4.52	5.27	4.76
Correlation coefficient	0.73	0.686	0.731	0.691
p-value	0.001***	0.001***	0.001***	0.001***

Note: IEQ = Indoor environmental quality, IAQ = Indoor air quality. ***p<0001.

Table 3.12 Evaluation of four care homes

	Factors	*Measure subjective evaluations*	*Correlation coefficient*
Activity room	Acoustic	4.59/1.845	0.717/0.000***
	Lighting	4.13/2.042	0.705/0.000***
	Thermal-Env	5.21/1.916	0.732/0.000***
	Indoor air quality	4.31/2.004	0.736/0.000***
Bedroom	Acoustic	3.82/1.794	0.695/0.000***
	Lighting	3.96/1.965	0.740/0.000***
	Thermal-Env	4.67/1.959	0.849/0.000***
	Indoor air quality	4.12/2.060	0.715/0.000***
Restaurant	Acoustic	5.28/1.992	0.784/0.000***
	Lighting	4.83/1.988	0.666/0.000***
	Thermal-Env	4.81/1.747	0.694/0.000***
	Indoor air quality	5.16/1.812	0.708/0.000***
Corridor	Acoustic	3.65/1.798	0.826/0.000***
	Lighting	3.40/1.946	0.701/0.000***
	Thermal-Env	4.96/1.935	0.849/0.000***
	Indoor air quality	3.45/1.837	0.664/0.000***
Consultation room	Acoustic	3.45/1.783	0.674/0.000***
	Lighting	4.76/1.953	0.726/0.000***
	Thermal-Env	5.20/1.895	0.851/0.000***
	Indoor air quality	4.57/1.864	0.658/0.000***

exceeding 4.5 points out of seven. Moreover, these four selected physical environment parameters exhibited a strong positive correlation with the overall indoor environmental quality evaluation, with all correlation coefficients close to or above 0.7 ($p < 0.001$).

Subsequently, the four indoor environmental quality factors were further analyzed to comprehensively evaluate the physical environmental parameters of care homes, as presented in Table 3.12. Column A in Table 3.12 lists the mean evaluation and standard deviation of the four factors among elderly residents in different types of rooms.

Activity rooms and restaurants received the highest ratings, approaching five points. Conversely, the corridor scored lower for acoustics, lighting, and indoor air quality, all falling below four points. This lower corridor evaluation, as indicated in Column B, could be attributed to poor acoustic and lighting environments, given their high correlation with indoor environmental quality evaluation, reaching 0.826 and 0.701, respectively ($p < 0.001$). The indoor environmental quality evaluations of the other five types of rooms exhibited a strong correlation with the four physical parameters, with correlation coefficients ranging from 0.66 *to* 0.85 $(p < 0.001)$.

Based on this analysis, it is evident that the four physical environment factors of care homes – acoustic, lighting, thermal, and indoor air quality – are highly correlated with indoor environmental quality evaluation ($p < 0.001$). Furthermore, significant correlations exist among the evaluations of various physical environmental elements, indicating an interactive relationship among these factors and their joint significant impact on the quality of life of the elderly.

3.6 Conclusion

This study conducted a comprehensive investigation of care homes in Northeast China, revealing that the elderly rated the acoustic environment of quiet areas the highest, followed by corridors, lounges, and small activity areas, with the lowest ratings for larger activity areas. Regarding building types, the elderly were most satisfied with the acoustic environment of non-reconstructed, large, or super-large care homes, while satisfaction was lower for small and medium-sized facilities. Seasonally, the highest perceived acoustic comfort was reported during winter. Geographically, the elderly exhibited the highest satisfaction with care homes in urban areas, followed by suburban areas, with the lowest satisfaction for facilities in rural and remote areas.

This chapter also explored the influence of the acoustic environment on elderly behavior. It was found that participation significantly affected satisfaction with the acoustic environment, with elderly participants experiencing greater satisfaction than observers. Under natural sound conditions, all three activity areas saw increased low-decibel activities ($p < 0.001$). Conversely, the proportion of high-decibel activities significantly increased with fast-paced instrumental music, indicating that the elderly are more inclined to participate in activities with a conducive musical environment.

Observations of activity spaces indicated that music increased crowd density, especially in environments featuring natural sounds, as the elderly preferred these acoustic settings without lyrical interference. As the duration of natural sound playback increased, the variety of activity types also rose. However, satisfaction decreased as crowd density increased during both low and high-decibel activities.

Furthermore, this chapter analyzed the influence of demographic and social backgrounds on acoustic environment assessment results. Gender differences did not significantly impact acoustic environment assessment, while marital status did. Age, education level, and length of residence all had significant effects on acoustic environment satisfaction ratings ($p < 0.001$).

The study also found a strong correlation between the acoustic environment and other indoor physical environments, collectively affecting the environmental comfort of the elderly. Analysis revealed that the correlation between the acoustic environment and temperature was stronger than that with humidity. Lighting, indoor temperature, and humidity all influence indoor acoustic environment comfort. Both the acoustic and lighting environments significantly impacted the physical environment of care homes, greatly affecting residents' assessments of their physical surroundings. Therefore, managing the acoustic environment in care homes may influence elderly residents' perceptions of the thermal environment. Additionally, the lighting environment also affects the comfort of the indoor acoustic environment. Ultimately, our research indicates that these three factors interact with each other, and balancing them may improve indoor comfort for the elderly.

References

[1] Winker MA. The aging global population: A call for papers (vol 276, pg 1758, 1996) [J]. *JAMA: The Journal of the American Medical Association*, 1997, 277(2):114–114.

[2] Leung MY, Wang C, Chan IYS. A qualitative and quantitative investigation of effects of indoor built environment for people with dementia in care and attention homes[J]. *Building and Environment*, 2019, 157(June):89–100.

[3] Huang YC, Chu CL, Lee SNC, et al. Building users' perceptions of importance of indoor environmental quality in long-term care facilities[J]. *Building & Environment*, 2013, 67(Sept.):224–230.

[4] Stansfeld SA, Matheson MP. Noise pollution: Non-auditory effects on health[J]. *British Medical Bulletin*, 2003(1):243.

[5] Kerns E, Masterson EA, Themann CL, et al. Cardiovascular conditions, hearing difficulty, and occupational noise exposure within US industries and occupations[J]. *American Journal of Industrial Medicine*, 2018, 61(6):477–491.

[6] Du X. Investigation of indoor environment comfort in large high-speed railway stations in Northern China[J]. *Indoor and Built Environment*, 2019, 29(1):1420326X1984229.

[7] Gao J, Barroso C, Zhang P, et al. N-terminal acetylation promotes synaptonemal complex assembly in C. elegans.[J]. *Genes and Development: A Journal Devoted to the Molecular Analysis of Gene Expression in Eukaryotes, Prokaryotes, and Viruses*, 2016, 30(21).

[8] Mu J, Kang J, Wu Y. Acoustic environment of comprehensive activity spaces in nursing homes: A case study in Harbin, China[J]. *Applied Acoustics*, 2021, 177(24):107932.

[9] Mu J, Kang J, Sui Z. Effect of music in large activity spaces on the perceptions and behaviours of older adults in China[J]. *Applied Acoustics*, 2022(Jan.):188.

[10] Bottiroli S, Rosi A, Russo R, Vecchi T, Cavallini E. The cognitive effects of listening to background music on older adults: Processing speed improves with upbeat music, while memory seems to benefit from both upbeat and downbeat music[J]. *Frontiers in Aging Neuroscience*, 2014, 6:284.

[11] Aletta F, Botteldooren D, Thomas P, et al. Monitoring sound levels and soundscape quality in the living rooms of nursing homes: A case study in Flanders (Belgium)[J]. *Applied Sciences,* 2017, 7(9):874.

[12] Aletta F, Mynsbrugge TV, Van de Velde D, et al. Awareness of 'sound' in nursing homes: A large-scale soundscape survey in Flanders (Belgium)[J]. *Building Acoustics*, 2018, 25(1):43–59.

[13] Wang L, Kang J. Acoustic demands and influencing factors in facilities for the elderly[J]. *Applied Acoustics*, 2020, 170:107470.

[14] Mu JY, Kang J, Zheng S. Evaluating the objective and subjective physical environments of residential care facilities[J]. *Indoor and Built Environment*, 2023, 23(5):1033–1050.

[15] Lundbeck M, Grimm G, Hohmann V, et al. Sensitivity to angular and radial source movements as a function of acoustic complexity in normal and impaired hearing[J]. *Trends in Hearing*, 2017, 21(4):2331216517717152.

[16] Shen CH, Wang YJ, Chen YG, et al. Suzhou Yangshan nursing home[J]. *Architectural Practice*, 2018, (05):18–23. (In Chinese)

[17] Zhou JM, Chen JW. An honest interpretation of the everyday in a philosophical way: Commenting on Suzhou Yangshan nursing home[J]. *Architectural Journal*, 2016, (01):82–85+76–81. (In Chinese)

[18] Liang XF, Chen Y. Xinbei, Taiwan, China Shuanglian Xinzhuang social welfare center[J]. *Archicreation*, 2020, (05):94–99. (In Chinese)

[19] Rockwood K, Song XW, MacKnight C, et al. A global clinical measure of fitness and frailty in elderly people[J]. *Canadian Medical Association Journal*, 2005, 173(5):489–495.

[20] Meng Q, Kang BJ. The influence of crowd density on the sound environment in commercial pedestrian streets[J]. *Science of the Total Environment*, 2015, 511:249–258.

[21] Barney D, Prusak KA. Effects of music on physical activity rates of elementary physical education students.[J]. *The Physical Educator*, 2015, 72:236–44.

[22] Bronwyn T, Jacques L, Dunbar RIM. Music and social bonding: "Self-other" merging and neurohormonal mechanisms[J]. *Frontiers in Psychology*, 2014, 5:1096.

[23] Sztubecka M, Skiba M. Noise level arrangement in determined zones of homogenous development of green areas on the example of the spa park in Inowrocaw[J]. *Nephron Clinical Practice,* 2016, 6(1):-.

[24] Lesiuk T. The effect of preferred music on mood and performance in a high-cognitive demand occupation[J]. *Music Therapy* 2010, 47(2):137–154.

[25] Cassidy G, Macdonald RAR. The effect of background music and background noise on the task performance of introverts and extraverts[J]. *Psychology of Music*, 2007, 35(3):517–537.

[26] Axelsson Ö. The ISO 12913 series on soundscape[J]. *Psykologi*, 2011.

[27] Ost LG, Jerremalm A, Johansson J. Individual response patterns and the effects of different behavioral methods in the treatment of social phobia[J]. *Behaviour Research and Therapy*, 1981, 19(1):1–16.

[28] Layard R. Happiness: Has social science a clue? Lecture 1: What is happiness? Are we getting happier?[J]. *Rethinking Economic Policy*, 2003.

[29] Van Dyck E, Moelants D, Demey M, Deweppe A, Coussement P, Leman M. The impact of the bass drum on human dance movement[J]. *Music Perception*, 2012, 30(4):349–359.

[30] Mu JY, Kang J. Indoor environmental quality of residential elderly care facilities in Northeast China[J]. *Frontiers in Public Health*, 2022, 10:860976.

[31] Lai ACK, Mui KW, Wong LT, et al. An evaluation model for indoor environmental quality (IEQ) acceptance in residential buildings[J]. *Energy & Buildings*, 2009, 41(9):930–936.

[32] Thomas P, Aletta F, Filipan K, et al. Noise environments in nursing homes: An overview of the literature and a case study in Flanders with quantitative and qualitative methods[J]. *Applied Acoustics*, 2020, 159:107103.

[33] Yu L, Kang J. Factors influencing the sound preference in urban open spaces[J]. *Applied Acoustics*, 2010, 71:622–33.

[34] Cui P, Zhang J, Li TT. Research on acoustic environment in the building of nursing homes based on sound preference of the elderly people: A case study in Harbin, China[J]. *Frontiers in Psychology*, 2010, 12:707457.

[35] Wu Y, Kang J, Zheng W, Wu Y. Acoustic comfort in large railway stations[J]. *Applied Acoustics*, 2020, 160:107137.

[36] Mu JY, Zhang SS, Yue W. The Influence of physical environmental factors on older adults in residential care facilities in Northeast China[J]. *Herd-Health Environments Research & Design Journal*, 2022, 15(1):131–149.

[37] Mulero R, Almeida A, Azkune G, et al. An IoT-aware Approach for Elderly-Friendly Cities[J]. *IEEE Access*, 2018:7941–7957.

[38] Liu F, Kang J. Relationship between street scale and subjective assessment of audio-visual environment comfort based on 3D virtual reality and dual-channel acoustic tests[J]. *Building & Environment*, 2018, 129:35–45.

[39] Xiong J., Ma T., Lian Z., De Dear R. Perceptual and physiological responses of elderly subjects to moderate temperatures[J]. *Building and Environment*, 2019, 156:117–122.

4 Influence of acoustic environment of care homes on well-being

4.1 The influence of sound source type on well-being

4.1.1 Introduction

As the world's population ages, the need for developing care homes becomes increasingly evident. The acoustic environment, a vital aspect of the spatial ambiance in these facilities, significantly impacts the health and well-being of the elderly [1]. Research indicates that excessive noise, particularly harmful noise, can disrupt the daily lives of elderly individuals, especially those with hearing impairments in care facilities [2]. Furthermore, prolonged exposure to sound levels exceeding 65 dB(A) can lead to severe health issues such as sleep disorders, hearing loss, tinnitus, hypertension, and cardiovascular diseases [3, 4]. Given that elderly individuals often have compromised health conditions, they are more vulnerable to the adverse effects of acoustic environmental factors. However, current research on the acoustic environment primarily focuses on landscape design, architectural layout, and music-related structures, with limited studies on the indoor acoustic environment of care homes [5].

In order to further explore the acoustic environment, some scholars have introduced the concept of "soundscape" to underscore the collection and planning of sounds [6, 7]. It is found that human behavior and perception are influenced by soundscapes, and acoustic comfort can reflect individuals' subjective evaluations of sounds and soundscapes [8]. Therefore, this study will investigate the soundscape of care homes based on acoustic comfort.

While various sound sources can affect acoustic comfort, interpersonal communication, and human activity, sounds are considered the primary factors influencing indoor acoustic environments. Scholars have scrutinized the impact of the acoustic environment on human perception and behavior, revealing that sound can lead to various negative effects, such as difficulties in verbal communication, sleep disturbances, agitation, and increased indifference [4]. Hence, creating a comfortable indoor acoustic environment is crucial. Some existing studies have explored the relationship between acoustic comfort and sound pressure levels, suggesting that reducing sound pressure levels can enhance comfort [9]. However, numerous

DOI: 10.1201/9781003407232-4

factors seem to affect acoustic comfort, including sound types [10] and noise levels. Previous research has demonstrated that reducing noise levels in care homes can alleviate the elderly's emotions and promote psychological well-being [11].

In studies exploring healthy acoustic environments, certain scholars have noted that sound serves as an inducing and restorative element in the physiology and psychology of older adults, while overly quiet environments may potentially detrimentally affect their mental state [12]. Moreover, to better gauge the impacts of various acoustic environments on health, health indicators such as electroencephalograms, heart rate, and heart rate variability have been employed in relevant studies. However, overall, there is relatively limited research utilizing physiological indicators for testing.

Care homes in China typically feature comprehensive halls that offer residents recreational spaces [13, 14]. With the diversification of activities for the elderly and the introduction of mechanical equipment in care homes, the range of sounds in these facilities has become increasingly complex, potentially causing discomfort among residents in noisy or poorly communicative environments [15]. Additionally, the speech of staff and the noise generated by mechanical equipment (such as central air conditioning) are also significant factors influencing the acoustic environment of care homes [16]. Although these sounds are part of familiar indoor environments, studies have indicated that they can reduce the comfort of elderly individuals and affect their satisfaction with the acoustic environment. Currently, research on mechanical noise primarily concentrates on large public places, with relatively limited studies on care homes. Background music also constitutes a familiar sound for the elderly, effectively enhancing the environment's appeal and boosting people's sense of well-being [17]. Overall, as intricate acoustic environments, the indoor acoustic characteristics of care homes should be thoroughly studied to enhance the comfort and health levels of the elderly.

This chapter aims to investigate the assessment of the acoustic environment in the activity spaces of older adults and the influence of different sound sources on their behavior and evaluations of the acoustic environment [18]. The research site is the activity hall of a care home in Harbin, China. The collected data include objective acoustic parameters, subjective behavioral observation data, questionnaire survey data, and physiological indicator data of the elderly. The main purposes of this chapter are as follows:

(1) Conduct a comprehensive assessment of the acoustic environment in the activity hall based on measurements of sound pressure level and reverberation time.
(2) Explore the impact of various sound types and sources on evaluations of the acoustic environment.
(3) Investigate the influence of elderly residents' activity types and behaviors on evaluations of the acoustic environment in different areas of the activity hall.
(4) Analyze personal and social factors that influence the acoustic environment evaluations of the elderly.
(5) Examine the relationship between elderly individuals' physiological indicators and activity types under the influence of the same sound source.

This chapter focuses on the influence of the acoustic environment on the behavior and evaluations of the elderly in large activity spaces in care homes, providing a reference for the construction and design of care homes.

4.1.2 Case study

Due to the rapid aging of society, the government places great importance on the construction of care homes. In the northern regions of China, where the climate is cold and heating primarily relies on coal, indoor environmental quality is crucial for the health of the elderly. This study selected Harbin, the provincial capital city of Northeast China, as the research location. According to the Harbin Statistical Yearbook 2022, by the end of 2021, the elderly population in Harbin had reached 2.344million, accounting for 24.9%of the total population. With the rapid increase in the elderly population, the demand for care homes from both the government and society continues to rise. Therefore, this study chose a representative super-large care home (with 2,000beds) in Harbin to investigate the perception of acoustic environments.

To control environmental variables, the study focused on the impact of different sound source types on the acoustic comfort, behavioral activities, and physiological indicators of the elderly within the lobby space of this particularly large care home. Given that the behavior of the elderly may vary across care homes of different sizes and types, this study also selected two additional types of care homes for case analysis. This approach provided a more comprehensive understanding of the acoustic environments in Chinese care homes. The basic information about these care homes is shown in Table 4.1.

4.1.2.1 Case 1-SA

Case 1-SA is located in the Qixia district of Nanjing City, covering a building area of approximately 3,080 square meters. This facility is a renovated elderly apartment, originally a three-story L-shaped frame structure sales office. Due to the increasing number of local elderly residents, it was converted into a nursing care center.

Table 4.1 Basic information on care homes

Code	*Project name*	*Location*	*Opening time*	*Beds*	*Area*	*Service object*
Case 1-SA	Jindi Xianlinhu nursing apartment	Nanjing	2020	125	3080m^2	Self-care, semi-independent/semi-disabled, non-self-care/bedridden disabled, special care, cognitive impairment
Case 2-RC	Yishou Jiayuan senior community	Beijing	2023	201	10640m^2	Self-care, semi-independent, disabled, cognitive impairment

Note: SA = Senior Apartment, RC = Retirement Community.

The building spans three floors and accommodates 130 beds. The design strategically places public areas in the central part of the building, benefiting from excellent sunlight conditions at the corners. The first floor, featuring the most open space, includes a lobby, reception area, rest area, and painting area, all divided by partitions to enhance spatial fluidity. The kitchen, medical area, and rehabilitation nursing area are concentrated on the south side, adjacent to the logistics entrance, to prevent interference with resident flow (Figure 4.1).

Unlike traditional care homes, the interior of this elderly apartment exudes a fresh and elegant ambiance. The color scheme features combinations of brown, blue, orange, and yellow (Figure 4.2), with each floor having distinct main color tones to enhance spatial recognizability. The material selection includes non-slip floor glue for most public space floors, and walls and ceilings painted with standard coatings, without special acoustic treatment. The indoor furniture is predominantly wooden, with some areas furnished with sofas and other soft furnishings. Overall, the public indoor spaces of the elderly apartment have not undergone special acoustic treatment.

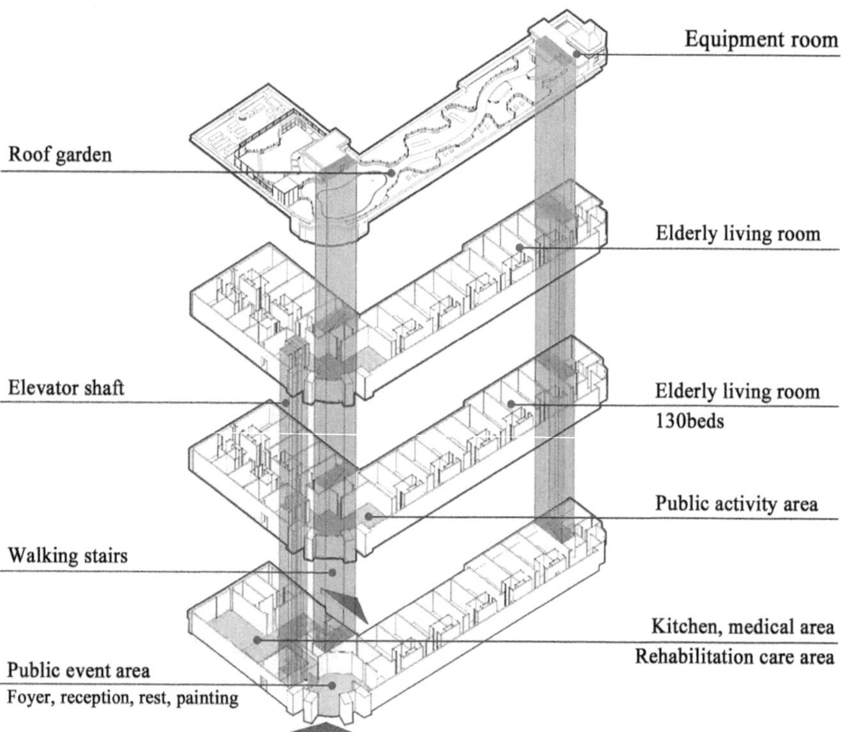

Figure 4.1 Exploded axonometric view

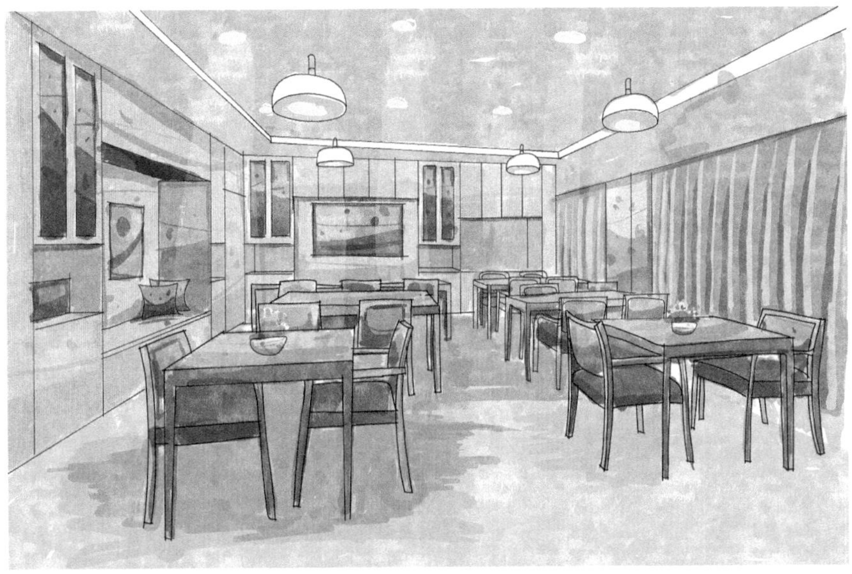

a) Activity room

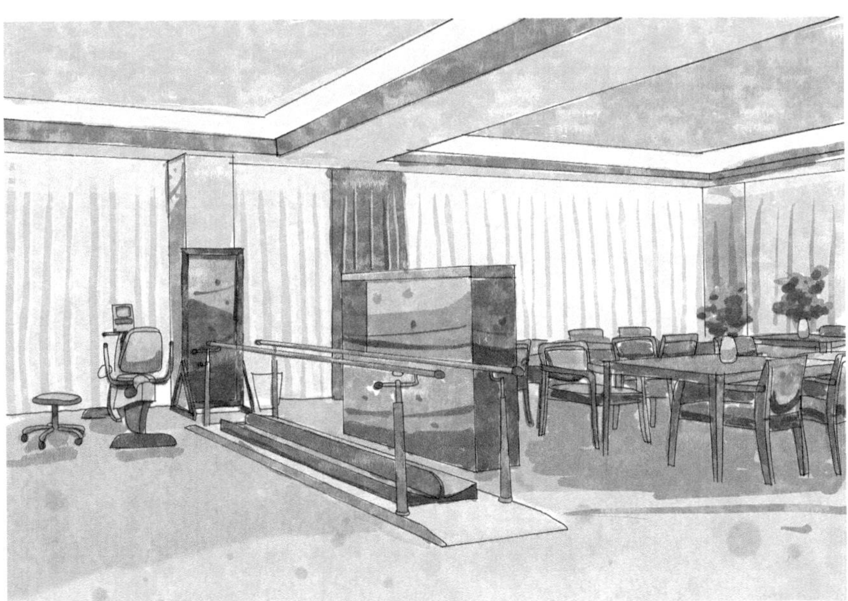

b) Rehabilitation area

Figure 4.2(a-f) Indoor public spaces in senior apartments

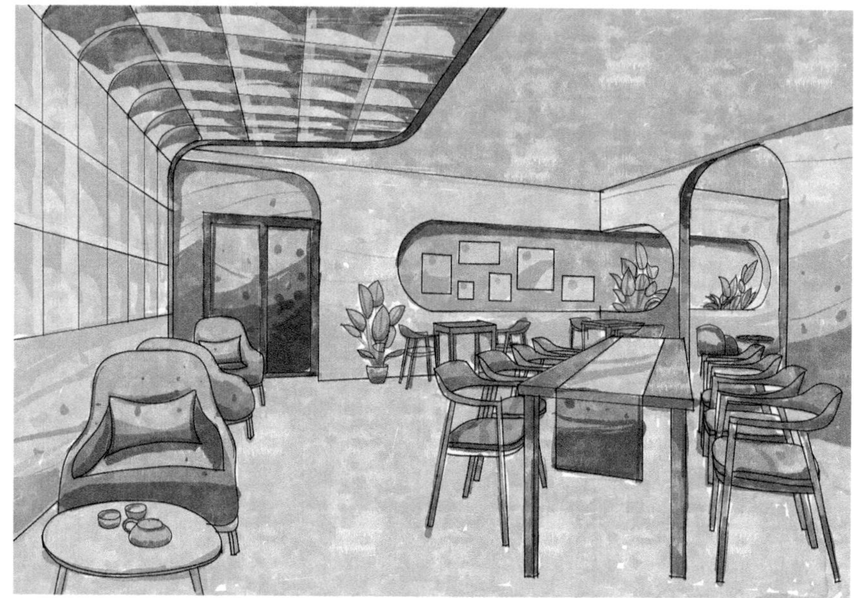

c) Painting and calligraphy room

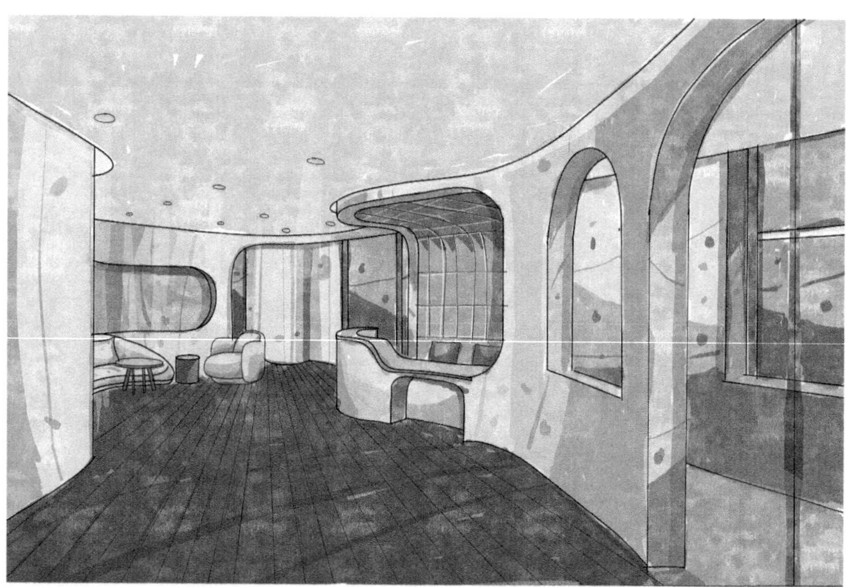

d) Lobby

Figure 4.2(a-f) (Continued)

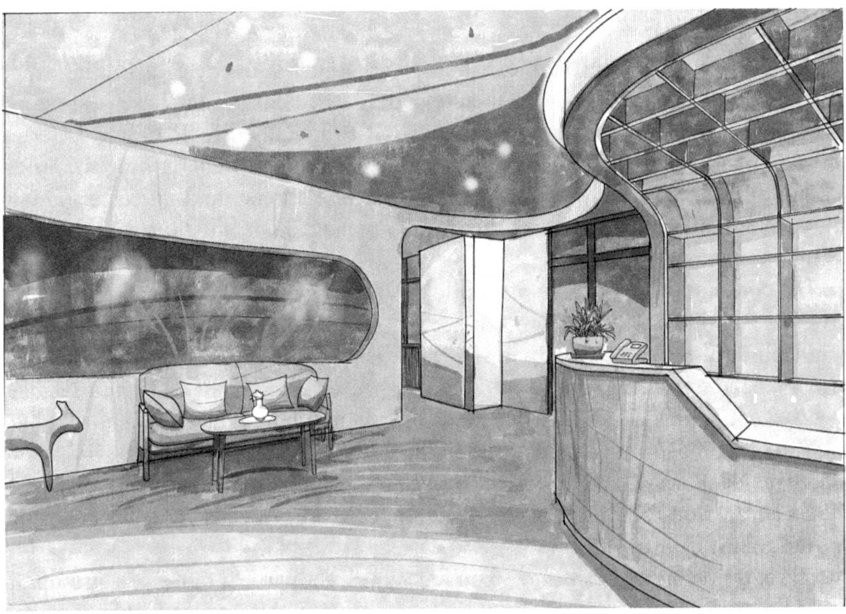

e) Nursing station

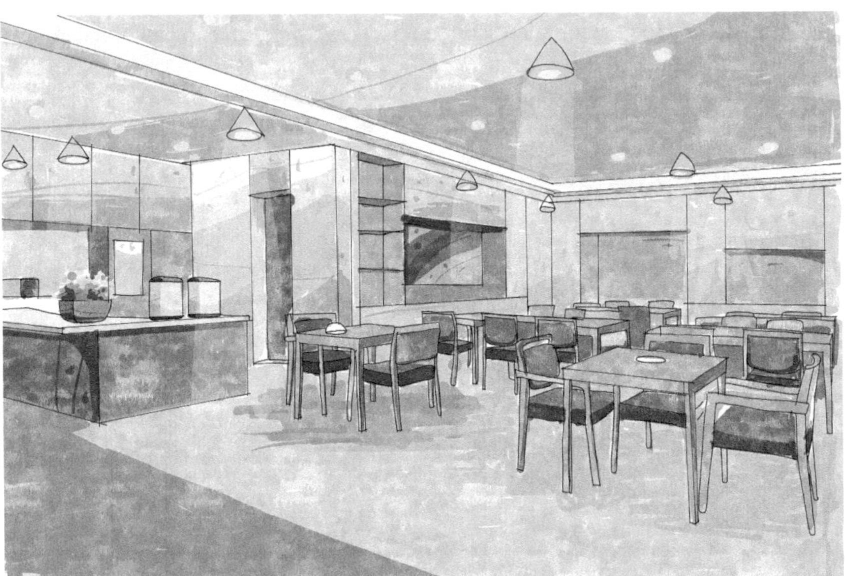

f) Dining room

Figure 4.2(a-f) (Continued)

4.1.2.2 Case 2-RC

Case 2-RC is a typical northern care home located in Shunyi district, Beijing. With a building area of 10, 640square meters and 201 beds, it primarily serves elderly individuals who are self-sufficient, semi-self-sufficient, disabled, and suffering from dementia. This community is a renovation project, transforming the original buildings, previously used as a municipal price bureau training center (Dongzhuyuan Hotel), into a care home due to poor management and the increasing local aging population.

The community consists of five buildings (Figure 4.3), each three stories above ground. Buildings 1 and 4 are connected and mainly serve self-sufficient and semi-self-sufficient elderly individuals, while Buildings 2 and 5 are independent and provide accommodation and rehabilitation spaces for disabled and semi-disabled elderly people. Building 3 is dedicated to elderly individuals with dementia, featuring single rooms forming small-scale living units. Each unit includes a living room where residents can converse, dine, and engage in recreational activities. Different themed colors on each floor of the dementia care area effectively enhance spatial recognizability.

The interior public spaces of the care home, shown in Figure 4.4, are dominated by warm colors. Apart from the tiled flooring in the entrance lobby, wooden flooring is used in other functional areas. Walls and ceilings are mostly painted with coatings, with some walls featuring wooden veneers. Most indoor furniture is made of wood with some sound-absorbing properties. Functional rooms,

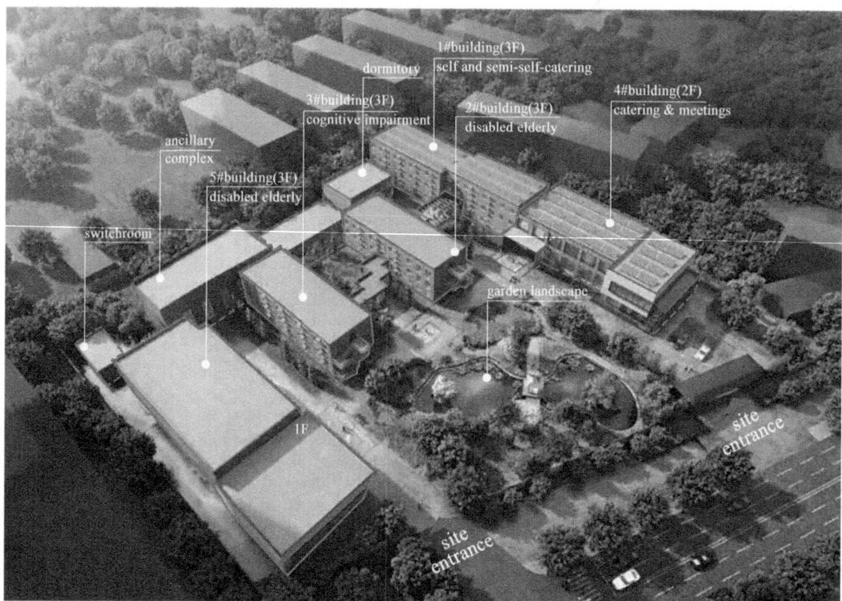

Figure 4.3 Aerial view of the retirement community

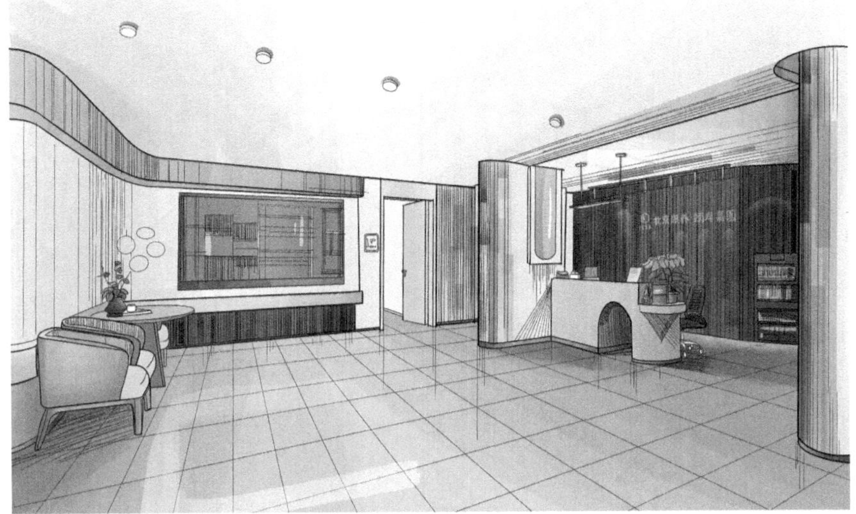

a) Lobby

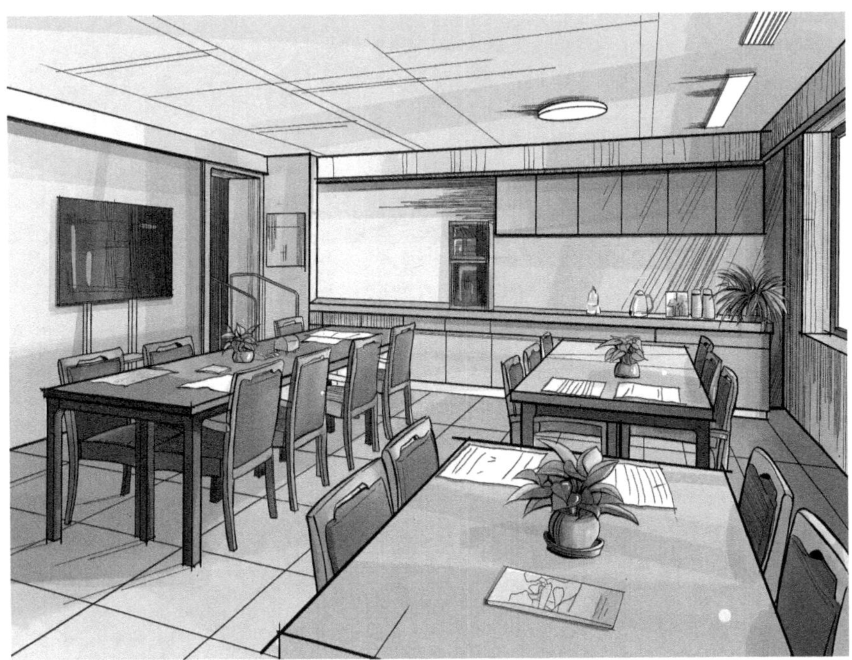

b) Public sitting room

Figure 4.4(a-f) Indoor public activity space

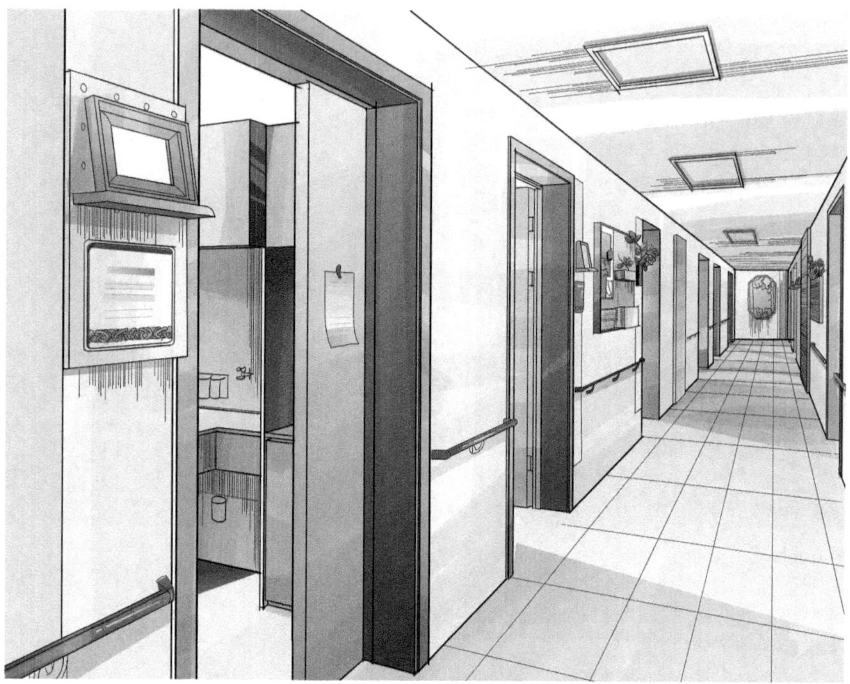

c) Corridor

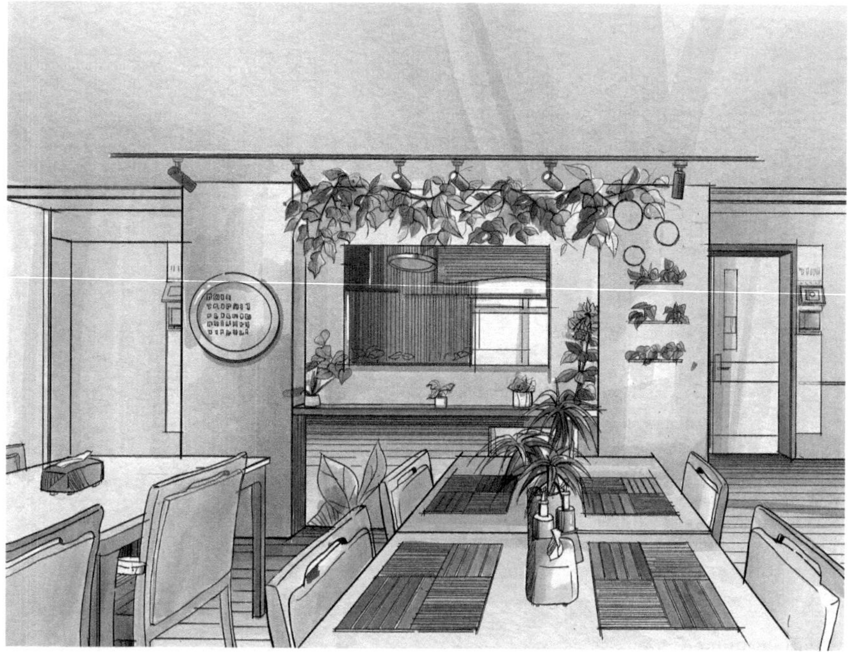

d) Cognitive unit living room

Figure 4.4(a-f) (Continued)

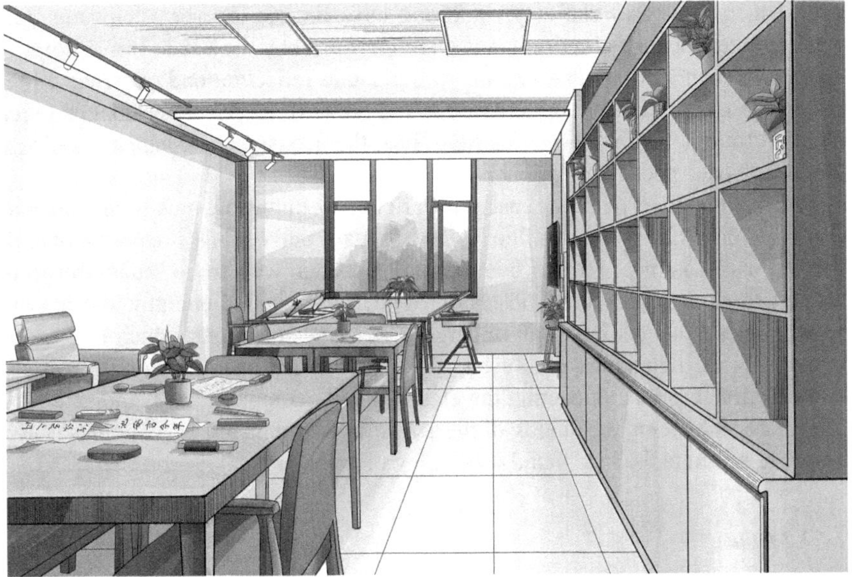

e) Painting and calligraphy room

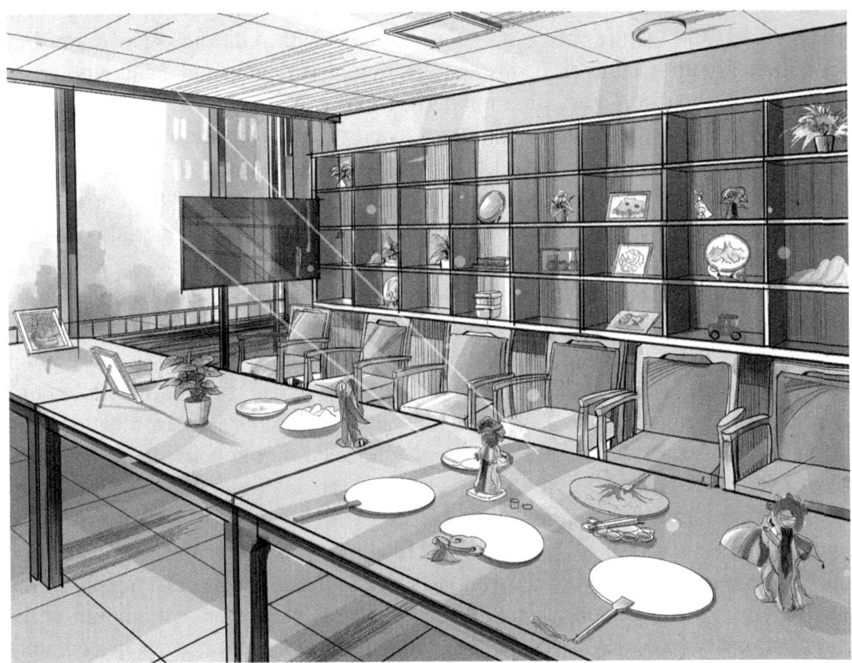

f) Public activity area

Figure 4.4(a-f) (Continued)

except the lobby, are relatively small and have limited reverberation time, suggesting better acoustic environment quality. The lobby, however, has decorative materials (such as tiles) that exhibit strong sound reflection and experience high pedestrian traffic, leading to increased sound pressure levels and prolonged reverberation time, affecting speech clarity. Thus, the acoustic environment quality of the lobby space needs improvement.

Overall, the floors of public spaces in various care homes are mostly covered with non-slip floor glue or wooden flooring, while walls and ceilings are predominantly painted with coatings. Furniture is primarily wooden with some sound-absorbing properties, though the sound absorption effect is limited. Generally, the internal spaces of care homes have not undergone acoustic treatment, which may result in excessively high sound pressure levels or prolonged reverberation time in certain functional rooms, impacting the elderly's daily communication and activities. Therefore, enhancing the quality of the acoustic environment of care homes is necessary to promote the health and well-being of the elderly.

4.1.3 Method

The study delved into research at a large-scale care home in Harbin, showcasing the layout of its comprehensive activity hall depicted in Figure 4.5. The activity hall encompasses two sections: the expansive fan-shaped sunshine hall (1700 m^2, 14m $high$) and the rectangular living area (850 m^2). The living area hosts various smaller activity spaces, including a calligraphy and painting room, chess room, and lecture room, totaling 1200 m^2. Within the fan-shaped sunshine hall, there are three main divisions: a quiet zone, a rest area, and an activity space. While there's no distinct demarcation between the rest and activity zones, the entire area can be flexibly utilized for different events. The quiet section, situated adjacent to the 14-meter-high glass curtain wall, benefits from ample natural light and outdoor vistas. Despite the absence of a clear partition between the corridor and the fan-shaped hall, differences in architectural structure and materials delineate distinct ambiance and functionality for each space.

The primary parameters influencing the acoustic ambiance are the sound pressure level and reverberation time [19], measured through the following methodologies. Figure 4.5 illustrates the measurement points, encompassing sound source points (S1-S5), sound pressure level measurement points (R1-R17), and reverberation time measurement points (T1-T41), all potentially impacting indoor sound evaluations [20].

Sound pressure level assessments were conducted during activity hall operation from 8:00 a.m. to 6:00 p.m. Sound level meters were configured to slow mode, and A-weighting Leq was measured and recorded every 10 seconds. To mitigate sound source discrepancies, sound pressure level readings were taken 10 times per hour at each measurement point, with the average value of these 10 sets of data representing the findings. Measurements at each location were collected from a minimum of five different points, spaced at least 3 meters apart to minimize measurement inaccuracies.

Reverberation time measurements were carried out during nighttime when the activity room was vacant and quiet. An OS002 omnidirectional sound source

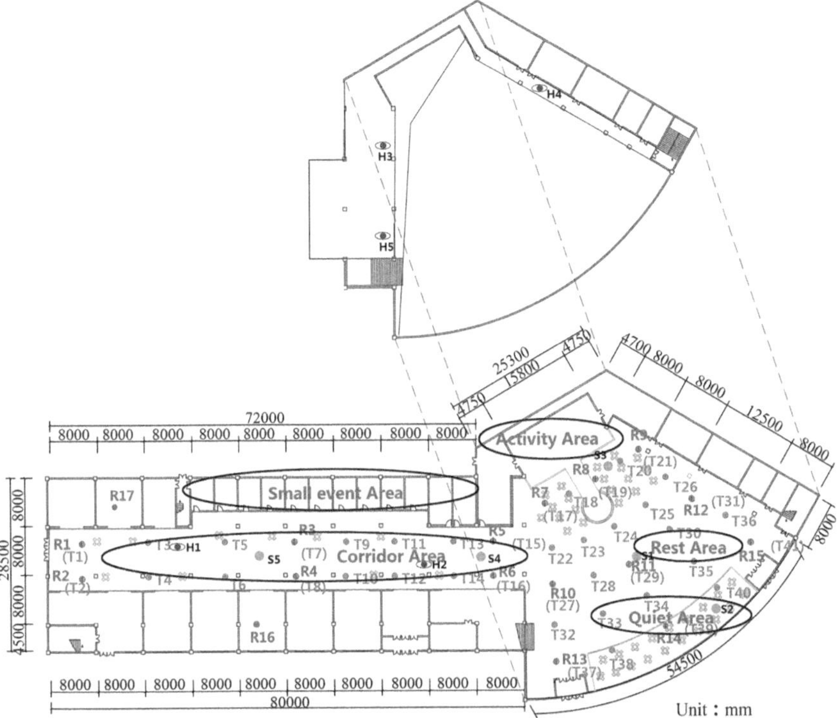

Figure 4.5 Floor plan of the comprehensive activity hall, with sound source points (S1–S5), sound pressure level monitoring points (R1–R17), and reverberation time test points (T1–41)

emitted white noise from the designated sound source points (illustrated in Figure 4.5, S1-S5) to minimize measurement biases. Upon reaching stability, the sound source was abruptly turned off, and the duration for the sound to decay by 30 dBA (referred to as T30) was recorded to ascertain the reverberation time, later extrapolated to 60 dBA. Due to the hall's spaciousness, T30 measurements were preferred over T60. Equipment selection and measurement procedures adhered to the guidelines stipulated in the ISO3382 standard.

Video recording serves as a pivotal method for analyzing human behavior. Cameras strategically positioned around the activity hall and on the second-floor circular corridor ensured minimal interference with the elderly's activities during the study. Recording sessions spanned from 8:00 a.m. to 6:00 p.m., capturing footage every 10 minutes, with each recording lasting 5 minutes. To ensure comprehensive coverage, each activity at recording points (H1-H5) was documented at least 15–20 times to ensure variability and randomness.

Following preliminary research on the care home's activity hall, elderly activities were categorized into three groups based on sound pressure level: 1) (near-) silent activities such as rest and reading, with sound pressure level < 35 dBA;

2) low-dBA activities like meetings, conversations, walking, and chess playing, with sound pressure level < 50 dBA; and 3) high-dBA activities including playing music, TV sounds, singing, and dancing, with sound pressure level > 60 dBA [21]. Observations and recordings of elderly activities were meticulously conducted for 15 minutes for each activity type during this period [22].

Given the widespread use of the seven-point Likert-type scale in subjective comfort surveys [23], the questionnaire (Table 4.2) in this study adopted this scale to measure the elderly's evaluation of the acoustic environment. The questionnaire's reliability coefficient was estimated at 0.81 (Cronbach's alpha).

Participation in the study involved 320 elderly individuals, with one-on-one questionnaire administration completed within 5 minutes per participant. Each survey point underwent at least 10 interviews, with individuals with hearing impairments excluded during the survey process, resulting in 307 valid questionnaires. SPSS 20.0 facilitated the establishment of a database encompassing subjective and objective results [24]. Pearson's correlation coefficient was harnessed to identify the factors and dominant sound sources influencing elderly comfort evaluations of the acoustic environment, while mean differences were explored to understand the impact of the presence or absence of dominant background sound sources on the elderly. Pearson's correlation and multiple regression analysis were subsequently employed to ascertain the factors influencing the acoustic comfort of the dominant sound sources based on their characteristics. Factors influencing the elderly's acoustic comfort evaluations were then examined from the perspective of their demographic and social factors.

Table 4.2 Questionnaire and scales

Category	*Questions*	*Scale*
Background information	Gender; age; education level; pension; length of residence; usage duration; usage frequency	
Subjective evaluation	Evaluation of the overall sound environment	1 being very noisy and 7 being very quiet
	Acoustic comfort of the overall sound environment	1 being very uncomfortable and 7 being very comfortable
	Subjective impression of reverberation	1 being very long and 7 being very short
	Acoustic comfort of various sound sources	1 being very uncomfortable and 7 being very comfortable
	Loudness of various sound sources	1 being very low and 7 being very high
	Intelligibility of various sound sources	1 being very clear and 7 being very unclear
	Noise level of various sound sources	1 being very noisy and 7 being very quiet
	Preference degree of various sound sources	1 being highly disliked and 7 being highly liked

4.1.4 Results

4.1.4.1 Effect of sound pressure level on acoustic comfort

Given the variances in sound pressure levels, identical sound types may elicit differing impacts on the acoustic comfort of the elderly. Consequently, this segment scrutinizes the correlation between comfort levels associated with distinct sound types and their respective sound pressure levels, illustrated in Figure 4.6. This graphical representation employs linear regression and correlation coefficients to delineate the evolving trend in comfort influenced by sound pressure level and the correlation between sound type and sound pressure level.

As elucidated in Figure 4.6, with the escalation of sound pressure level, all evaluation indicators witness a decrement. Notably, indicators linked to activity sound, loudness, intelligibility, and noise level evince robust correlations with sound pressure level. Specifically, as the measured sound pressure level ascends, the noise level of speech sounds declines (0.55). Conversely, indicators associated with speech sound, loudness, intelligibility, and preference degree demonstrate feeble correlations with sound pressure level. Mechanical and activity sounds yield akin outcomes, with solely the preference degree exhibiting a feeble correlation with sound pressure level; however, other indicators (noise level, loudness, and

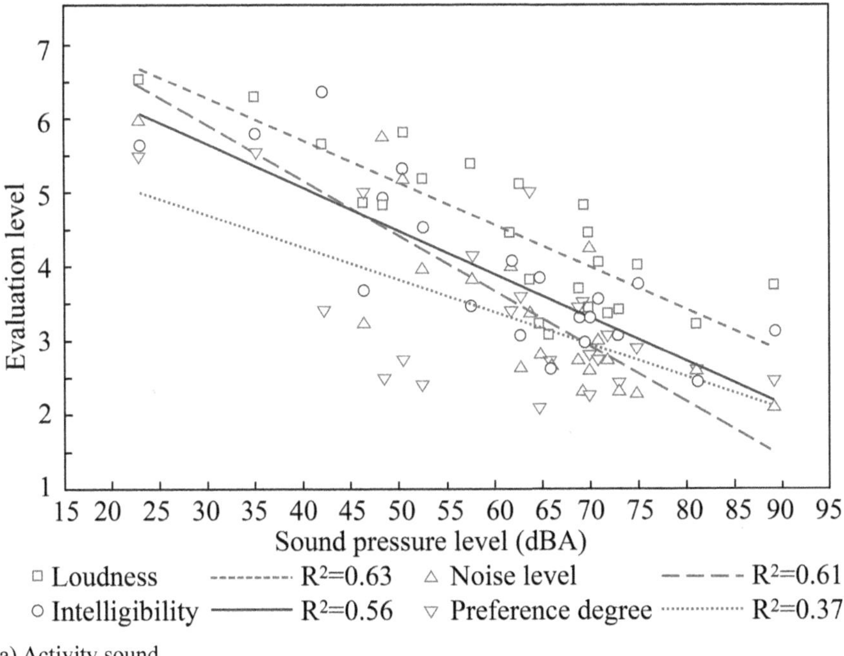

a) Activity sound

Figure 4.6(a-e) Relationship between sound pressure level and sound characteristics of the dominant sound types

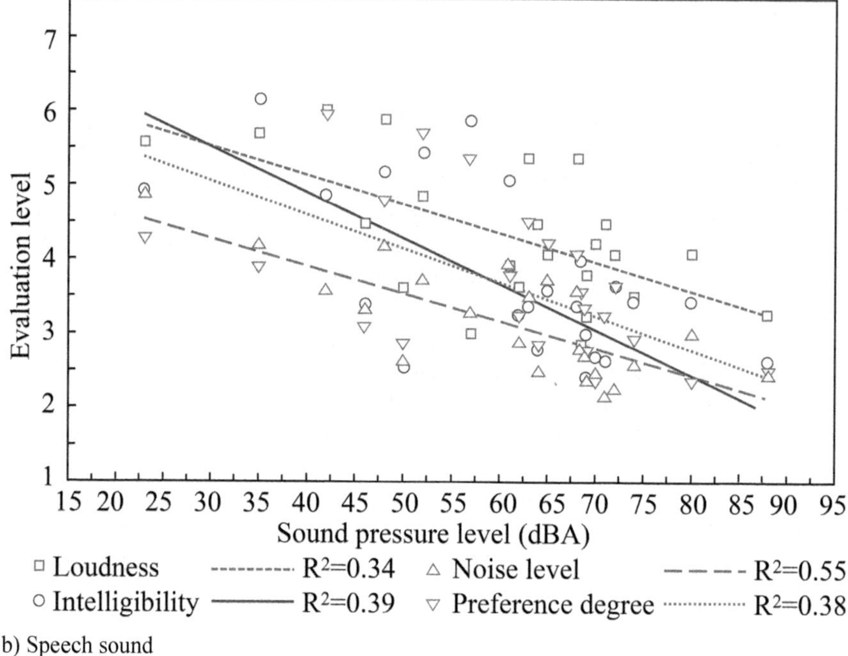

b) Speech sound

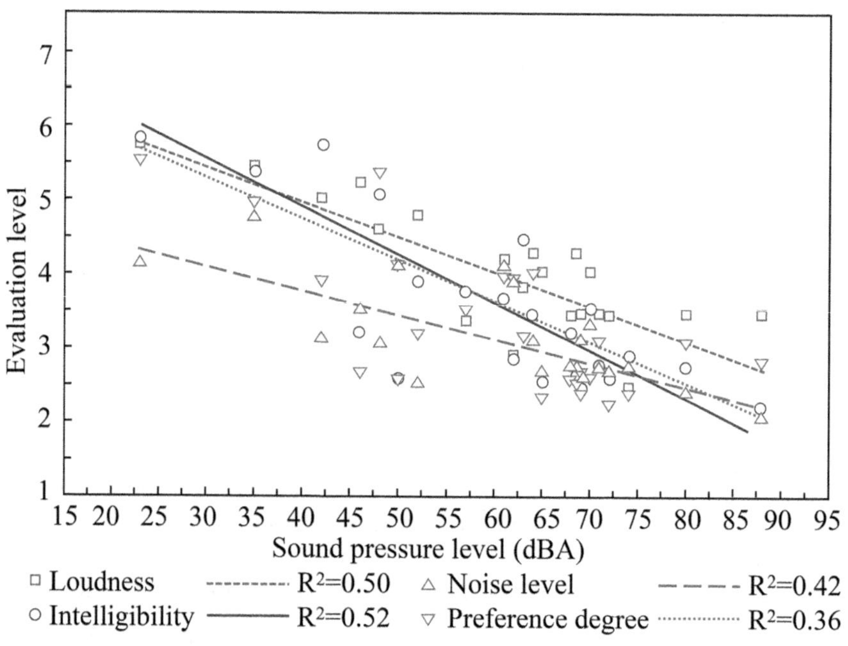

c) Mechanical sound

Figure 4.6(a-e) (Continued)

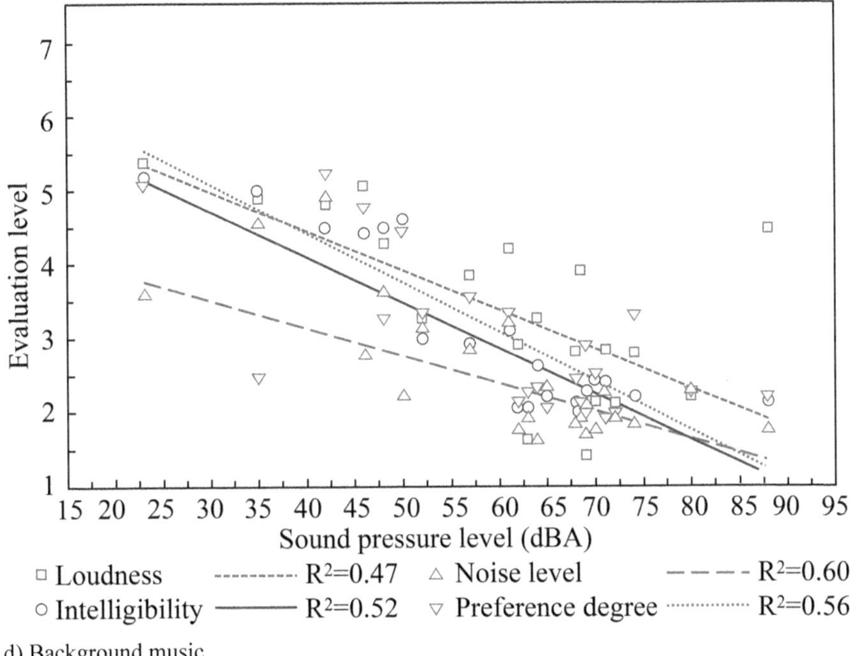

d) Background music

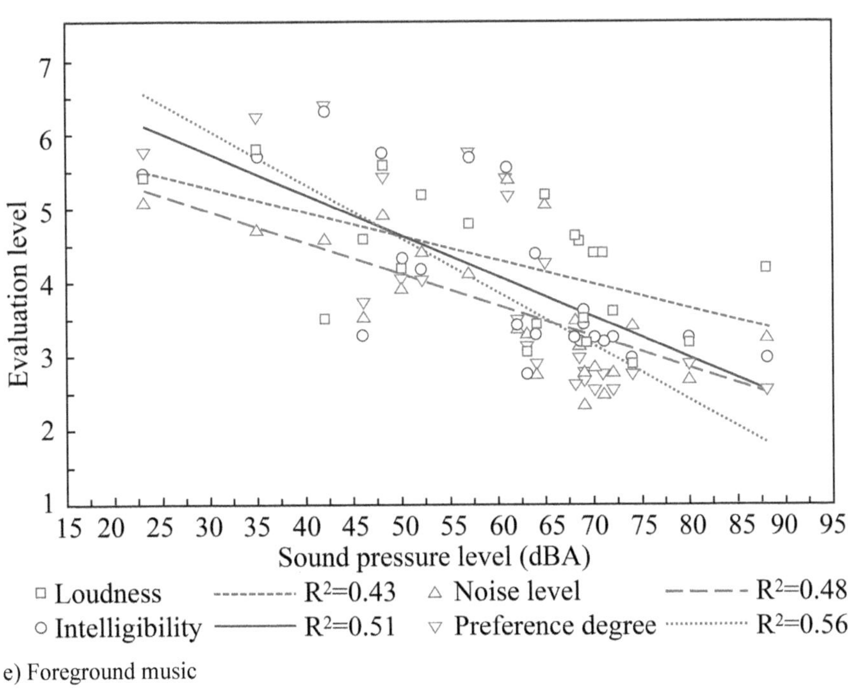

e) Foreground music

Figure 4.6(a-e) (Continued)

intelligibility) manifest a stronger correlation. The correlation between background music, foreground music, and sound pressure level mirrors each other; barring weak correlation with noise levels, all indicators (loudness, intelligibility, and preference degree) exhibit correlation. These findings elucidate a decline in participants' satisfaction with the acoustic environment as the sound pressure level escalates. Notably, the deceleration in satisfaction with music is more gradual than with other sound types, with participants expressing greater satisfaction and preference for music sounds compared to others.

Generally, the evaluation of most sound types demonstrates either a weak correlation or no correlation with acoustic comfort (<0.5), as delineated in Figure 4.7. However, a reduction in loudness evaluation aligns with an increase in acoustic comfort, with the most conspicuous example being foreground music (= 0.61). This underscores that elderly individuals do not favor foreground music when it exceeds a certain loudness threshold.

4.1.4.2 Correlation between acoustic rating and sound source in different areas of care homes

The study delved into how the elderly perceive different sound sources in various areas of the activity hall to scrutinize the correlation between the acoustic environment evaluations of each area and sound types [18]. The analysis results are laid out in Table 4.3.

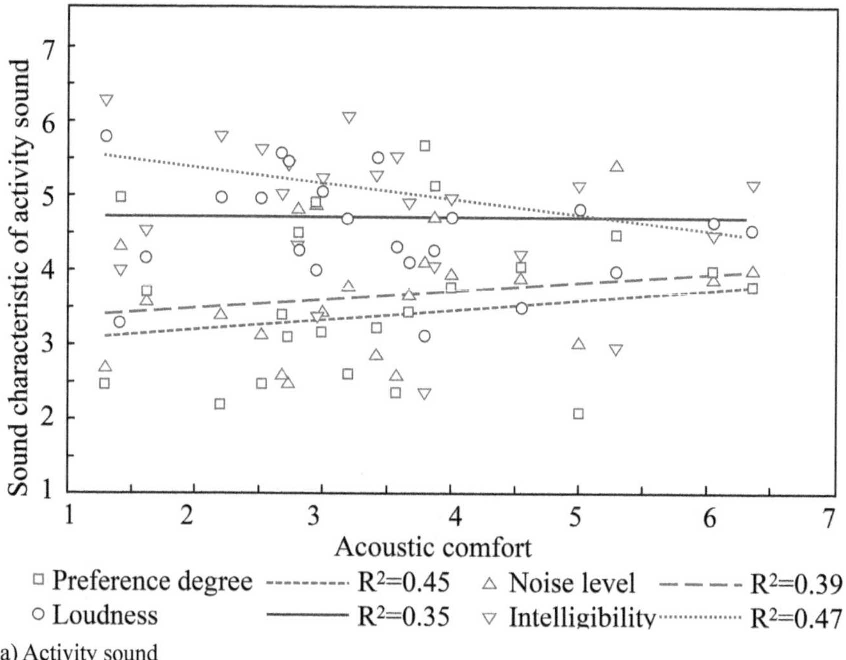

a) Activity sound

Figure 4.7(a-e) Relationship between acoustic comfort and the sound characteristics of the dominant sound types hall

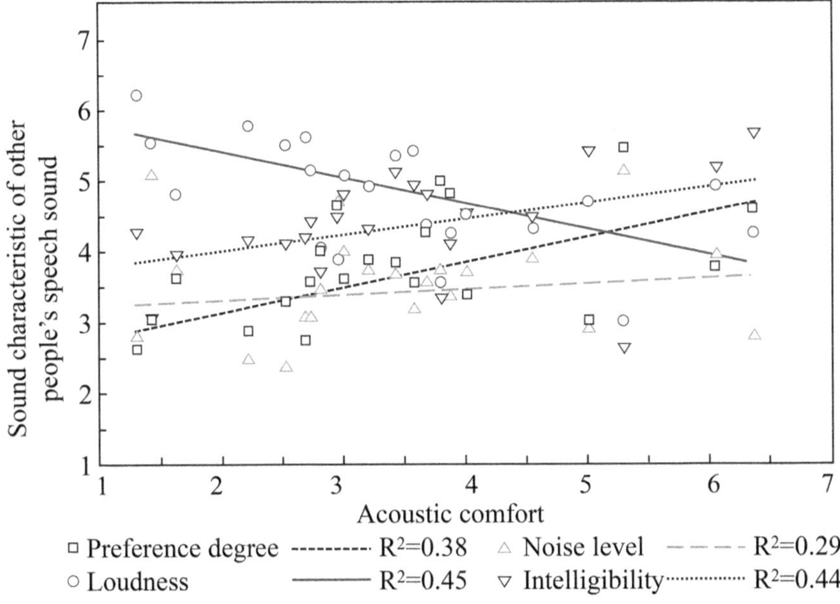

b) Speech sound

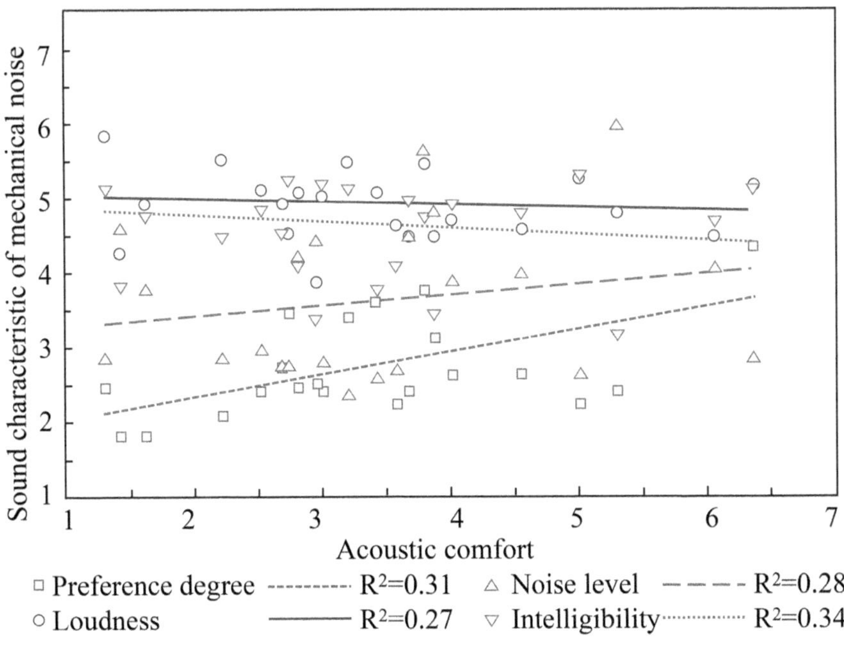

c) Mechanical sound

Figure 4.7(a-e) (Continued)

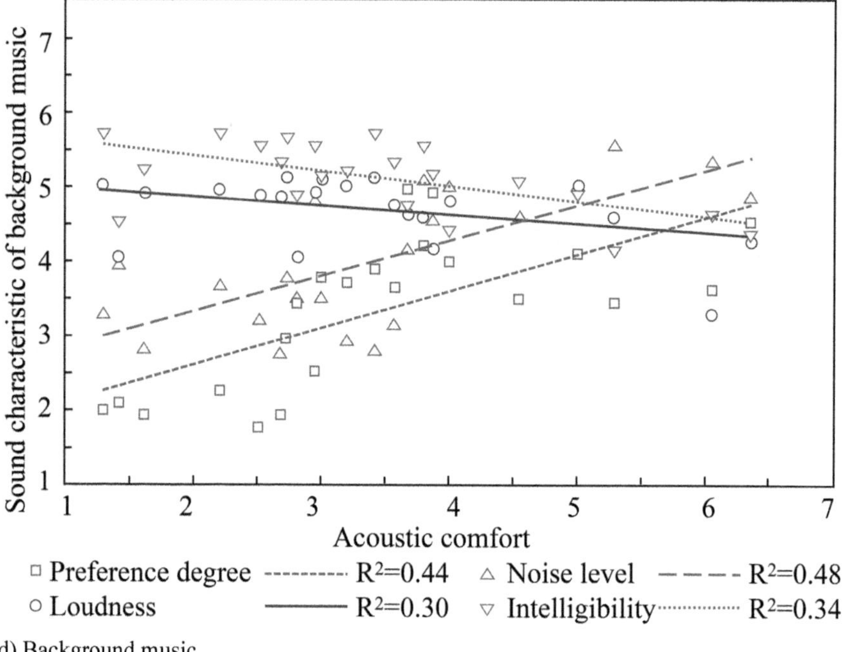

d) Background music

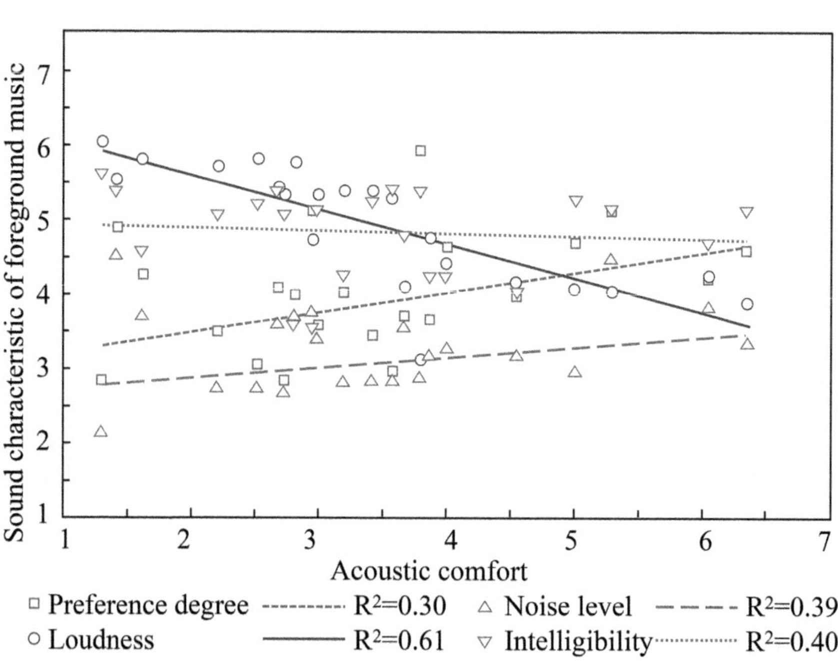

e) Foreground music

Figure 4.7 (Continued)

Column A in Table 4.3 delineates the mean and standard deviation of the elderly residents' evaluations concerning acoustic comfort. Remarkably, the quiet area garnered higher ratings compared to all other areas across all sound types, averaging close to four points. This preference could stem from the fact that elderly individuals

Table 4.3 Correlation between sound sources and acoustic comfort

Name of area	*Sound types*	*Sound sources*	*A: Average value/ variance*	*B: Correlation coefficient/p value*
Rest area	Activity sound		3.060/1.348	0.596/0.000***
		Playing card sounds	3.262/1.701	0.342/0.006**
		Seat and table moving sounds	2.962/1.746	−0.023/0.815
		Dancing sounds	3.01/1.943	−0.036/0.718
		Chess sounds	2.933/1.224	0.335/0.001**
	Speech sound		3.167/1.511	0.539/0.000***
		Talking sounds	3.644/1.645	0.206/0.000***
		Explanation sounds	2.869/1.674	−0.209/0.033*
		Talking sounds of staff	2.923/1.863	0.031/0.757
		Talking sounds of onlookers	2.933/1.829	0.098/0.323
	Mechanical sound		2.703/1.328	0.245/0.113
		Air conditioning sounds	3.058/1.683	0.017/0.863
	Background music		2.77/1.638	0.494/0.001**
		Background music	3.172/1.448	0.452/0.000***
		TV sounds	2.262/1.779	−0.095/0.340
	Foreground music		3.542/1.401	0.541/0.000***
		Dance music	3.748/1.585	0.269/0.002**
		Singing sounds	3.462/1.689	0.351/0.000***
Activity area	Activity sound		2.956/1.032	0.187/0.172
		Walking sounds	2.926/1.885	0.17/0.063
		Dancing sounds	3.841/1.637	0.426/0.000***
		Chess sounds	2.917/1.860	0.066/0.047
	Speech sound		3.162/1.411	0.588/0.000***
		Talking sounds	3.273/1.812	0.145/0.112
		Talking sounds of onlookers	3.066/1.252	0.19/0.000***
	Mechanical sound	Trolley sounds	3.033/1.288	0.342/0.09*
	Background music	Background music	2.63/0.924	0.222/0.104
	Foreground music		2.846/1.278	0.624/0.000***
		Dance music	3.725/1.544	0.319/0.000***
		Singing sounds	1.982/0.683	0.119/0.193

(*Continued*)

Table 4.3 (Continued)

Name of area	*Sound types*	*Sound sources*	*A: Average value/ variance*	*B: Correlation coefficient/p value*
Quiet area	Activity sound		3.365/1.765	0.459/0.000***
		Seat and table moving sounds	3.570/1.296	0.395/0.000***
		Walking sounds	2.860/1.823	0.227/0.003**
		Chess sounds	3.041/1.923	0.276/0.000***
		Using computer sound	2.959/1.733	0.272/0.000***
		Dancing sounds	2.959/1.829	0.154/0.054
	Speech sound		3.147/2.028	0.640/0.000***
		Talking sounds of staff	2.591/1.731	0.225/0.000***
		Talking on the phone sounds	3.281/1.763	0.155/0.003**
		Talking sounds	3.058/1.651	0.044/0.565
	Mechanical sound		3.352/1.704	0.350/0.000***
		Trolley sounds	3.547/1.641	0.220/0.000***
		Air conditioning sounds	3.041/1.646	0.175/0.022*
	Background music	Background music	3.362/2.028	0.440/0.000***
	Foreground music		3.062/2.073	0.615/0.000***
		Singing sounds	3.170/1.766	0.258/0.001**
		Dance music	3.023/1.598	0.261/0.000***
Corridor	Activity sound		2.765/1.255	0.324/0.021*
		Walking sounds	3.197/1.031	0.315/0.014*
		Seat and table moving sounds	2.297/1.433	0.222/0.086
		Playing card sounds	3.049/1.784	0.149/0.003**
	Speech sound		2.386/1.077	0.188/0.186
		Talking sounds	2.195/1.764	0.008/0.952
		Talking sounds of staff	1.966/0.636	0.226/0.08
		Talking sounds of onlookers	2.731/1.836	0.151/0.009*
	Mechanical sound		2.451/1.246	0.420/0.002**
		Air conditioning sounds	2.470/1.287	0.058/0.655
		Trolley sounds	2.547/1.241	0.220/0.004**
	Background music	Background music	2.41/1.344	0.426/0.002**
	Foreground music		2.296/0.999	0.409/0.003**
		Music from electronic devices	3.023/1.598	0.261/0.001**
		Singing sounds	1.728/0.557	0.223/0.084

(*Continued*)

Table 4.3 (Continued)

Name of area	*Sound types*	*Sound sources*	*A: Average value/ variance*	*B: Correlation coefficient/p value*
Small event space	Activity sound		2.236/0.826	0.133/0.566
		Walking sounds	2.331/0.839	-0.037/0.713
		Playing billiards sounds	2.165/0.880	-0.045/0.653
	Speech sound		1.973/0.915	0.411/0.030*
		Talking on the phone sounds	1.902/0.510	-0.069/0.487
		Talking sounds of onlookers	2.123/1.066	-0.242/0.013*
	Mechanical sound	Air conditioning sounds	2.50/1.036	0.663/0.000***
	Background music	Background music	2.46/1.401	0.691/0.000***
	Foreground music	Music from electronic devices	2.14/1.044	0.359/0.061

predominantly engage in quiet or near-silent activities in this area, such as reading, resting, and savoring the outdoor scenery through glass, which serves as a stress-relief mechanism. Notably, speech sounds were deemed most irksome by the elderly, with a minimum rating of 1.86points across all areas. Residents in the corridor expressed discomfort with speech sounds, describing them as pervasive, clamorous, and causing extreme discomfort. This perception could be attributed to the intricate structural design of the corridor and its walls, resulting in sound refraction and creating a sensation of amplified sound emanating from various directions [25].

The suboptimal acoustic environment in the activity hall necessitates elevated voice projection by care home managers and staff to ensure effective communication and operational efficiency. Some elderly residents expressed discontent with loud speaking by managers, citing headaches and discomfort in the heart region as a consequence. Activity sounds present a more intricate scenario due to multiple sources, leading to ambiguous descriptions by the elderly. Consequently, overall evaluations of activity sounds ranked higher compared to other sound types, second only to mechanical sounds, which were rated slightly uncomfortable with an average exceeding three points. Notably, talking and singing sounds received the lowest ratings in certain areas, with scores falling below three points. Various sections of the activity hall, including the rest area, activity area, corridor, and small event space, were affected by speech sounds, while louder noises stemmed from activities such as talking, singing, and dancing. Despite the aversion to speech sounds, the elderly exhibited greater tolerance toward mechanical sounds and activity sounds. Interestingly, low-frequency mechanical sounds received more favorable evaluations compared to activity sounds, possibly indicating reduced sensitivity to low-frequency stimuli [26]. The negative appraisal of activity and speech sounds suggests a potential adverse impact on elderly residents' activities and emotional well-being. Overall, the elderly rated the acoustic environment of the activity hall unfavorably.

Column B in Table 4.3 reveals that the acoustic comfort evaluation of the rest area is influenced by activity sound, speech sound, background music, and foreground music. Conversely, mechanical sounds are nearly absent in this area. Notably, TV sounds received the worst evaluation, while dancing sounds garnered the best.

In the activity area, foreground music and speech sounds emerge with the strongest correlations with sound satisfaction (0.624 [$p < 0.01$] and 0.588 [$p < 0.01$], respectively). This discovery is attributed to the interactive nature of these activities, which necessitate communication through speech sounds among participants and observers. Music, especially foreground music, acts as an enhancer for elderly individuals engaging in exercises and leisure activities. Given the focused engagement of residents in the activity area, they tend to allocate lesser attention to external activity and background sounds, resulting in a lower correlation between these sound types and overall satisfaction. Notably, dancing sounds and music during dance sessions emerge as the most preferred sound sources in this area, whereas singing is perceived less favorably, likely due to its potential to disrupt other activities.

The quiet area, characterized by a higher overall evaluation of the acoustic environment, experiences influence from all sound sources, with speech (0.64, $p < 0.01$) and foreground music (0.615, $p < 0.01$) exhibiting the strongest correlations. Intriguingly, respondents in the quiet area rated all sound sources at a moderate level, with most sources receiving ratings above three points. Evidently, participants demonstrate a degree of accommodation or acceptance towards these sound sources.

Given the limited time spent in the corridor and the multi-directional nature of sound sources, the elderly may struggle to discern sounds effectively. Consequently, survey results indicate a low correlation between activity and speech sound sources and satisfaction with the corridor. Mechanical sounds and sustained musical sounds, such as trolley noises and electronic device music, exert a more pronounced influence on the corridor area.

In the small event space, mechanical sounds and background music exhibit the strongest correlations with sound satisfaction. This phenomenon arises from the subjective perception of the elderly engaging in high-decibel activities within this space. Conversely, speech sounds are rated lowest in this area, suggesting that the small event space is characterized by noisy acoustics.

In general, elderly residents expressed a subdued assessment of the acoustic environment in the activity hall of the care home, signaling discomfort with the prevailing auditory surroundings. Various factors could contribute to this discontent, including the building materials and interior decor of the activity hall, which may not adequately cater to the diverse needs of residents [23]. Age-related hearing decline has been demonstrated to affect individuals' perception of speech, particularly in noisy settings [27]. In this study, the interplay of voices with background music impacted the elderly's ability to perceive and distinguish sounds [26]. Moreover, the overall appraisal of music received a lower rating, possibly due to the size of the space. It's conceivable that in a spacious, multifunctional area, a medley of sounds blends together, making it challenging to recognize and discern sound content, thus inducing unease and diminishing comfort levels. Consequently, the evaluation of sound sources within the rectangular living area (encompassing the corridor and small activity room) was lower compared to the fan-shaped sunshine hall (comprising the activity area, quiet area, and rest area).

While air-conditioning sounds and background music permeate all areas, they are marginally louder in the fan-shaped hall than in the living area. As a result, areas with relatively higher noise levels display slightly greater tolerance and appraisal of sound compared to quieter areas, even when exposed to the same sound source.

4.1.4.3 Sound characteristics of different activity types

In this section, activity sounds will be classified to distinguish the impact of different sound pressure levels on the evaluation of the acoustic environment. Building upon the preceding discussion, the elderly's activity types will be categorized into three groups based on sound pressure level: (near-) silent, low-dBA, and high-dBA activities.

Despite the activity hall's division into distinct areas, elderly individuals often engage in similar activities across these spaces. Figure 4.8 illustrates the subjective evaluation of the overall acoustic environment comfort in the activity hall by the elderly. Figure 4.8a demonstrates that the overall evaluation of the acoustic environment in the activity hall is low. The average evaluation on quiet area, activity area, corridor, and small event space are all below 3-point. With the exception of the four-point average in quiet areas, considered 'neither comfortable nor uncomfortable,' evaluations of the acoustic environment in other areas generally fall below three points. Figure 4.8b displays the subjective evaluations of the acoustic environment during different types of activities. The evaluation of the acoustic environment for (near-) silent activities is significantly higher than that for low-dBA and high-dBA activities.

Table 4.4 presents the variations in acoustic comfort evaluations for different activity types ($F = 28.280$, $p < 0.001$). The mean value of acoustic comfort for (near-) silent activities (3.8 points) is significantly greater than that for low-dBA activities (2.28 points) and high-dBA activities (2.31 points). Apart from acoustic comfort, the evaluation of low-dBA activities based on other characteristics is also significantly higher than that for the other two sound pressure levels. This suggests that the elderly prefer quiet activities and surroundings. However, it is noteworthy that the evaluation of low-dBA activities is lower than that of high-dBA activities. This discrepancy may be attributed to the prevalence of speech sounds in low-dBA activities; previous surveys have indicated that elderly individuals tend to give poor evaluations of speech and singing sounds. Among these, the evaluation of the loudness and intelligibility of low-dBA activities exceeds 4.5 points, indicating that the elderly perceive low-dBA activities as noisy. High-dBA activities such as dancing and playing music capture the attention of the elderly and receive higher evaluations. While research by Meng and Kang has suggested that

Table 4.4 Comparison of acoustic environment evaluations of the three activity sounds

	(Near-) Silent activities	*Low-dBA activities*	*High-dBA activities*	*F*	*p*	η_p^2
Acoustic comfort	3.80	2.28	2.31	28.280	0.000	0.157
Loudness	3.65	4.50	3.92	8.932	0.000	0.056
Noise level	3.53	2.77	2.92	8.124	0.000	0.051
Intelligibility	3.78	4.76	4.45	11.540	0.000	0.071
Preference level	3.36	2.72	3.06	5.826	0.003	0.037

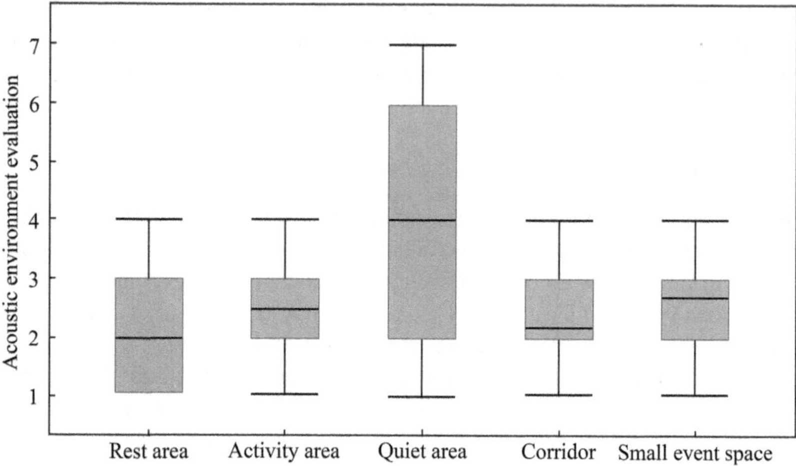

a) Evaluation of the acoustic environment in different space

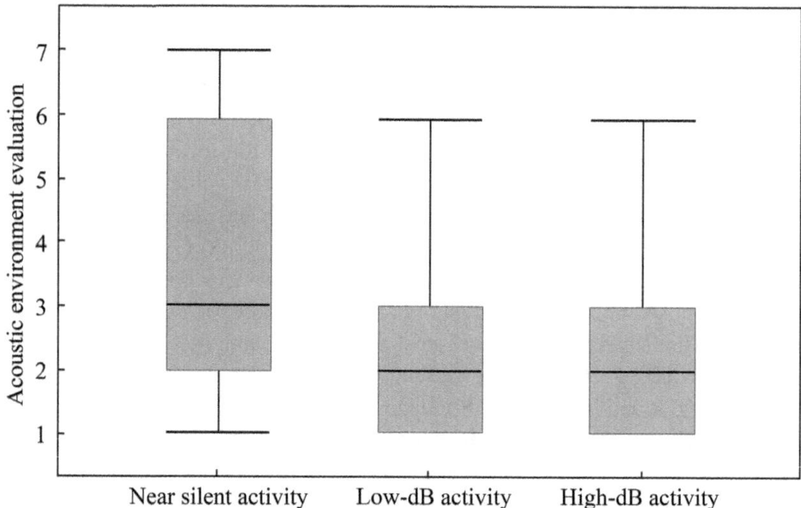

b) Evaluation of the acoustic environment for different types of activities

Figure 4.8(a-b) Evaluation of the acoustic environment in the activity hall

music can enhance concentration and comfort [28], this study found that care home residents prefer (near-) silent activity sounds, whereas their evaluation of low- and high-dBA activity sounds depends on the level of engagement and personal preference.

4.1.4.4 Influence of participation degree on acoustic comfort

In some activities, elderly participants and observers may have different evaluations of acoustic comfort. This section selects the four most participated activities in the care home for acoustic environment analysis [18], as depicted in Table 4.5.

Table 4.5 demonstrates that, barring chess-playing ($p = 0.131 > 0.05$), notable disparities exist in the acoustic comfort experienced by participants and observers across all other activities. Onlookers generally exhibit lower levels of acoustic comfort compared to participants, with activities involving music (singing and dancing) being more conducive to comfort than those involving predominantly vocal interaction (e.g., playing chess and cards). Notably, the noise level during chess-playing surpasses that of other activities, indicating participants' susceptibility to ambient sound interference. This phenomenon likely stems from the requisite concentration and need for a tranquil environment to mitigate distractions inherent in chess gameplay.

Regarding card-playing, participants rate loudness and intelligibility higher than observers ($p < 0.05$), indicating a more relaxed atmosphere among observers conducive to interpersonal communication. However, the speech emanating from observers may impinge upon participants, thereby compromising their acoustic comfort. It is noteworthy that participants express a heightened preference for card-playing, with an average rating of 4.583 points, surpassing all other activities. Subjective affinity for this particular activity may contribute to the elevated comfort levels experienced by participants. With regard to noise levels, disparities exist between the evaluations of dance participants and observers ($p < 0.05$), with participants being particularly susceptible to interference from external sounds.

In summary, disparities in acoustic comfort among the elderly are primarily associated with their level of participation, whether as active participants or observers. The elderly residents who engage in music-related activities tend to report higher levels of acoustic comfort compared to those participating in other activities. However, for observers, the type of activity has minimal impact on acoustic comfort. Observers typically prefer engaging in conversation with each other and are generally unaffected by loudness and sound pressure levels; only participants may experience disturbance from surrounding sounds.

4.2 Relationship between different sound source responses and individual differences

Studies have illustrated the significant correlation between acoustic evaluations and individuals' backgrounds [28, 29]. These backgrounds encompass various factors, including physiological aspects such as gender and age, social factors like education and pension, and adaptation to the environment, such as length of residence, duration of use, and frequency of use. This section will delve into the impact of these factors on the elderly's evaluation of the acoustic environment [18].

4.2.1 The elderly's life experiences

Figure 4.9 visually demonstrates the impact of the length of the elderly residence on acoustic evaluation, unveiling a negative correlation between prolonged residency in the care home and satisfaction levels. This implies that newcomers initially perceive the care home environment favorably but encounter acoustic challenges that diminish their comfort over time. The elderly with extended usage of the activity

Table 4.5 Acoustic comfort of participants and onlookers in different activities

Playing chess	*Participants*	*Onlookers*	*t*	*p*	$\cdot^2_p$
Acoustic comfort	2.973	2.222	1.532	0.131	0.042
Preference level	3.243	2.500	2.141	0.037	0.051
Loudness	2.784	2.278	1.217	0.229	0.019
Noise level	3.568	2.333	3.482	0.001	0.127
Intelligibility	3.000	2.111	2.334	0.023	0.059
Playing cards	*Participants*	*Onlookers*	*t*	*p*	$\cdot^2_p$
Acoustic comfort	3.583	2.167	2.550	0.021	0.289
Preference level	4.583	1.667	6.667	0.000	0.735
Loudness	3.417	2.000	3.400	0.006	0.259
Noise level	3.833	2.500	2.126	0.049	0.220
Intelligibility	4.500	2.500	2.579	0.020	0.294
Dancing	*Participants*	*Onlookers*	*t*	*p*	$\cdot^2_p$
Acoustic comfort	4.143	2.571	2.696	0.01	0.134
Preference level	3.457	2.714	1.434	0.161	0.033
Loudness	4.086	3.000	1.823	0.075	0.066
Noise level	4.057	2.714	2.49	0.016	0.117
Intelligibility	3.514	2.357	2.205	0.035	0.075
Singing	*Participants*	*Onlookers*	*t*	*p*	$\cdot^2_p$
Acoustic comfort	4.080	3.038	2.408	0.020	0.106
Preference level	3.520	3.077	0.812	0.421	0.013
Loudness	3.800	2.577	2.964	0.005	0.152
Noise level	3.480	2.654	1.556	0.126	0.047
Intelligibility	3.760	3.231	1.098	0.278	0.024

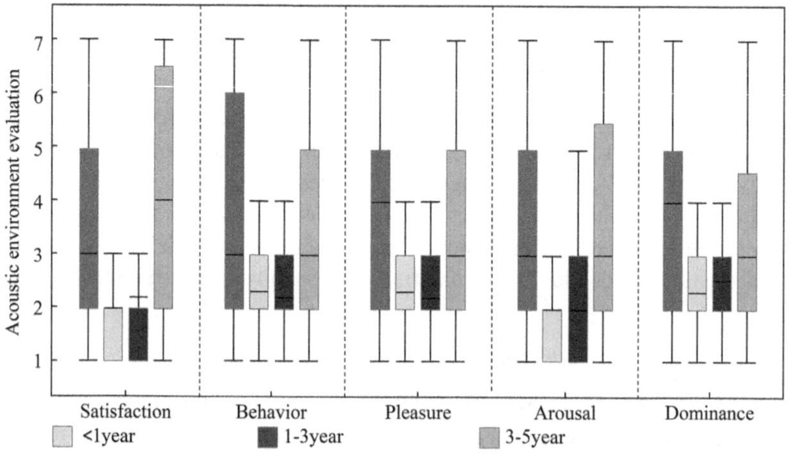

a) Length of residence

Figure 4.9(a-c) Relationship between acoustic assessment and life experiences of older people

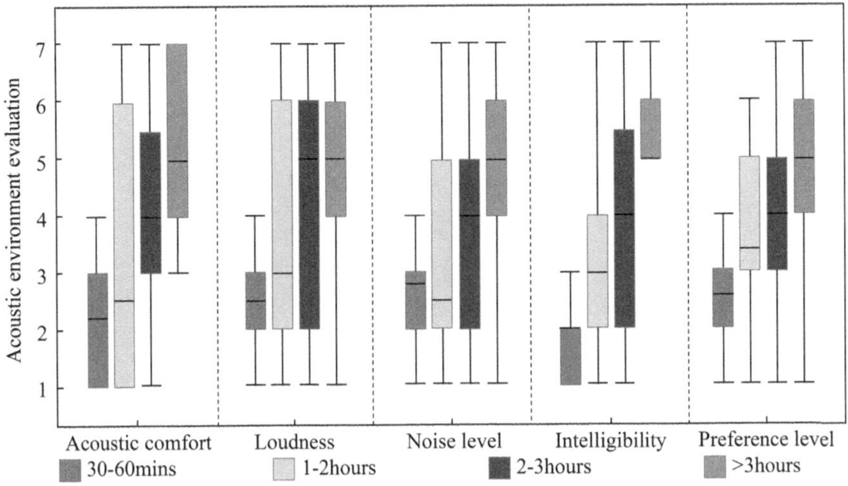

b) Usage duration

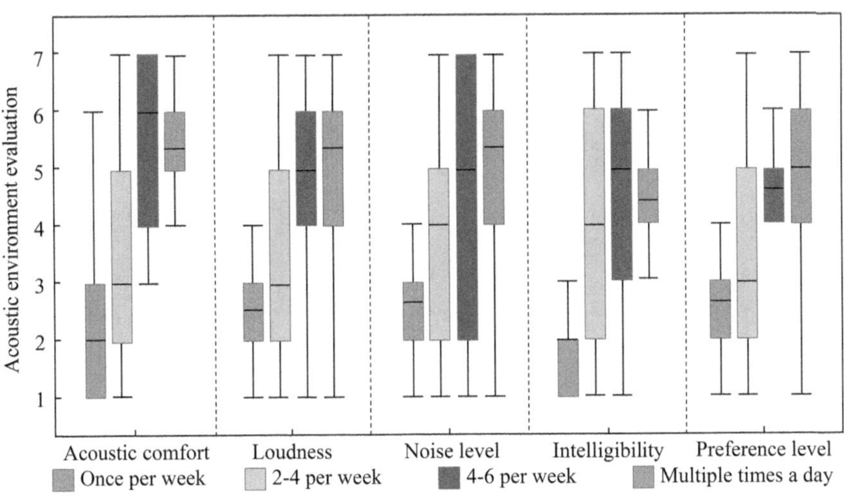

c) Usage frequency

Figure 4.9(a-c) (Continued)

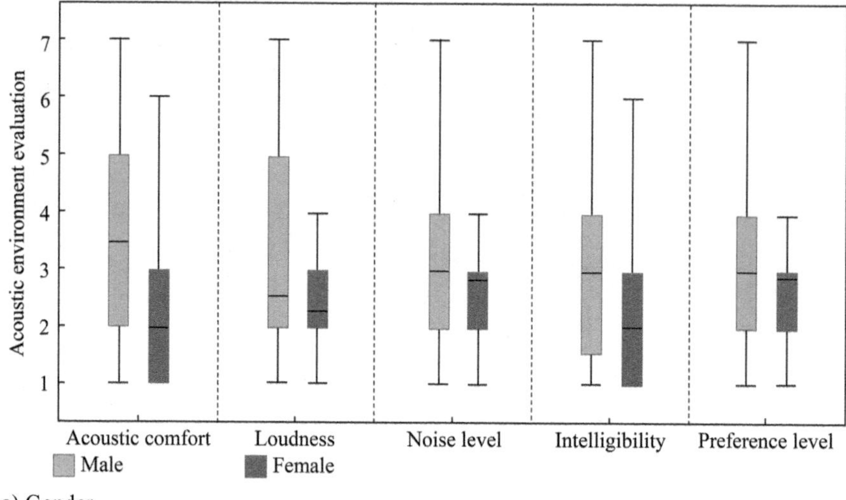

a) Gender

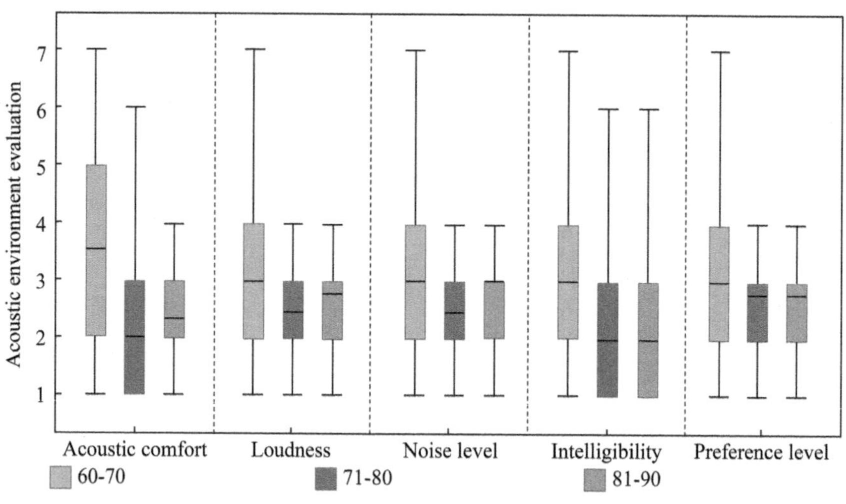

b) Age

Figure 4.10(a-d) Relationship between acoustic assessment and elderly population factors

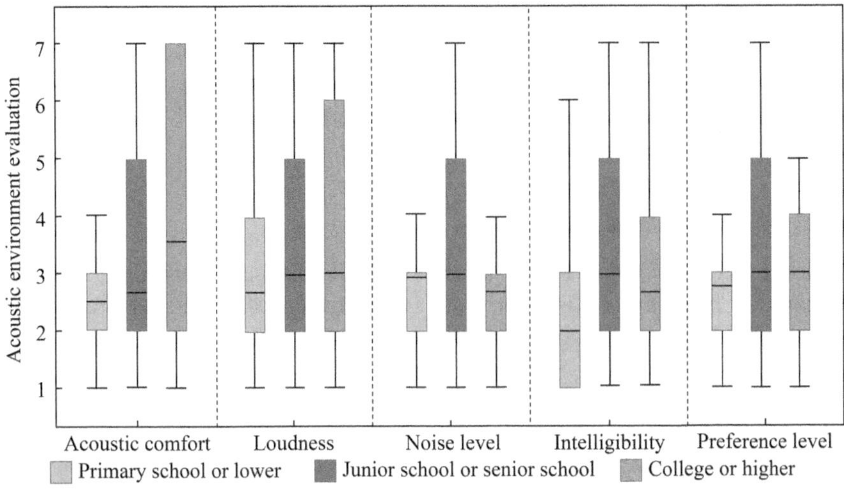

c) Education

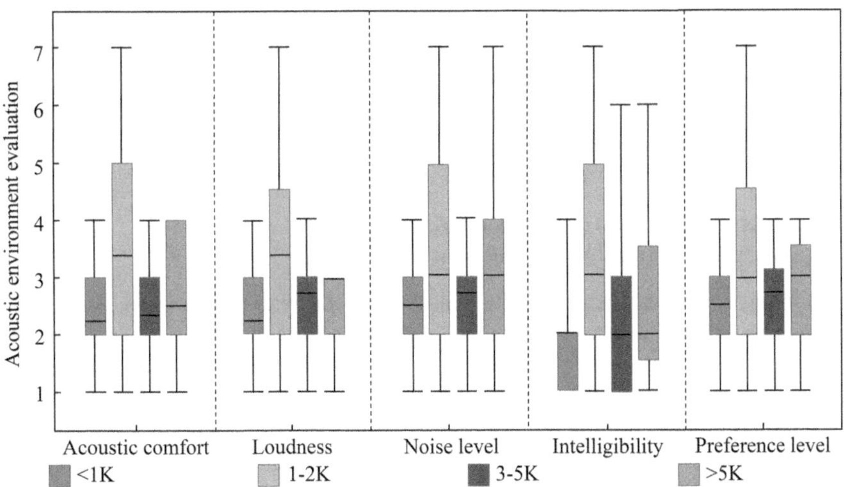

d) Pension

Figure 4.10(a-d) (Continued)

hall exhibit higher acoustic satisfaction compared to those with shorter usage durations, indicating a gradual adaptation to the hall's noisy acoustic ambiance with increased usage time. Notably, evaluations based on frequency and duration of usage are congruent, with higher evaluations reported among high-frequency users relative to their low-frequency counterparts.

4.2.2 The elderly's demographic factors

Acoustic evaluations also unveil discernible gender differences among the elderly, as depicted in Figure 4.10. Elderly men consistently exhibit higher preferences across all indicators, particularly regarding acoustic comfort. This aligns with the findings of Meng and Kang [30], who noted that men tend to be more comfortable with acoustic conditions while engaging in their preferred activities. This study corroborates these findings, suggesting that recreational activities in care homes may better cater to the preferences of older elderly men, who consequently rate their acoustic comfort more favorably during participation in such activities. Regarding age, younger elderly individuals (aged 60–70 years) report higher comfort levels compared to their older counterparts (aged over 70 years), likely due to better hearing function in the former group. Conversely, older elderly may experience heightened anxiety and frustration stemming from gradual declines in hearing ability [31]. Moreover, the elderly with a junior high school education exhibit the highest-rated sound evaluations, while those with pensions ranging between 1000 and 3000 yuan per month tend to rate the acoustic environment more favorably compared to their counterparts.

4.3 Relationship between physiological indicators and activity types under the same sound source

The impact of the acoustic environment on the elderly extends beyond subjective evaluations; it is intricately linked with physiological parameters. Physiological indicators offer an intuitive insight into the restorative effect of soundscapes and their influence on the emotions of the elderly. Research has demonstrated that following heightened stress levels, the sympathetic nervous system recuperates more swiftly from natural sounds compared to noise. However, as the sound pressure level escalates, the nervous system's recovery slows down [32]. Moreover, natural sounds have been found to decrease heart rate, respiratory rate, and respiration depth while augmenting heart rate variability and EEG and other physiological indicators [33], underscoring their efficacy in promoting physiological recovery in the human body.

The array of sound types indoors in nursing homes, ranging from speech to mechanical air conditioning noise, background music, and activity sounds, significantly impacts the physical and mental well-being of the elderly. Physiological indicators serve as indirect reflections of the health status of the elderly. Thus, this subsection delves into the ramifications of indoor acoustic environments in care homes on the elderly based on physiological indicators.

Preliminary research revealed that younger elderly individuals are primarily inclined to partake in various activities organized by care homes. Additionally, socialization serves as a crucial avenue for the elderly to assuage loneliness. Therefore, this subsection primarily explores the relationship between the physiological indicators of the elderly and activity types under the same sound source. Three types of activities were selected for the study: chess, table tennis, and billiards, with sitting serving as the control. The measured physiological indicators include skin conductance, skin temperature, αbrain waves, βbrain waves, heart rate, R wave amplitude, and heart rate variability. The BIOPAC MP160 physiological recorder was employed to measure the physiological indicators of the elderly every 30 seconds, with each experiment lasting for 510 seconds.

4.3.1 Skin conductivity and skin temperature

Figure 4.11 elucidates the relationship between skin conductance, skin temperature, and activity types among the elderly under the same sound source. From Figure 4.11a, it is discernible that except for sitting and playing chess, the skin conductance of the elderly engaging in billiards and table tennis exhibits a gradual

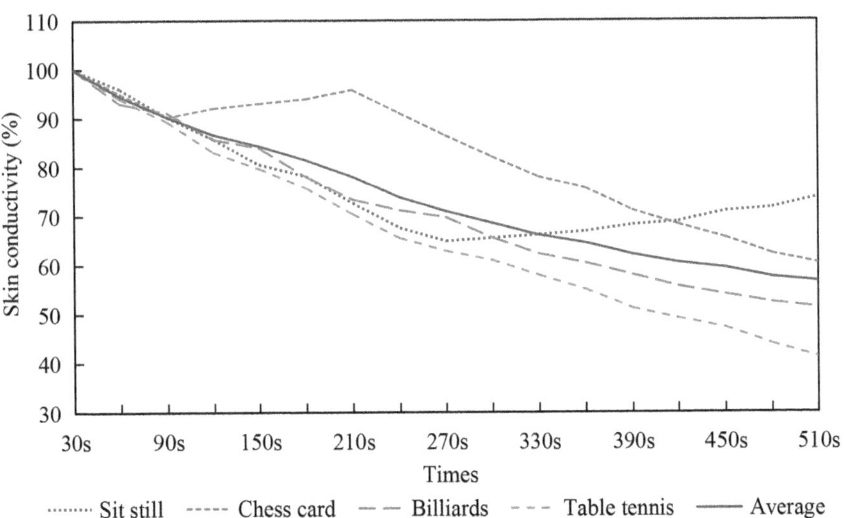

a) Skin conductivity

Figure 4.11(a-b) Skin conductivity and skin temperature test data

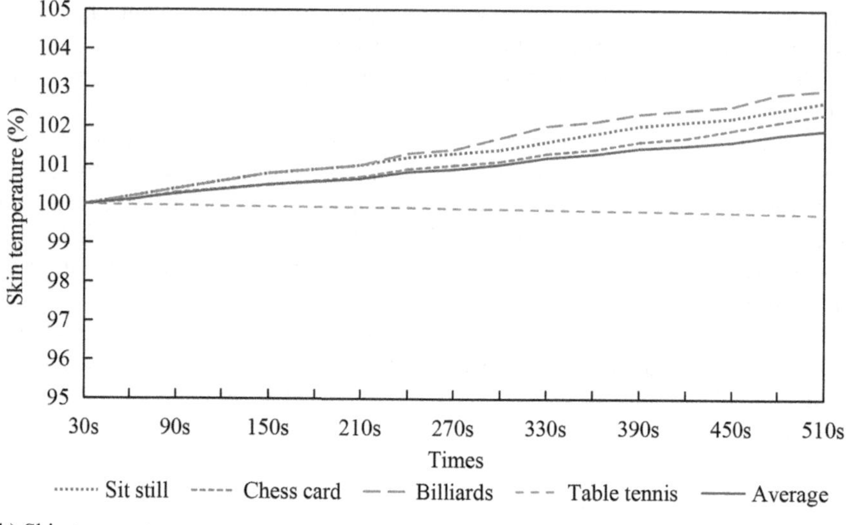

b) Skin temperature

Figure 4.11(a-b) (Continued)

decline, with table tennis demonstrating a swifter decline. The fluctuation in skin conductance of elderly individuals engaged in chess is more intricate, showing a gradual decrease around 0 – 90 seconds, followed by a slow rise, and then decreasing again around 210 seconds. The skin conductance of elderly individuals sitting gradually decreases for 0 – 270 seconds, followed by a gradual increase after 270 seconds. Overall, the skin conductance of elderly individuals participating in all activity types demonstrates a downward trend, although the data for those sitting vary, warranting further investigation.

Figure 4.11b unveils that, barring table tennis, the skin temperature of elderly individuals engaged in other activities gradually rises. Billiards witnessed the most rapid increase, succeeded by sitting and playing chess, whereas the skin temperature of elderly individuals playing table tennis declined steadily.

4.3.2 Brain waves

In Figure 4.12, the α and β brain wave data of elderly individuals participating in different activities are presented. Both brain waves exhibit a trend of fluctuating increase. Concerning α brain waves, elderly individuals immersed in chess display the most rapid escalation, trailed by billiards and table tennis, with sitters registering the slowest rise in α brain waves during the latter stages. The α brain waves of elderly individuals engaged in table tennis exhibit a swift surge around 0–100 seconds, a gradual decline around 100–330 seconds, and then another rapid increase

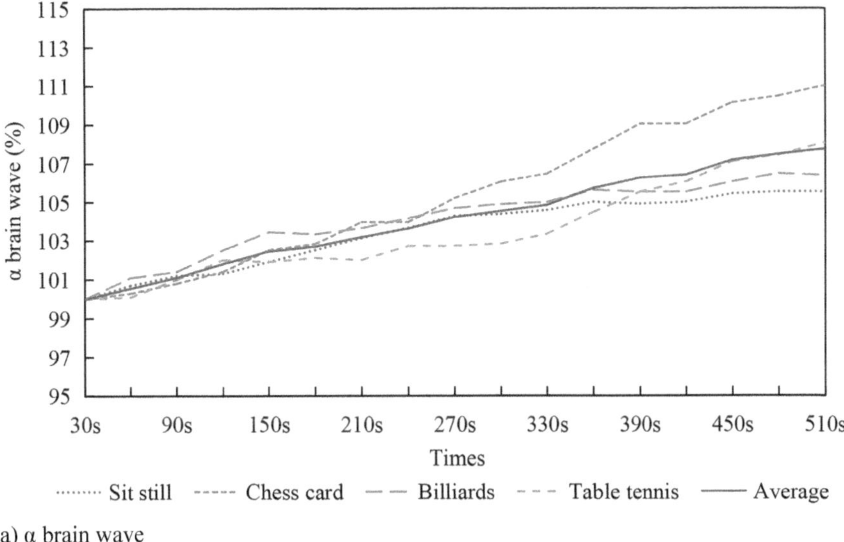

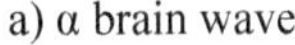
a) α brain wave

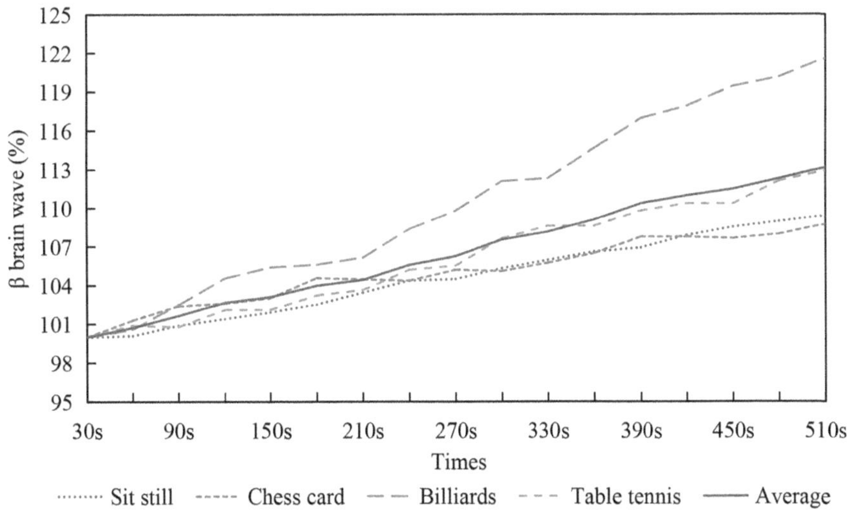

b) β brain wave

Figure 4.12(a-b) Brainwave test data

from 330–510 seconds. Overall, the α brain waves of elderly individuals involved in various activities display a gradual uptick.

Figure 4.12b delineates that the β brain waves of elderly individuals also demonstrate a gradual increase, with those partaking in billiards experiencing the swiftest elevation, followed by table tennis, while sitters and chess players exhibit

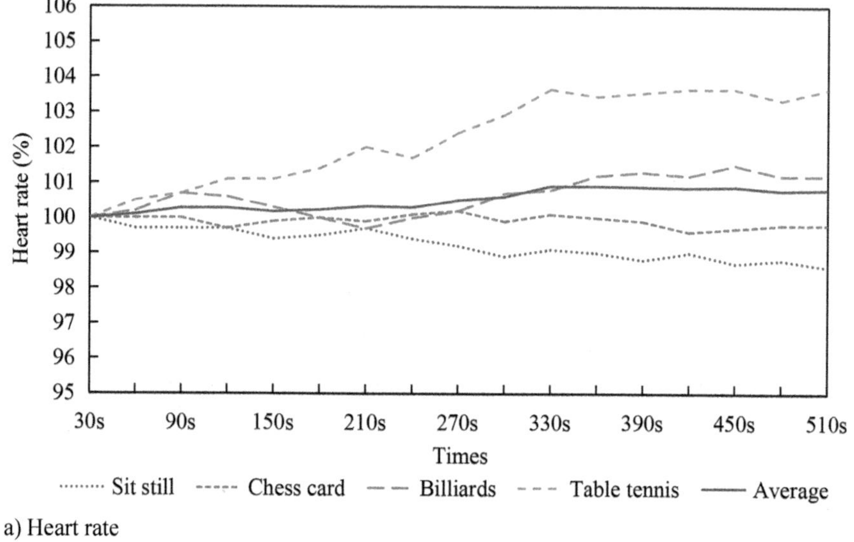

a) Heart rate

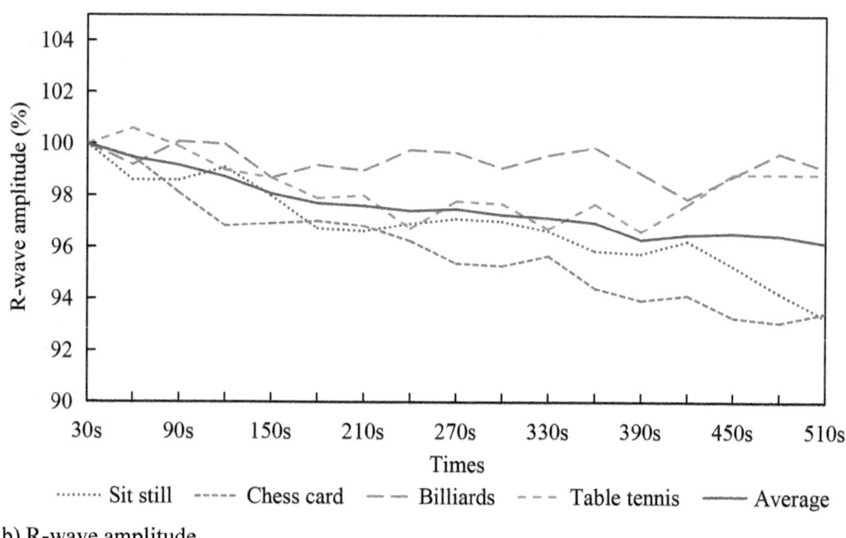

b) R-wave amplitude

Figure 4.13(a-c) Test data for ECG-related indicators

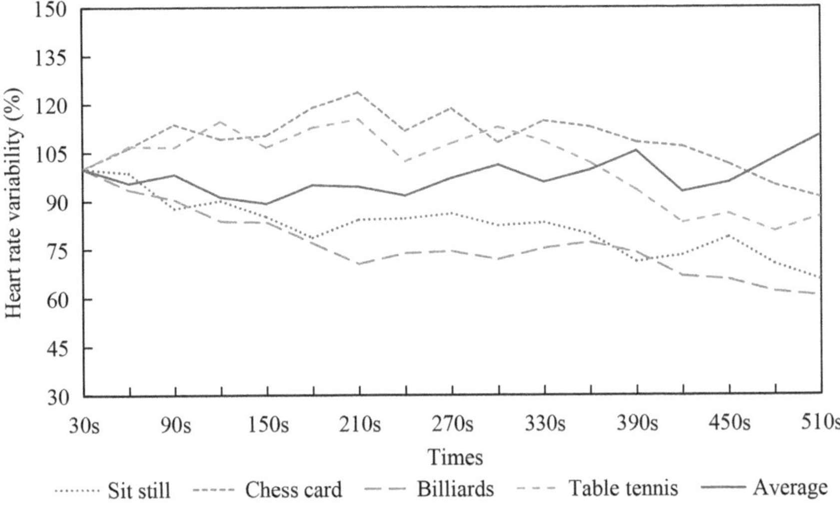

c) Heart rate variability

Figure 4.13(a-c) (Continued)

comparable trends and values. This phenomenon may stem from elderly individuals engaging in these two activities predominantly maintaining a sitting posture, resulting in values akin to those playing table tennis and billiards.

4.3.3 Electrocardiogram-related indicators

Figure 4.13 depicts the electrocardiogram-related indicators of elderly individuals engaged in various activities under identical sound conditions, encompassing heart rate, R wave amplitude, and heart rate variability. Significant disparities in physiological indicators among elderly participants are evident. As shown in Figure 4.13a, the heart rate of elderly individuals engaged in table tennis experiences an initial rapid surge, plateauing after 330 seconds. Conversely, those playing billiards witness a gradual increase from 0 – 90 seconds, followed by a decrease from 90 – 210 seconds, subsequent fluctuations from 210 – 360 seconds, and stabilization post 390 seconds. Meanwhile, individuals seated and engaged in chess observe a fluctuating downward trend in heart rate, with chess players experiencing a more gradual transition, while the heart rate of seated individuals exhibits a more pronounced decrease.

In comparison to heart rate, the shifts in R wave amplitude and heart rate variability among elderly individuals are more intricate. Figures 4.13b-c reveal a general decline in R wave amplitude among most elderly individuals, with chess players demonstrating the most rapid decrease, followed by seated participants. The R wave amplitude of elderly individuals engaged in table tennis decreases from 0 – 210 seconds and fluctuates from 240 – 390 seconds before stabilizing. Conversely, heart rate variability tends to decrease among seated and billiards players, with the latter experiencing the most substantial decline. The heart rate variability of chess players fluctuates upward from 0 – 300 seconds before decreasing post 330 seconds. Similarly, individuals engaged in table tennis exhibit heart rate variability akin to billiards players, with values fluctuating upward from 0 – 300 seconds and decreasing thereafter. In summary, the diverse shifts in physiological indicators among elderly individuals partaking in various activities underscore the need for further research into the influence of sound on their physiological well-being.

4.4 Conclusion

The objective of this study was to delve into the influence of specific environmental factors on the responses of older adults within a defined space. Specifically, the study scrutinized how different types of music impacted personal satisfaction and emotional and behavioral responses, aiming to control audio variables within the designated space meticulously. Furthermore, this chapter delved into the interplay between sound influences, physiological indicators, and activity types among the elderly. The principal research findings are outlined below:

(1) Through a comparative analysis of the behavioral impacts of various acoustic environments on older adults, it was discerned that they did not exhibit strong preferences for environments with or without music. However, the elderly showcased a penchant for slow-paced instrumental music in terms of music rhythm and evinced a preference for natural sounds concerning music type.
(2) A significant positive correlation was observed between the education level of older adults and slow-rhythmed music ($p < 0.001$), indicating that highly educated the elderly expressed greater satisfaction with slow-paced instrumental music.
(3) The influence of acoustic environments on the psychological well-being of the elderly chiefly manifests in how music affects individual behaviors, reflecting the elderly's generally favorable evaluation of the acoustic environment and heightened satisfaction compared to onlookers. Notably, environments featuring natural sounds witnessed a notably higher frequency of low-decibel activities across all three activity areas ($p < 0.001$). Conversely, the introduction of fast-paced instrumental music led to a significant increase in the proportion of the elderly engaging in high-decibel activities. These findings underscore the elderly's inclination to participate in activities when accompanied by suitable music environments.
(4) Observations of activity spaces revealed that the presence of music correlated with increased crowd density, particularly in environments featuring natural sounds, as the elderly favored a natural sound environment devoid of lyrical

interference. Moreover, with prolonged exposure to natural sounds, the proportion of various activity types also increased. However, satisfaction levels exhibited a decline during both low- and high-decibel activities as crowd density increased.

(5) The investigation into the relationship between physiological indicators and activity types among elderly individuals exposed to the same sound source unveiled distinct trends in physiological indicators among those engaged in different activities. For example, significant differences in heart rate variation were observed between elderly individuals playing table tennis and those sitting quietly during the experiment. However, the underlying reasons for these differences remain unclear and warrant further investigation.

In this chapter, it was concluded that while the care home boasts a commendable overall environment and facilities characterized by its expansive comprehensive activity hall, the acoustic environment in the event hall is suboptimal. Despite designated areas within the lobby, such as rest and activity zones, sounds tend to interfere with each other, resulting in 'bleeding across' these areas. This highlights that large spaces and a diverse range of activities cannot entirely mitigate the adverse effects of sound. Respondents may experience nervousness and irritability due to the intricate acoustic environment in such expansive spaces. Hence, it is recommended that when designing facilities for the elderly, large activity spaces should be reconsidered. Furthermore, the questionnaire revealed that the elderly held a higher-rated evaluation of both background and foreground music. Therefore, future research could explore incorporating music more suited to older adults, as music that irks them could prompt an instantaneous negative evaluation, shedding light on their assessment of large spatial acoustic environments. Additionally, in terms of physiological health, the relationship between music, activity type, and physiological indicators of older individuals remains unclear, necessitating further in-depth research in this domain to furnish a scientific basis for enhancing the living environment and well-being of the elderly.

References

[1] Devos P, Aletta F, Thomas P, et al. Designing supportive soundscapes for nursing home residents with dementia[J]. *International Journal of Environmental Research and Public Health*, 2019, 16(24):4904.

[2] Wang L, Kang J. Acoustic demands and influencing factors in facilities for the elderly[J]. *Applied Acoustics*, 2020, 170:107470.

[3] Stansfeld SA, Matheson MP. Noise pollution: Non-auditory effects on health[J]. *British Medical Bulletin*, 2003(1):243.

[4] Kerns E, Masterson EA, Themann CL, et al. Cardiovascular conditions, hearing difficulty, and occupational noise exposure within US industries and occupations[J]. *American Journal of Industrial Medicine*, 2018, 61(6):477–491.

[5] Sharaf FM. An approach to improve acoustic performance in multipurpose halls[J]. *Journal of American Science*, 2014, 10(3s):9–15.

[6] Schafer RM. *The soundscape: Our sonic environment and the tuning of the world*[M]. New York, NY: Simon and Schuster, 1993.
[7] Brown AL, Kang JA, Gjestland T. Towards standardization in soundscape preference assessment[J]. *Applied Acoustics*, 2011, 72(6):387–392.
[8] Gao J, Barroso C, Zhang P, et al. N-terminal acetylation promotes synaptonemal complex assembly in C. elegans.[J]. *Genes and Development: A Journal Devoted to the Molecular Analysis of Gene Expression in Eukaryotes, Prokaryotes, and Viruses*, 2016(21).
[9] Yang W, Kang J. Acoustic comfort evaluation in urban open public spaces[J]. *Applied Acoustics*, 2005, 66(2):211–229.
[10] Chen X, Kang J. Acoustic comfort in large dining spaces[J]. *Applied Acoustics*, 2017, 115:166–172.
[11] Thomas P, Aletta F, Mynsbrugge TV, et al. Evaluation and improvement of the acoustic comfort in nursing homes: A case study in Flanders[C]. *11th European Congress and Exposition on Noise Control Engineering (Euronoise 2018).* Belgium: European Acoustics Association (EAA); Hellenic Institute of Acoustics (HELINA), 2018, 405–412.
[12] Long XJ, Din NC, Lei YL, et al. The restorative effects of outdoor soundscapes in nursing homes for elderly individuals[J]. *Building and Environment*, 2023, 242:110520.
[13] Chu LW, Chi I. Nursing homes in China[J]. *Journal of the American Medical Directors Association*, 2008, 9(4):239–245.
[14] Wu M, Li SX, Zhang NJ, et al. Nursing home research in Jinan, China: A focus group approach[J]. *International Journal of Public Policy*, 2012, 8(1–3).
[15] Büchler M, Allegro S, Launer S, et al. Sound classification in hearing aids inspired by auditory scene analysis[J]. *EURASIP Journal on Advances in Signal Processing*, 2005, 2005(18):2991–3002.
[16] Joosse LL. Sound levels in nursing homes[J]. *Gerontological Nursing*, 2011, 37(8):30–35.
[17] Yi F, Kang J. Effect of background and foreground music on satisfaction, behavior, and emotional responses in public spaces of shopping malls[J]. *Applied Acoustics*, 2019, 145(Feb.):408–419.
[18] Mu J, Kang J, Wu Y. Acoustic environment of comprehensive activity spaces in nursing homes: A case study in Harbin, China[J]. *Applied Acoustics*, 2021, 177(24):107932.
[19] Tavossi HM. Traffic noise attenuation by scattering, resonance, and dispersion[J]. *Acoustical Society of America*, 2003, 114(4):2353–2353.
[20] Zannin PHT, Marcon CR. Objective and subjective evaluation of the acoustic comfort in classrooms[J]. *Applied Ergonomics*, 2007, 38(5):675–680.
[21] Berglund B, Lindvall T, Schwela DH, et al. Guidelines for community noise[J]. *World Health Organization – WHO*, 1999.
[22] Meng Q, Liu SS, Kang J. Effect of children on the sound environment in fast-food restaurants[J]. *Applied Acoustics*, 2020, 162:107201.
[23] Liu F, Kang J. Relationship between street scale and subjective assessment of audio-visual environment comfort based on 3D virtual reality and dual-channel acoustic tests[J]. *Building & Environment*, 2018, 129:35–45.
[24] Zhang X, Ba MH, Kang J, et al. Effect of soundscape dimensions on acoustic comfort in urban open public spaces[J]. *Applied Acoustics*, 2018, 133:73–81.
[25] Lam YW. A comparison of three diffuse reflection modeling methods used in room acoustics computer models[J]. *The Journal of the Acoustical Society of America*, 1996, 100(4):2181–2192.
[26] Hannes M. *Aging and sound perception: Desirable characteristics of entertainment audio for the elderly*[C]. New York, NY: Audio Engineering Society, 2008.
[27] Frisina DR, Frisina RD. Speech recognition in noise and presbycusis: Relations to possible neural mechanisms[J]. *Hearing Research*, 1997, 106(1–2):95–104.
[28] Meng Q, Kang J. Effect of sound-related activities on human behaviours and acoustic comfort in urban open spaces[J]. *Science of the Total Environment*, 2016, 573:481–493.

[29] Liu F, Kang J. Relationship between street scale and subjective assessment of audio-visual environment comfort based on 3D virtual reality and dual-channel acoustic tests[J]. *Building & Environment,* 2018, 129:35–45.
[30] Meng Q, Kang BJ. The influence of crowd density on the sound environment in commercial pedestrian streets[J]. *Science of the Total Environment*, 2015, 511:249–258.
[31] Lacerda CF, Silva LO, de Tavares Canto RS, et al. Effects of hearing aids in the balance, quality of life and fear to fall in elderly people with sensorineural hearing loss[J]. *International Archives of Otorhinolaryngology*, 2012, 16(2).
[32] Li ZKJ. Sensitivity analysis of changes in human physiological indicators observed in soundscapes[J]. *Landscape and Urban Planning*, 2019, 190.
[33] Alvarsson JJ, Wiens S, Nilsson ME. Stress recovery during exposure to nature sound and environmental noise[J]. *International Journal of Environmental Research and Public Health*, 2010, 7(3):1036–1046.

5 Case study and acoustic environment simulation of care homes

5.1 Case study

5.1.1 Introduction

Since 2010, in tandem with the escalating challenges of population aging and the rise in the number of empty-nest elderly, China's eldercare industry has witnessed substantial growth, leading to a diversification of eldercare building types. Alongside this expansion, various facilities such as nursing homes, care homes, senior apartments, community senior day care centers, and elderly service stations have emerged.

In the initial phases of eldercare building development, domestic scholars embarked on extensive foundational research concerning existing eldercare facilities. They meticulously summarized and analyzed the needs of the elderly population alongside the prevailing conditions of eldercare buildings. Recognizing the pivotal role of early architectural designs in shaping the spatial ambiance of care homes, scholars primarily concentrated on design methodologies and strategies for eldercare buildings. Their investigations delved into aspects like site planning, functional arrangements, layout optimization, and circulation design [1].

Over the past decade, propelled by the rapid expansion of eldercare facilities, the research landscape has expanded significantly. Scholars have broadened their exploration, scrutinizing the architectural characteristics and prevalent challenges of eldercare facilities from multifaceted perspectives, including early-stage planning, spatial attributes, management protocols, age-friendly design principles [2], and integrated eldercare facilities. Consequently, a more nuanced comprehension of spatial environment design for eldercare facilities has emerged.

Presently, in architectural design discourse, attention has shifted from mere functional layouts to intricate designs aimed at enriching the spatial quality for the elderly through meticulous architectural detailing and interior embellishments. Moreover, scholars have begun to emphasize the creation of interior atmospheres and emotional experiences tailored to the needs of the elderly, prioritizing their comfort and emotional well-being. Concurrently, research endeavors pertaining to smart aging and age-friendly renovations are on the rise.

DOI: 10.1201/9781003407232-5

In contrast to the wealth of architectural design research, there exists a relative dearth of studies on the physical environment of care homes within the domestic landscape. Nonetheless, empirical evidence suggests that indoor physical environments significantly influence individuals' sense of well-being and overall quality of life. Among these environmental factors, the acoustic environment stands out as a critical component, exerting a profound impact on the health, emotions, and behaviors of the elderly [3, 4]. Moreover, indoor acoustic environments in eldercare facilities tend to be complex, featuring a myriad of sound types such as speech, HVAC equipment noise, background music, and activity noise, all of which can shape the physical and mental well-being and quality of life of the elderly population. Hence, there is a pressing need for research dedicated to the acoustic environment of care homes.

This chapter aims to illustrate the current state of care homes in China by selecting representative cases for in-depth exploration of spatial layout and interior design while scrutinizing the characteristics and prevalent issues pertaining to the acoustic environment of these facilities. Additionally, software simulation methods are introduced. Leveraging Odeon, which is recognized as the most comprehensive architectural acoustics performance assessment software, simulations are conducted to measure the indoor acoustic effects of care homes. Accordingly, three-dimensional models of care homes are constructed using Sketchup and imported into the Odeon software for architectural acoustic environment simulation. Parameters such as sound pressure level, speech intelligibility, and reverberation time are simulated, and based on the results, existing issues in the acoustic environment of care homes are analyzed, with proposed strategies for enhancing their acoustic environment through adjustments to interior materials and furniture.

5.1.2 Case study and method

Drawing from the prevailing landscape of care homes in China, three archetypal building types are singled out for scrutiny: nursing homes, senior service centers, and dementia care centers. Nursing homes, ubiquitous and widespread across China, constitute the most prevalent form of eldercare establishments. Typically, they offer a gamut of services encompassing meals, recreational activities, and medical rehabilitation. Senior service centers, on the other hand, cater to a similar spectrum of needs but often serve as more communal hubs, doubling as community activity centers, thereby boasting more open spatial designs compared to nursing homes. In contrast, dementia care centers, although fewer in number and with a briefer developmental trajectory, assume critical significance owing to China's burgeoning population of dementia-afflicted elderly [5], positioning the nation at the apex of global dementia prevalence. Consequently, some scholars prognosticate that dementia patients will emerge as the focal demographic for eldercare establishments in the future [6]. Moreover, the demographic shifts induced by the "one-child policy" have spurred a surge in demand for dementia care facilities, necessitating innovative spatial layouts, often characterized by cluster-based designs. Given these dynamics, these three paradigmatic eldercare facility types are chosen for comprehensive case analyses and acoustic environment simulations in this study.

This section meticulously selects seven representative cases, encompassing three nursing homes, two senior service centers, and two dementia care centers (as delineated in Table 5.1). These nursing homes exhibit marked divergences in their architectural blueprints and are geographically dispersed across various regions of China, thereby affording insights into the multifaceted developmental trajectories of care homes nationwide. Situated in key cities such as Beijing, Tianjin, Qingdao, Chengdu, and Guangzhou, these care homes span climatic zones classified under the <Code for thermal design of civil building> (GB50176–2016) [7] as cold, hot-summer and cold-winter, and hot-summer and warm-winter regions, respectively. The analysis of indoor acoustic environment simulations in these diverse

Table 5.1 Basic information of care homes

Code	*Project name*	*Type*	*Location*	*Opening time*	*Beds*	*Area*	*Service object*
Case1-NH	Taiyichun Elderly Care Center	Nursing Home	Beijing	2017	190	7704	Disabled, semi-disabled, and self-dependent elderly
Case2-NH	Oriental Yiniang Xiangshan Nursing Center	Nursing Home	Chengdu	2017	148	4150	Assistance, care, disability, dementia
Case3-NH	Le Shanju Nursing Home	Nursing Home	Foshan	2014	130	5400	Semi-disabled, disabled, and mentally retarded elderly
Case4-ESC	Yiyuan Elderly Service Center	Elderly service center	Tianjin	2018	206	8000	Disabled, semi-disabled, and self-dependent elderly
Case5-ESC	Zhonghai Jinnian Fuku	Elderly service Zcenter	Qingdao	2020	520	28000	Self-reliant, semi-disabled, disabled, and mentally retarded elderly
Case6-DCC	Zhangyou Huiyuan Memory Care Center	Dementia care center	Beijing	2019	114	8212	Cognitive elderly
Case7-DCC	Langshi Ever-green Ivy – Wuma Ferry Station	Dementia care center	Nanjing	2018	170	6588	Healthy, semi-self-reliant, disabled, mentally retarded elderly

Note: NH = Nursing Home, ESC = Elderly Service Center, DCC = Dementia Care Center.

locales serves as a potent adjunct to on-site investigations of care homes, enriching our understanding of their acoustic environment.

5.2 Nursing home

5.2.1 Case 1-NH

Case 1-NH, situated in the bustling Fengtai District of Beijing, boasts convenient transportation links and a plethora of urban amenities. Its selection as an elder-care building site stemmed from the region's pronounced aging population and the pressing need for additional elderly care facilities. The facility primarily caters to elderly individuals requiring nursing care, including those grappling with disabilities and dementia, alongside a smaller cohort of independently functioning seniors.

Architecturally, the building adopts a square-shaped layout with a central courtyard, a strategic choice that optimizes natural lighting and fosters an efficient internal circulation network [8]. The courtyard, serving as an expansive communal area, naturally facilitates elderly engagement in activities and social interactions. Spanning a total of seven floors, it includes five above ground and two below; the infrastructure is meticulously organized to cater to diverse needs. The subterranean levels house administrative offices, bathrooms, recreational spaces, dining areas, staff quarters, and equipment facilities, while the above-ground floors accommodate living quarters for the elderly, communal activity spaces, medical zones, and dining facilities.

The ground floor, characterized by its expansive openness, hosts a versatile restaurant/multi-function hall, rehabilitation zone, clustered living area, reception zone, kitchen, logistics training area, and a smattering of elderly living quarters. Floors 2 to 5 serve as residential hubs, outfitted with clustered communal living areas, nursing stations, circulation zones, and logistical support spaces (Figure 5.1). Each floor comprises two nursing units, each catering to approximately 25 elderly individuals, and is meticulously designed to streamline daily life services for the residents. The elderly living quarters are strategically positioned on either side of the communal living spaces within each unit.

Figure 5.1 showcases snapshots of the public activity zones and elderly bedrooms within the nursing home, revealing a harmonious blend of warm hues and verdant tones that aid in distinguishing between different spatial domains. While most public spaces lack sound-absorption treatments on their walls and ceilings, the wooden flooring and indoor soft furnishings offer a degree of sound absorption, albeit not exhaustive. Notably, the Four Seasons Lounge, with its expansive dimensions, exudes a cozy ambiance with its yellow-painted walls and stone flooring. However, the latter's reflective properties may exacerbate indoor sound levels and prolong reverberation times, warranting improvements in the lounge's acoustic environment.

Within each residential cluster, a range of accommodations are available, including single, double, and quadruple rooms, catering to the diverse needs of the elderly residents. While single rooms afford the highest degree of privacy and are

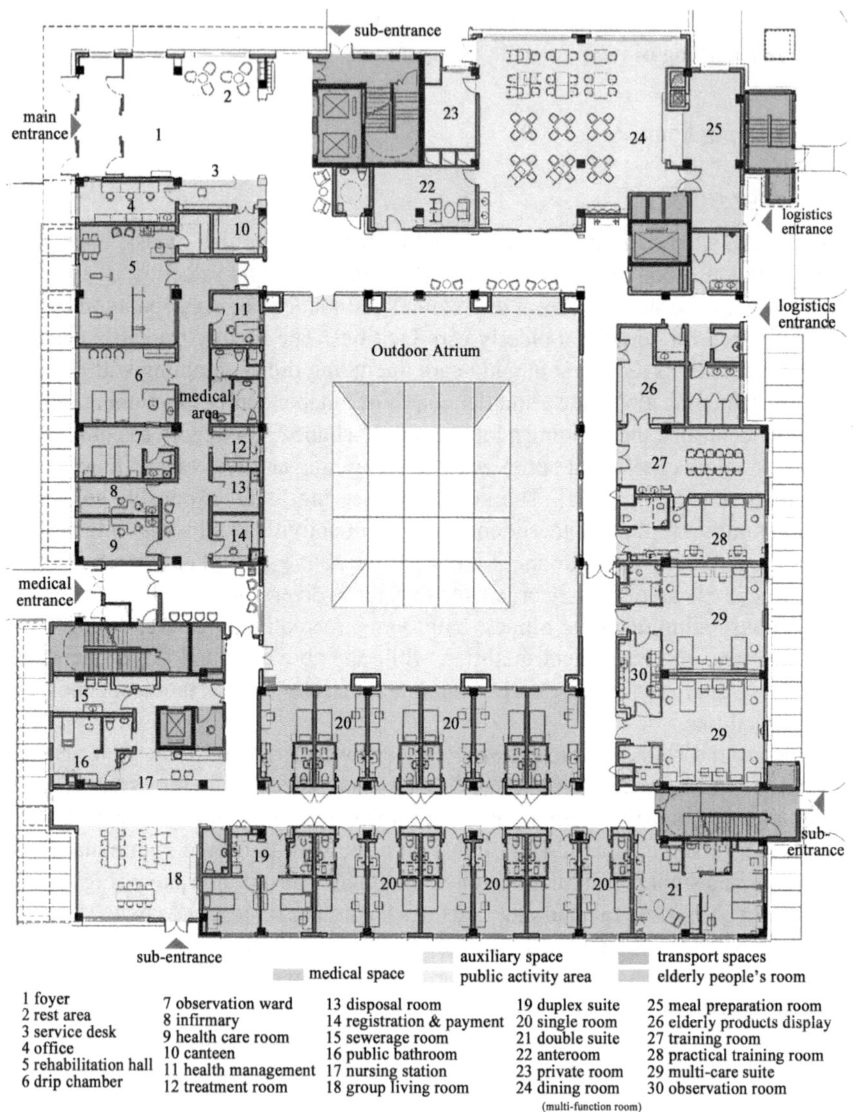

Figure 5.1 First floor plan and interior scene photograph

favored by many seniors, the design predominantly emphasizes single and double rooms to ensure the facility's financial viability. As illustrated in Figure 5.1, the wooden flooring and predominantly white walls and ceilings across all accommodation types lack specialized acoustic treatments, potentially leading to extended reverberation times, especially in larger spaces such as quadruple rooms.

5.2.2 Case 2-NH

Case 2-NH, nestled in the heart of Nanjing City's Gulou district, enjoys close proximity to residential neighborhoods and medical facilities. Originally a social welfare institute, the establishment sprawls across a generous expanse of 4150 square meters. It caters primarily to the needs of semi-disabled, disabled, and dementia-afflicted elderly individuals, with specialized care zones delineated within the premises.

Comprising four floors with a central courtyard, the structure adopts an enclosed layout, with public areas encircling the tranquil courtyard oasis. The ground floor, depicted in Figure 5.2, serves as the focal point of public engagement, featuring a welcoming lobby, dining enclave, communal living spaces, art exhibition area, and essential medical and logistical facilities. Notably, to optimize spatial efficiency, double rooms for elderly residents are strategically positioned on the ground floor's southern and northern extremities.

In terms of resident distribution, the ground floor accommodates independent seniors, while the second floor is tailored for the needs of disabled and semi-disabled individuals. The third floor is dedicated to dementia care, while the fourth floor provides specialized intensive care services, ensuring round-the-clock nursing attention for severely disabled residents. Public activity areas are thoughtfully dispersed throughout the building, with dining and living zones adjacent to the courtyard on the ground floor, a tranquil reading sanctuary on the second floor, and a contemplative chess enclave on the third floor. This deliberate allocation ensures that each floor offers residents ample spaces for engagement and social interaction, thus deviating from the conventional 'accommodation + corridor' spatial archetype. However, it may inadvertently inconvenience residents due to longer travel distances between different zones.

Figure 5.2 also offers a glimpse into the indoor public spaces of the Elderly Care Center, where warm hues dominate, imbuing the environment with a sense of comfort and homeliness. Most public areas feature anti-slip rubber flooring, painted walls and ceilings, and select wall surfaces are adorned with wooden veneers. The indoor furnishings, predominantly crafted from solid wood, exude a timeless elegance, complemented by plush sofas and soft furnishings. Despite the absence of specialized acoustic design, the interconnected nature of these public spaces around the central atrium poses challenges, as elevated sound pressure levels in one area may reverberate and affect adjacent spaces. Moreover, ambient sounds such as staff conversations, mechanical HVAC noise, and background music, while subtle, may collectively impact the acoustic comfort of the elderly, potentially undermining their physical and mental well-being.

The residential quarters within the care center primarily consist of double rooms, with a few floors featuring triple accommodations. As depicted in the diagram (Figure 5.2), the bedrooms boast wooden flooring, painted walls and ceilings, and minimal acoustic treatment. While the beds and furnishings contribute to sound absorption, the large size of the bedrooms, coupled with the presence of triple and multiple occupancy rooms, may inadvertently prolong reverberation times. The absence of specialized acoustic materials could exacerbate indoor sound pressure levels, particularly during activities such as television viewing or group conversations.

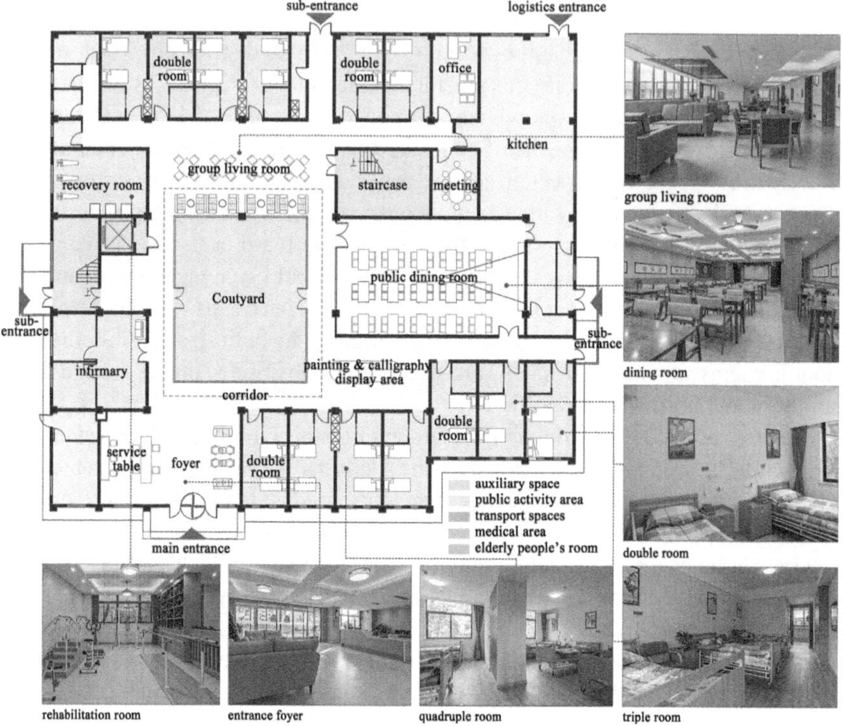

Figure 5.2 First floor plan

5.2.3 Case 3-NH

Case 3-NH, nestled in Shunde district, Foshan city, Guangdong province, originally housed a medical supplies warehouse. However, in response to the burgeoning elderly population and the dearth of accommodation-based elderly care institutions, the decision was made to repurpose it into a nursing home. This transformation aimed to provide essential medical rehabilitation and elderly care services while simultaneously relieving the strain on hospital beds.

The building, initially boasting four floors, underwent a comprehensive renovation. Post-renovation, the ground floor was earmarked for the emergency and radiology departments, featuring a separate elevator hall for direct access to the nursing home's entrance lobby on the third floor [1]. The second floor retained its original function as a medical supplies repository. The third and fourth floors were ingeniously reimagined into the nursing home, with a picturesque rooftop garden designed to foster daily interactions and activities among the elderly residents.

In terms of service allocation, the third floor primarily caters to semi-disabled elderly individuals, while the fourth floor is tailored for the disabled elderly. Both floors share similar functional layouts, encompassing communal spaces such as a common living room, family gathering area, card and board game room, public bathrooms, nursing stations, medication dispensary, and doctor's office. The third floor boasts additional amenities, including a rehabilitation training room, emergency department, and a tranquil Buddhist shrine, while the fourth floor features a traditional Chinese medicine facility.

Given the building's original warehouse configuration, its expansive length and depth posed challenges, hindering adequate lighting and potentially prolonging indoor traffic flow lines, thus impeding nursing efficiency. To mitigate these issues, towering atriums were strategically inserted on the east and west sides of the structure to enhance lighting and ventilation conditions [9]. Leveraging this design intervention, elderly residential clusters were strategically positioned around the atriums, with nursing stations strategically placed to optimize service routes and streamline nursing operations. To further augment illumination, residential units were situated along the outer walls, with public spaces nestled in the building's core, flanked by the two atriums (Figure 5.3).

Figure 5.3 also offers glimpses into various public spaces within the nursing home, including the living room, card and board game area, and activity hall. These communal hubs are ingeniously centered around naturally lit atriums to maximize exposure to natural light. While corridors and rehabilitation zones feature anti-slip rubber flooring, other areas boast tiled floors. Predominantly painted in white, the indoor walls and ceilings lack specialized acoustic treatments. The tiled flooring and wall surfaces, being poor sound absorbers, can lead to excessive reverberation and compromised auditory comfort. Therefore, there's an imperative need to enhance the acoustic quality of these public spaces.

Residential quarters within the nursing home predominantly comprise single and double rooms, alongside a few quadruple rooms and one-bedroom suites (Figure 5.3). The interior finishes across all room types remain consistent, with wooden flooring, painted walls or wallpaper, and white-painted ceilings devoid of specific sound-absorbing treatments. Soft furnishings like beds and sofas play a pivotal role in sound absorption within these spaces. While the acoustic environment might be tolerable in single and double rooms owing to their compact size, larger quadruple rooms, accommodating more residents, may experience heightened indoor sound pressure levels and prolonged reverberation times, potentially compromising the auditory comfort of the elderly occupants.

5.2.4 Simulation analysis

To further explore the intricacies of indoor sound environments in various care homes, the study utilized Odeon software to simulate the acoustic landscapes of care homes. Given the significance of sound pressure level and reverberation time in gauging sound quality, these parameters took center stage during the simulation phase. Initial case analyses uncovered striking similarities in bedroom environments across different nursing homes, characterized by wooden floors, solid wood furniture, and painted ceilings and walls devoid of sound absorption treatment. Conversely, public spaces within care homes exhibited notable variations, warranting a focused examination in this section. Since these spaces typically boast open layouts with seamless connectivity between functional zones and are interconnected with corridors and circulation spaces, the simulation process encompassed public areas, including corridors, for comprehensive analysis. Given the

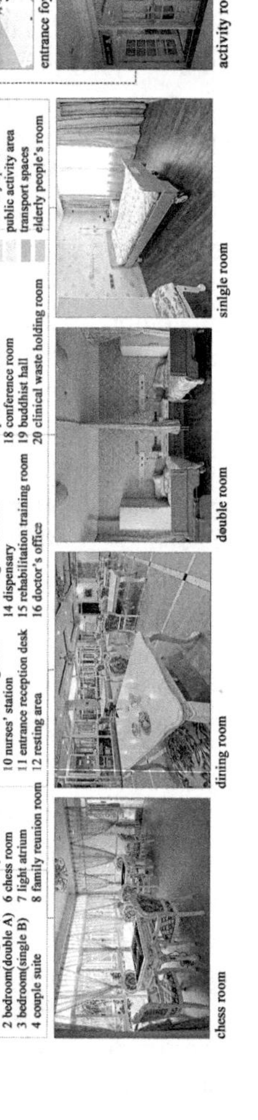

Figure 5.3 Third floor plan and interior scene photograph

Table 5.2 List of sound absorption coefficients for indoor materials in public spaces of care homes

Area	*Odeon material type*	*63Hz*	*125Hz*	*250Hz*	*500Hz*	*1000Hz*	*2000Hz*	*4000Hz*	*8000Hz*
Floor	linoleum or vinyl stuck to concrete	0.02	0.02	0.02	0.03	0.04	0.04	0.05	0.05
Glass	glass, ordinary window	0.35	0.35	0.25	0.18	0.12	0.07	0.04	0.04
Walls/ Ceiling	painted plaster surface	0.02	0.02	0.02	0.02	0.02	0.02	0.02	0.02
Seats	moderatelly upholstered chairs	0.44	0.44	0.56	0.67	0.74	0.83	0.87	0.87
Wooden furniture	solid wooden furniture	0.48	0.48	0.77	0.38	0.27	0.65	0.35	0.35
Wooden veneer	Plywood paneling, 1 cm thick	0.28	0.28	0.22	0.17	0.09	0.1	0.11	0.11
Wooden flooring	Thin plywood paneling	0.44	0.44	0.56	0.67	0.74	0.83	0.87	0.87
Tile/Stone	marble	0.01	0.01	0.01	0.01	0.01	0.02	0.02	0.02

resemblance in the types of materials employed in public spaces across various nursing homes, a standardized approach was adopted for indoor materials, with material sound absorption coefficients detailed in Table 5.2.

Incorporating an atrium or courtyard at the heart of the care homes natural lighting and ventilation. Spatially, Case 1-NH situates public areas at the building's corners, with spaces adjacent to the atrium primarily adopting a 'corridor + bedroom' configuration. In contrast, the other two nursing homes predominantly position public spaces around the atrium/courtyard, resulting in distinct spatial arrangements and sound environments. As depicted in Figure 5.4, high-traffic public zones (like common living rooms and dining areas) typically register elevated sound pressure levels, whereas corridors and similar areas exhibit lower sound pressure levels, leading to pronounced disparities in indoor sound pressures across the nursing home, potentially impacting the elderly adversely. Furthermore, the more open and dispersed the foot traffic in a space, the more balanced the distribution of indoor sound pressure levels tends to be. Hence, measures such as augmenting sound-absorbing and soundproofing materials and evenly dispersing public areas can be implemented to enhance the quality of the indoor sound environment in concentrated sound zones.

Reverberation time, crucial for assessing sound environment quality, denotes the duration for the sound pressure level to diminish by 60 dBA after the sound source ceases in an enclosed space. Analysis results of reverberation time for each nursing home are showcased in Figure 5.5. Notably, considerable disparities exist

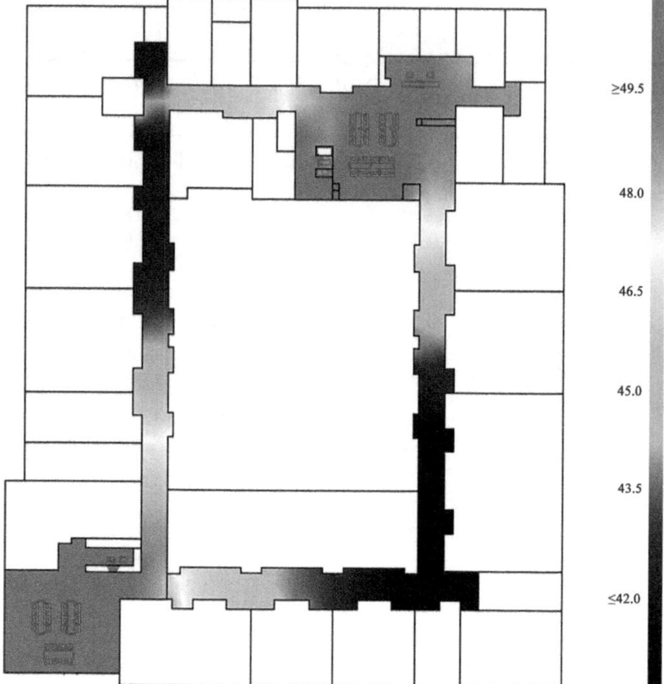

a) Case 1-NH

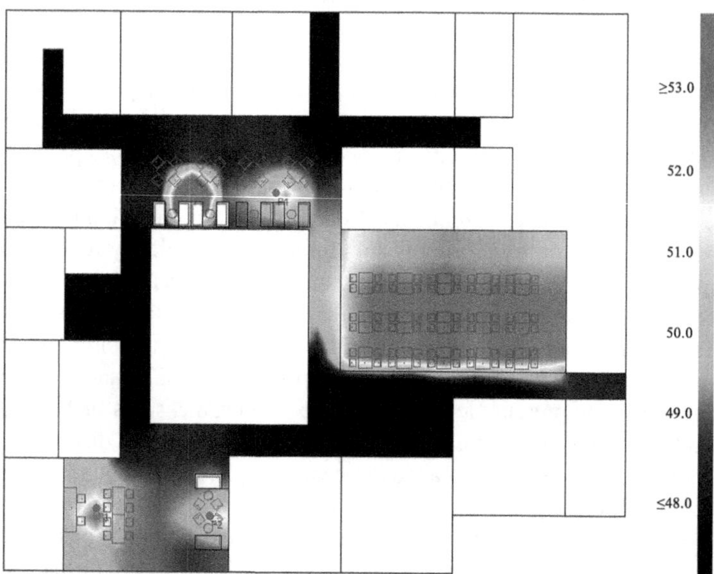

b) Case 2-NH

Figure 5.4(a-c) Sound pressure level(dB)

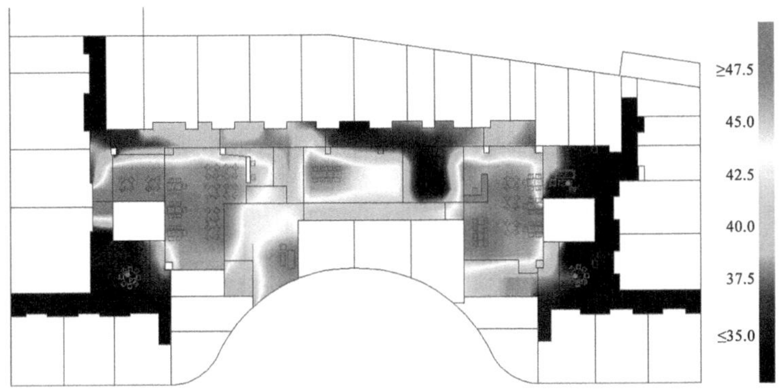

c) Case 3-NH

Figure 5.4(a-c) (Continued)

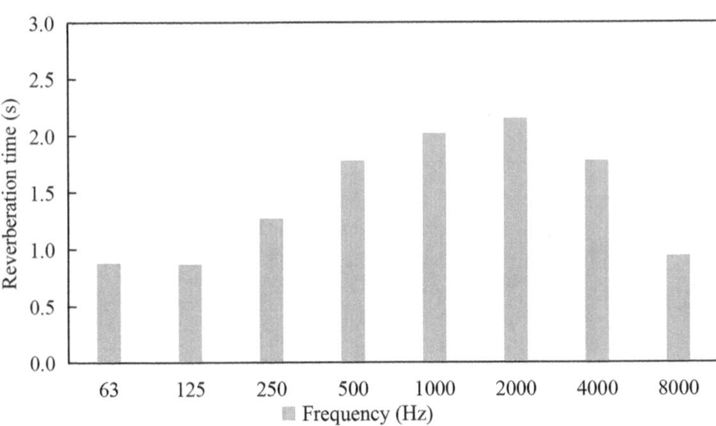

a) Case 1-NH

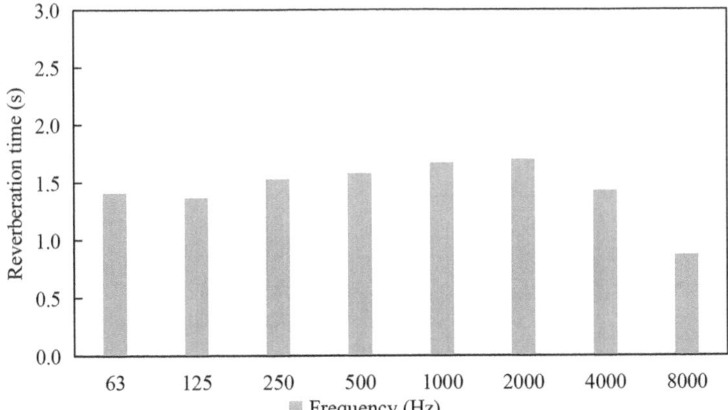

b) Case 2-NH

Figure 5.5(a-c) Reverberation time in nursing homes

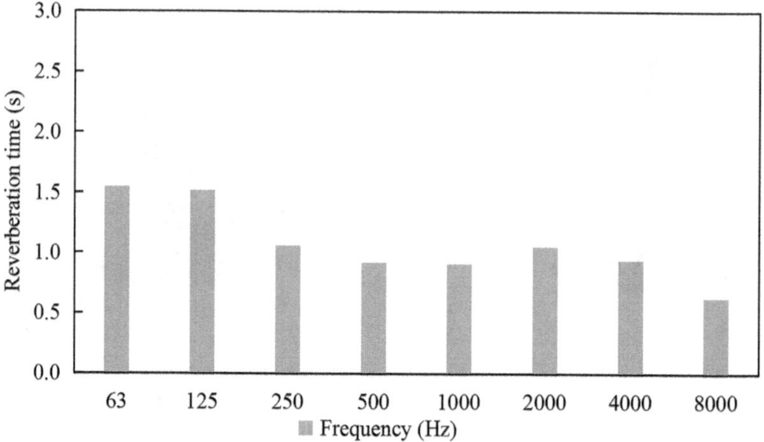

c) Case 3-NH

Figure 5.5(a-c) (Continued)

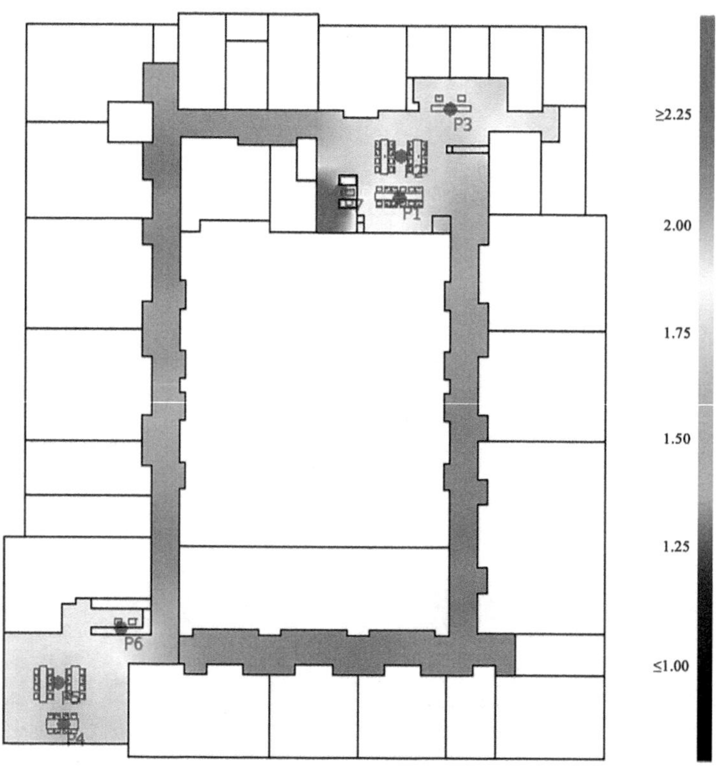

a) Case 1-NH

Figure 5.6(a-c) Spatial distribution of reverberation time in nursing homes

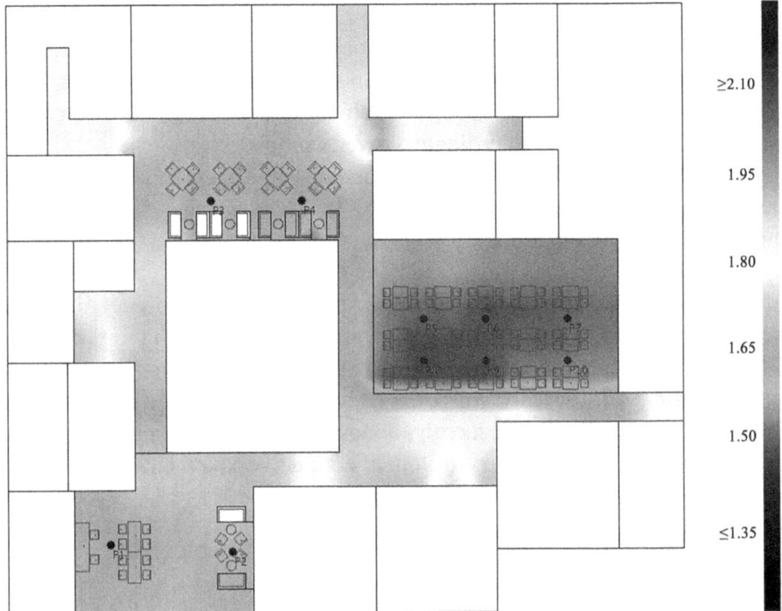

b) Case 2-NH

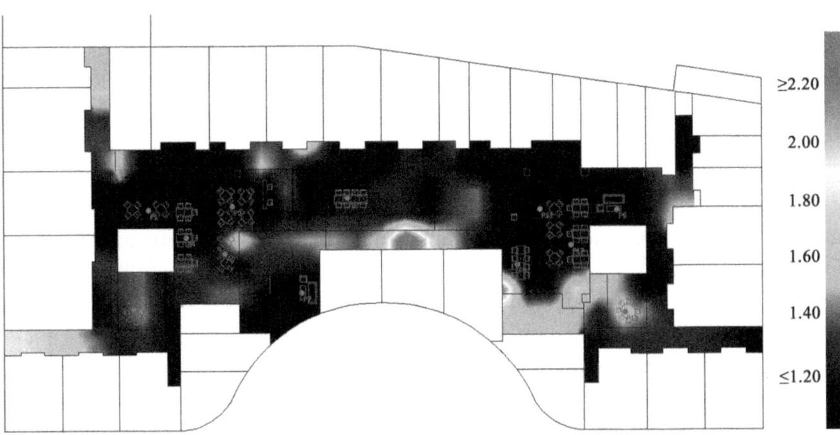

c) Case 3-NH

Figure 5.6(a-c) (Continued)

in reverberation times among the nursing homes, with Case 3-NH boasting the shortest duration. Save for low-frequency sounds, reverberation time for other frequency sounds approximates 0.9 seconds, offering heightened sound clarity albeit potentially affecting sound quality. Case 2-NH registers a reverberation time of around 1.6 seconds, characterized by a relatively balanced distribution across various frequency bands. Conversely, reverberation time in Case 1-NH exhibits significant variability, ranging from approximately 0.8 seconds for low-frequency sounds to 1.2 to 2.2 seconds for mid-frequency sounds. This variation may be due to the limited square-shaped spaces, the prevalence of corridor spaces, and the larger scale of the building in Case 1-NH. In long and narrow spaces, excessive sound reflections can result in prolonged reverberation times.

Figure 5.6 illustrates the reverberation time distribution in indoor public spaces of nursing homes at a frequency of 1000Hz, showcasing notable differences among the facilities. Case 3-NH displays the shortest reverberation time, typically below 1.2 seconds, whereas Case 1-NH and Case 2-NH feature relatively higher durations. Corridors, compared to activity spaces, exhibit prolonged reverberation times, attributed to their narrow and elongated spatial configuration fostering excessive sound reflections during propagation, thereby extending sound duration within the room. Additionally, indoor reverberation time is intricately linked to the materials employed. Consequently, adopting suitable measures is imperative to cultivate an indoor acoustic environment conducive to the elderly's comfort.

5.3 Elderly service center

5.3.1 Case 4-ESC

Case 4-ESC stands in the bustling districts of Xiqing and Taizhen in Tianjin, sprawled across an expansive 8000 square meters [10]. Formerly a five-story idle reinforced concrete frame office building, it underwent a metamorphosis into a contemporary elderly care center. Recognizing the original building's shortcomings in lighting, ventilation, facade design, and internal column grid, the renovation orchestrated facade enhancements, the integration of atriums to augment illumination, and the repositioning of existing columns into bedroom spaces to minimize structural modifications.

Spanning five floors, the ground level facing the urban streets, susceptible to external disruptions, wasn't earmarked for elderly care functions. Instead, it accommodates shops, a lobby, equipment rooms, and a rehabilitation medical area. The second through fourth floors comprise the elderly living quarters, with atriums central to floors 3 to 5, inviting sunlight through skylights adorning the roof (Figure 5.7). These lush atriums host verdant trees and serene leisure spots encircled by communal zones like reading nooks, dining areas, game parlors, and fitness centers (Figure 5.8). Resting alcoves and nursing stations nestle between the atriums and the more secluded elderly living spaces, facilitating seamless transitions

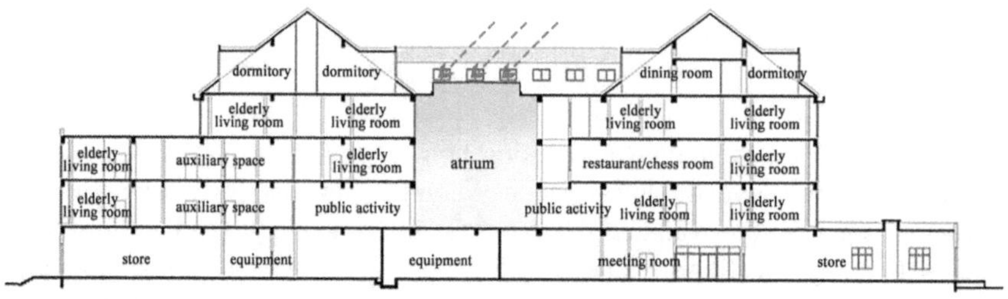

Figure 5.7 Section

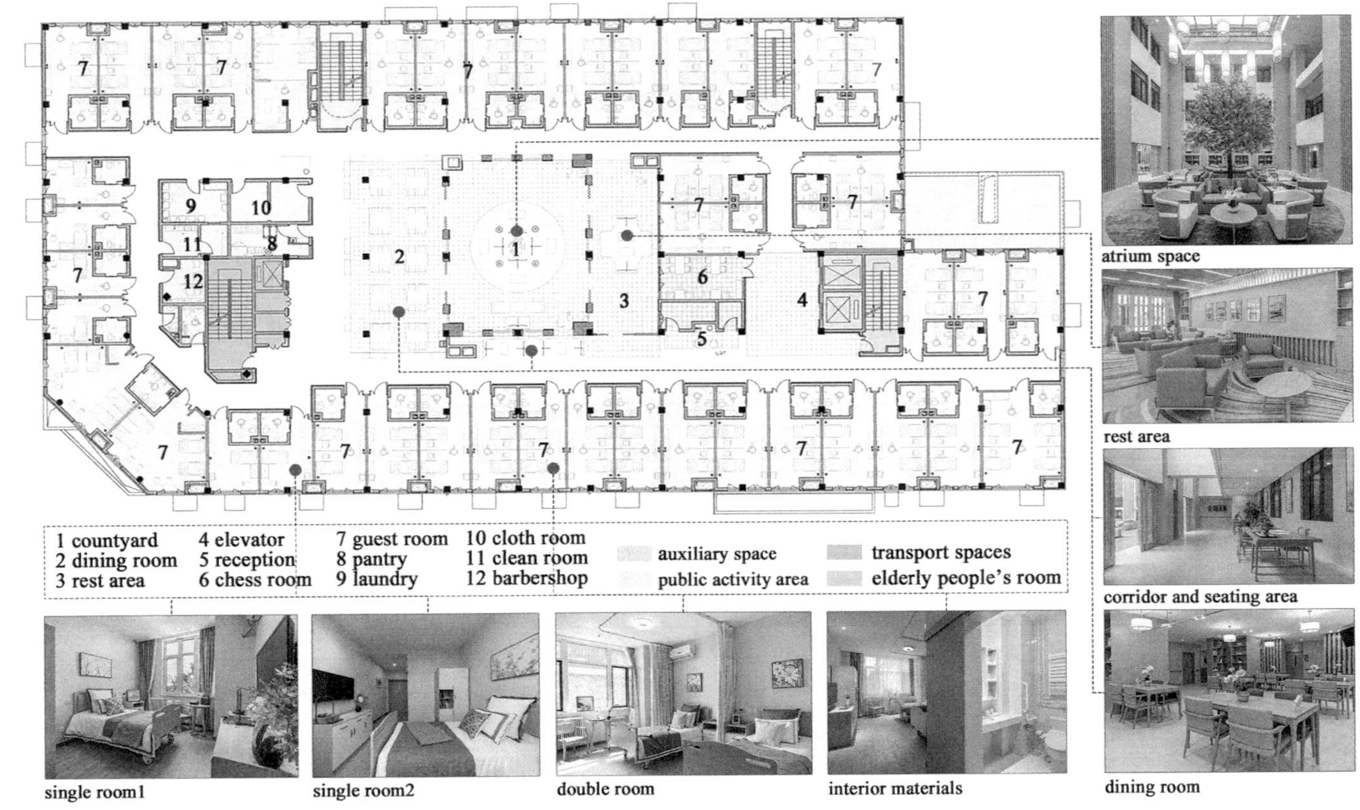

Figure 5.8 Second floor plan and interior scene photograph

and ensuring an optimal service radius for prompt caregiving. Elevated slightly on the fifth floor are offices and staff quarters.

Figure 5.8 encapsulates the frequently frequented spaces by the elderly within the nursing home. Ivory white hues interplay with warm orange tones in the interior design, complemented by solid wood furnishings. Exuding age-friendly sensibilities, furniture boasts rounded corners, while corridors boast a width of 2.1 meters, accommodating unhindered wheelchair mobility in both directions and significantly enhancing elderly safety during locomotion. Interior materials feature ceilings and walls adorned with coatings sans acoustic enhancements. Flooring predominantly comprises anti-slip rubber and wooden panels interspersed with carpeted sections. Wood dominates the indoor furniture, offering inherent sound-absorbing properties. However, owing to the nursing home's expansive scale and the towering three-story atrium, delineating distinct functional public spaces becomes challenging. Consequently, indoor reverberation time may be prolonged, potentially compromising sound clarity and acoustic comfort.

Elderly residential units, available in single, double, and four-person configurations, cater to diverse elderly demographics. Double rooms prevail, with sporadic single rooms scattered throughout the premises, as captured in the vivid scene of Figure 5.8. Infused with warm, vibrant color palettes accentuated by gray and brown hues, the elderly living spaces exude coziness. Bedroom entryways, fashioned as double-leaf doors, accommodate nursing bed passage, facilitating swift emergency responses. Each bedroom boasts an independent bathroom adorned with tiled finishes, while walls and ceilings sport coatings. Though devoid of specific acoustic treatments, the generally compact size of the bedrooms mitigates any substantial impact on the daily lives of elderly residents.

5.3.2 Case 5-ESC

Case 5-ESC nestles in the Binhu district of Wuxi city, a nursing home seamlessly integrated with the surrounding elderly community. Embraced by robust transportation, medical, and commercial amenities, its close proximity to the scenic Taihu Lake adds to its allure. Comprising three principal sections – supporting service facilities spanning floors 1–3, elderly apartments spanning floors 4–23, and nursing wards spanning floors 4–9 – the nursing home caters to a diverse elderly population. The elderly apartments cater primarily to healthy and semi-disabled individuals, while the nursing wards cater to disabled and cognitively impaired elderly individuals. Two tower buildings stand independently yet interconnected by supporting facilities on the ground floor (Figure 5.9).

This nursing home boasts 200 elderly apartments (340 beds) and 100nursing rooms (180 beds), accommodating up to 520 elderly residents. Floors 1–3 serve as sprawling public spaces, spanning approximately 7000 square meters. The ground floor hosts a welcoming lobby, negotiation room, restaurant, multifunctional hall, medical room, and health management center (Figure 5.10). The second floor is dedicated to the restaurant and logistical support areas like the laundry room, air conditioning room, storage room, and kitchen. Meanwhile, the third floor offers a

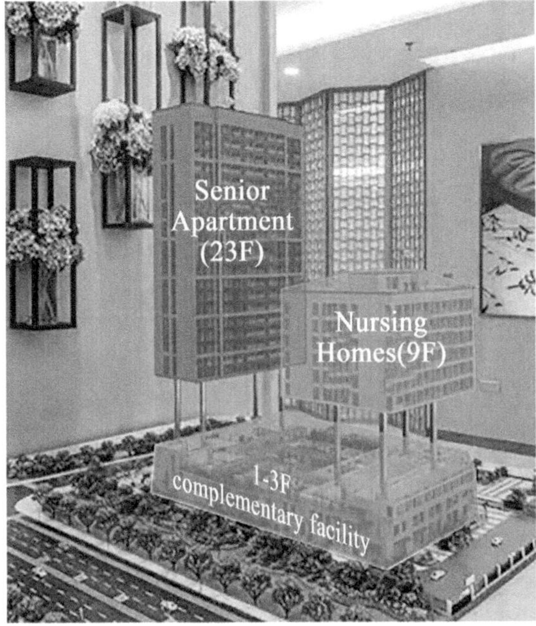

a) Functional distribution

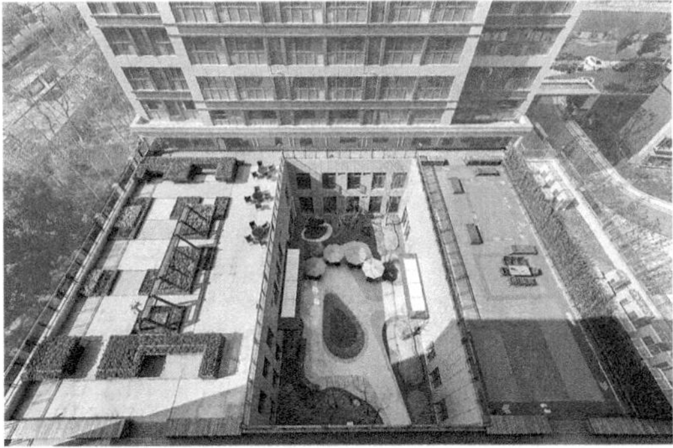

b) Supporting facilities rooftop garden

Figure 5.9(a-b) Functional zoning of the elderly service certer with roof garden

plethora of functional spaces, including a billiard room, reading room/small theater, tea tasting area, music bar, hair salon, religious room, game room, handicraft workshop, and gym. Additionally, a medical service area comprising internal medicine, end-of-life care, psychological counseling room, rehabilitation medicine, and rehabilitation therapy room is provided (Figure 5.11).

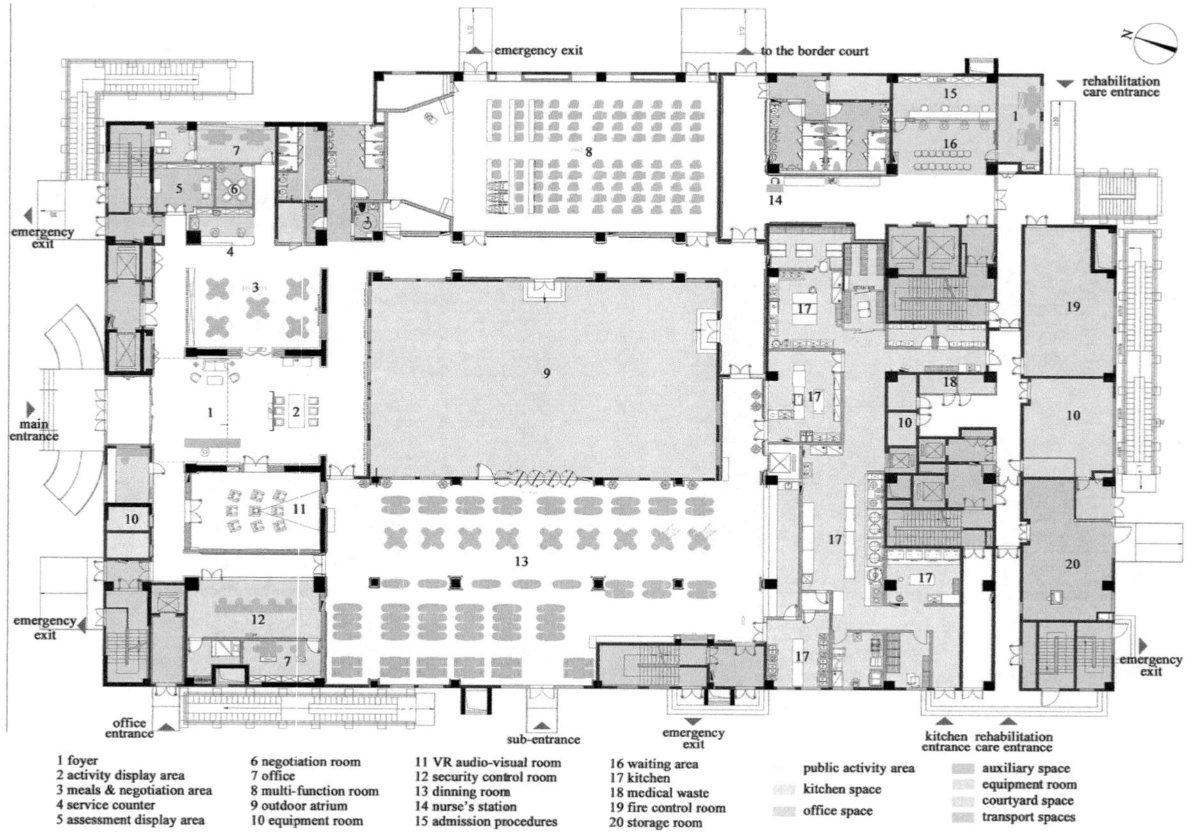

Figure 5.10 First floor plan

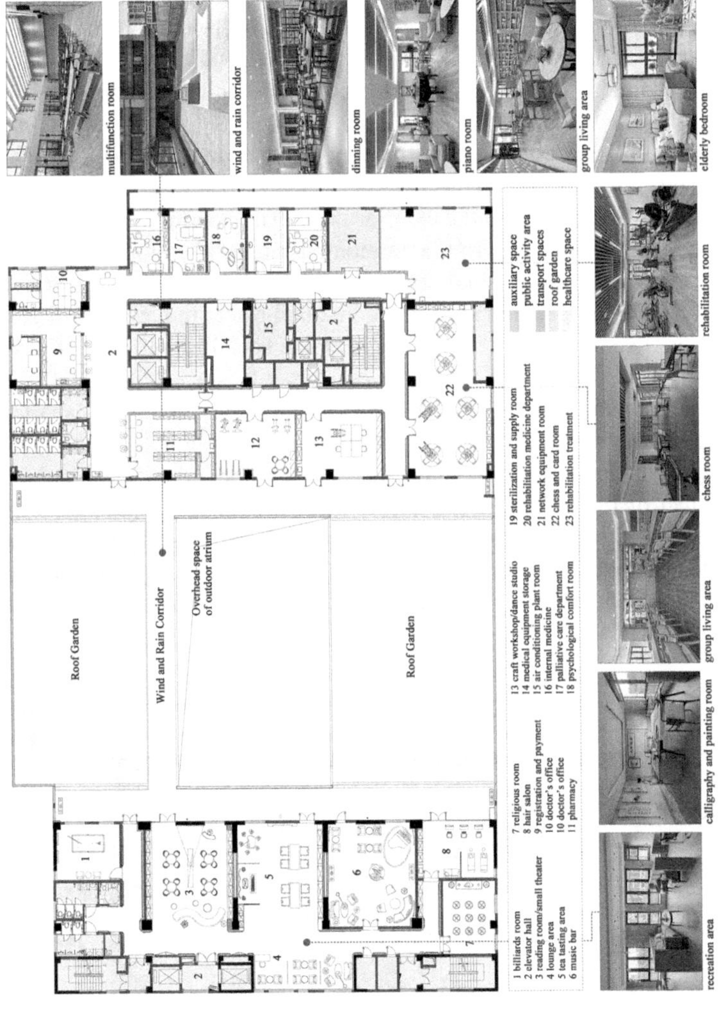

Figure 5.11 Third floor plan and interior scene photograph

Figure 5.11 encapsulates a typical public space within the nursing home, where warm colors dominate the interior ambiance. The expansive dining area is adorned with wooden veneer-clad walls and columns, while the flooring is a mix of anti-slip rubber and wooden panels, both contributing to sound absorption. Similar interior layouts and materials are echoed across other public spaces, with wooden flooring being the preferred choice, distinguished by varying hues. Wooden veneers envelop most walls and columns, complemented by wall-mounted cabinet-style furniture. Some rooms boast ceilings coated with paint, while others feature suspended wooden ceilings. Wooden chairs, upholstered with soft cushion fabrics, populate the indoor furniture ensemble, offering additional sound-absorbing properties.

Among all public spaces, the multifunctional hall boasts a meticulous acoustic design. Thoughtfully crafted ceilings facilitate sound refraction and reflection, with wooden veneer panels adorning the exterior walls. The flooring maintains consistency with wooden panels, ensuring a harmonious acoustic environment throughout. Equipped with a professional stage, sound control room, lifting projection screen, and lifting curtains, the multifunctional hall caters to a myriad of cultural and recreational activities, fostering a comfortable socialization and activity hub for the elderly.

Elderly residential units are available in two configurations: elderly apartments and nursing bedrooms, predominantly featuring single and double rooms spanning 50 to 75 square meters, complete with small kitchens and independent bathrooms. The floor plan of the elderly residential units is depicted in Figure 5.12. Bathrooms are outfitted with wet and dry separation, safety handrails, bathing chairs, and 24-hour emergency call ropes. Sporting a double-door design, the bathrooms accommodate wheelchair entry seamlessly, fulfilling the varied needs of the elderly.

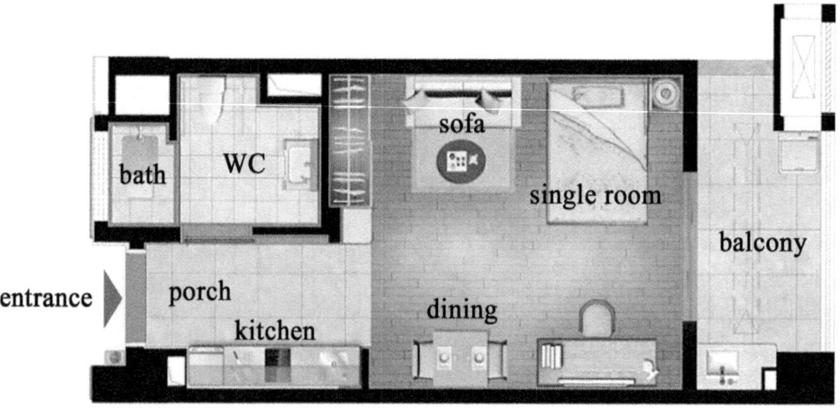

a) Single room (61 m^2)

Figure 5.12(a-b) The elderly's living room suite and accompanying bathroom

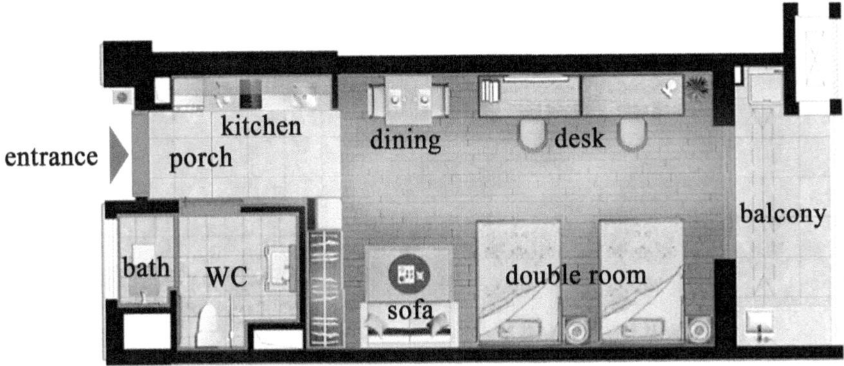

b) Double room (75 m²)

Figure 5.12(a-b) (Continued)

Figure 5.11 also offers glimpses into the interior scenes of the elderly residents' rooms, showcasing varying color palettes while maintaining material uniformity. Wooden flooring graces all rooms, complemented by walls and ceilings adorned with paint. Catering to the needs of healthy and semi-independent elderly individuals, standard beds furnish the single and double rooms in the senior apartments, while nursing beds grace the nursing rooms. Variations in furniture arrangements across spaces may yield differences in sound-absorbing effects, thereby influencing the overall quality of the indoor acoustic environment.

5.3.3 Simulation analysis

In comparison to conventional nursing homes, the communal areas in senior service centers typically boast a more expansive and open layout. Figure 5.13 presents the distribution of indoor sound pressure levels for Case 4-ESC and Case 5-ESC. Notably, areas of congregation such as lobbies, dining spaces, and public lounges register higher sound pressure levels, potentially causing discomfort to the elderly residents. Conversely, corridor spaces exhibit comparatively lower sound pressure levels, with sound intensity decreasing progressively farther from public zones. This discrepancy may arise from the function of corridors primarily as thoroughfares, while leisure and recreational activities predominantly occur in service-oriented areas like activity rooms.

Figure 5.14 details the reverberation times of public spaces within the senior service centers. A marked disparity is evident between the two centers. Case 4-ESC exhibits reverberation times of up to approximately 3.4 seconds, with longer reverberation times recorded for lower-frequency sounds. Conversely, Case 5-ESC displays maximum reverberation times of around 1.8 seconds, with mid-frequency sounds registering the longest reverberation times and both low and high-frequency sounds experiencing relatively shorter reverberation times. The substantial contrast

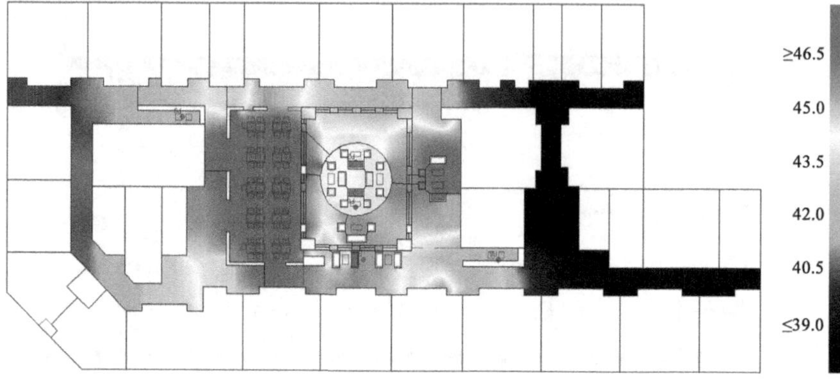

a) Case 4-ESC

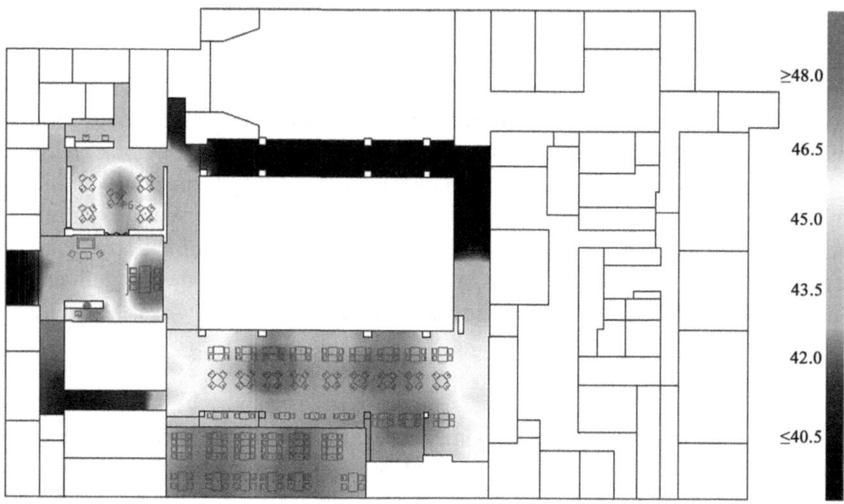

b) Case 5-ESC

Figure 5.13(a-b) Sound pressure level(dBA)

in reverberation times between the two centers may be attributed to differences in interior materials and spatial dimensions. Case 4 features a three-story atrium with a glass ceiling, optimizing natural lighting and ventilation. Moreover, the central courtyard space in Yiyuan employs more tiles on its walls, which are known for their sound reflective properties and inadequate sound absorption capabilities, potentially prolonging reverberation times. In contrast, Case 5 integrates a courtyard into the building's design instead of a lofty atrium and predominantly employs wooden materials known for their superior sound absorption properties, resulting in shorter indoor reverberation times.

Figure 5.15 delineates the spatial distribution of reverberation times within the senior service centers. Notably, activity spaces in both centers exhibit shorter reverberation times compared to narrower spaces like corridors. This phenomenon

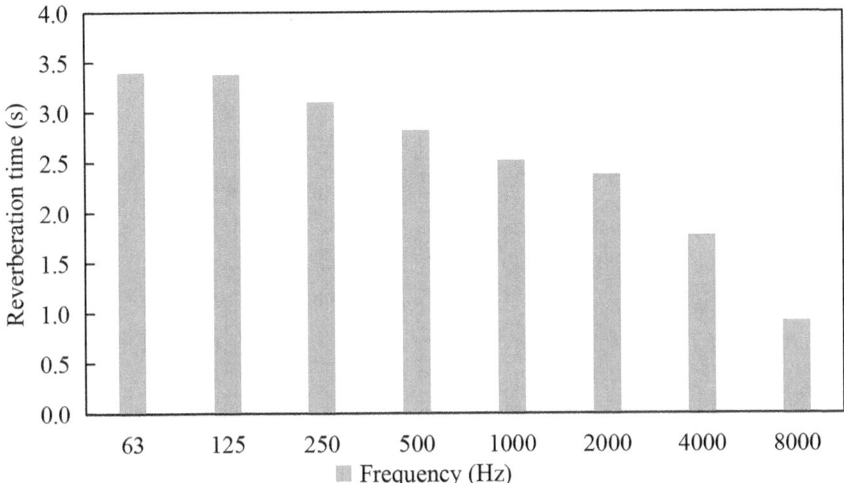

a) Case 4-ESC

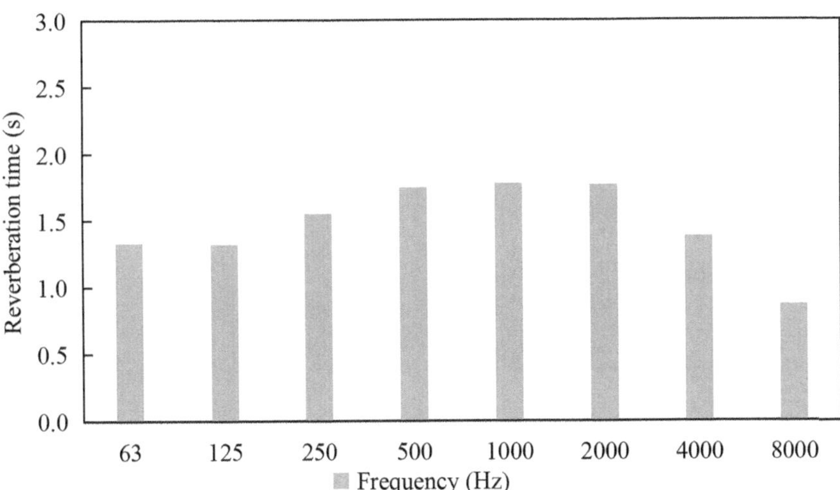

b) Case 5-ESC

Figure 5.14(a-b) Reverberation time in elderly service center

can be attributed to sound traveling greater distances in corridors, facilitating increased reflection and diffusion, consequently delaying sound attenuation. The predominantly square shapes of activity spaces engender relatively fixed patterns of sound propagation and reflection, contributing to reduced reverberation times. Furthermore, the size of public spaces also influences reverberation times, with larger spaces facilitating greater sound diffusion, while smaller rooms curtail sound propagation, resulting in shorter reverberation times.

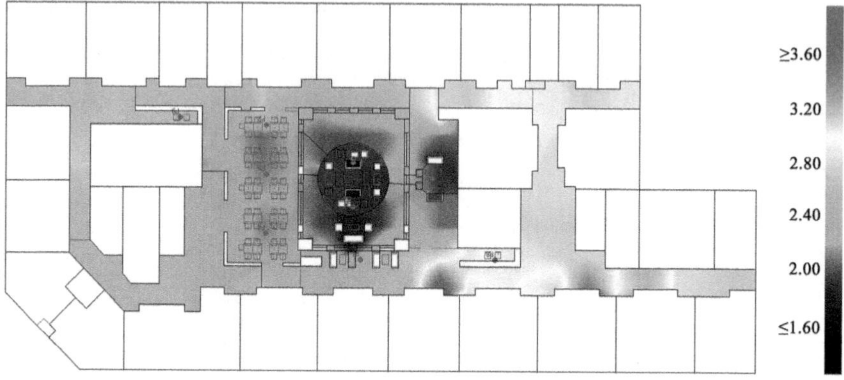

a) Case 4-ESC

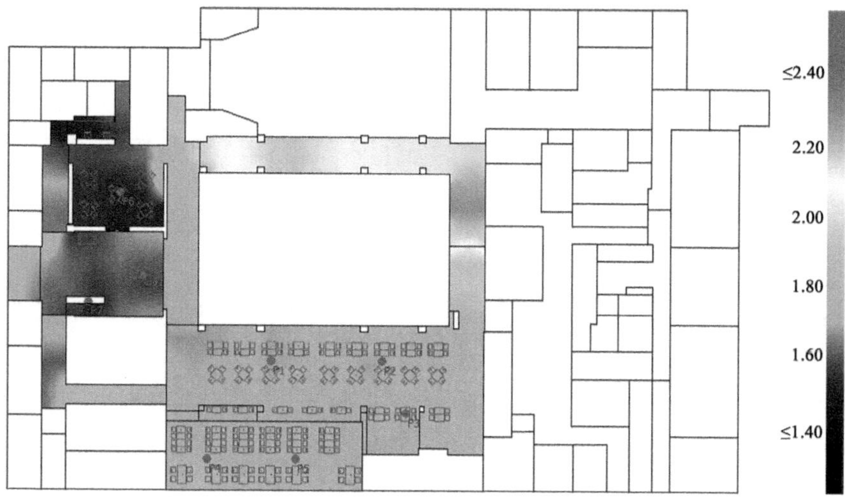

b) Case 5-ESC

Figure 5.15(a-b) Distribution of reverberation time in elderly service center

5.4 Dementia care center

5.4.1 Case 6-DCC

Case 6-DCC, nestled in Beijing's Chaoyang district, caters specifically to the elderly grappling with cognitive impairments. Originally, the structure boasted a circular design reminiscent of Hakka earthen buildings, setting the stage for a clustered layout inspired by these traditional dwellings, thus fostering a familial care model for dementia patients (Figure 5.16). With three floors at its disposal, accommodating 114 dementia care beds, the first floor was repurposed into a community service hub complete with a restaurant, supermarket, and medical facilities, while the second and third floors were dedicated to the residence and activities of dementia patients [11].

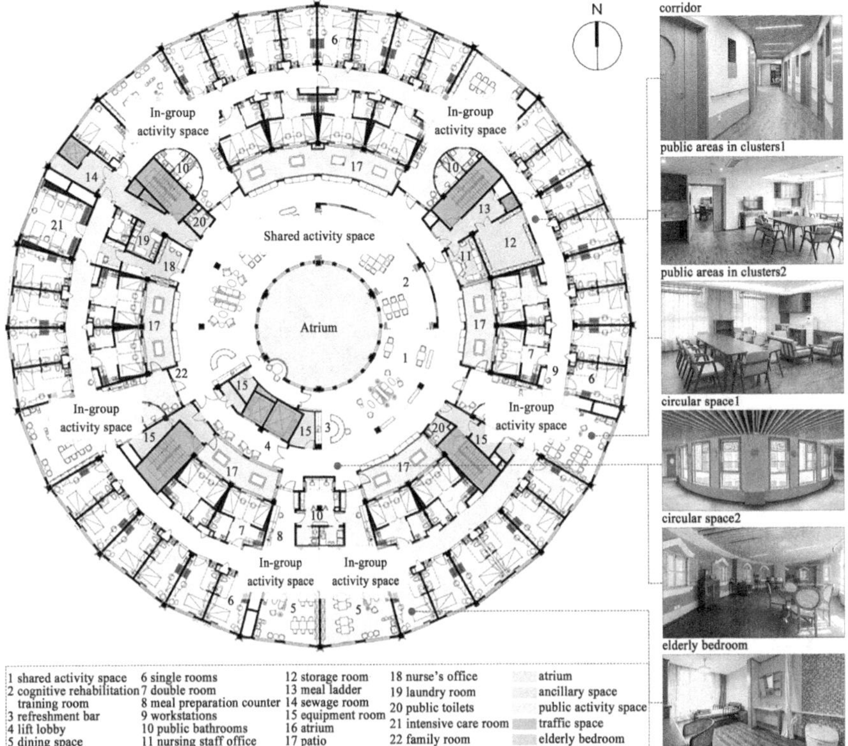

Figure 5.16 Second and third floor plan

Given the original building's substantial volume and deep floor plan, meeting the daylighting needs of eldercare facilities posed a significant challenge. Hence, a towering atrium was introduced at the building's core during renovations to address internal daylighting and ventilation concerns. Shared spaces, including open activity areas and cognitive rehabilitation training rooms, were strategically arranged around this central atrium.

To foster social engagement among dementia patients and mitigate cognitive decline, the clustered spaces within the building embraced the concept of duplex units. Here, two units could merge for collaborative use under the supervision of nursing staff. Each unit was assigned a distinct theme color, with color-coded interior walls aiding spatial recognition. Illustrated in Figure 5.17a, the floor plan of the unit space showcased accommodations for 10 individuals, facilitating their acclimatization to the surroundings. Equipped with nursing stations, dining areas, communal bathrooms, and more, each unit was meticulously designed to cater to the care and dining needs of the elderly. Owing to the fan-shaped partitioning of the original building, curved walls adorned auxiliary spaces near unit entrances, mitigating congestion and ensuring seamless transitions.

The living quarters for the elderly primarily comprised single and double rooms featuring parent-child doors to accommodate wheelchairs and nursing beds with

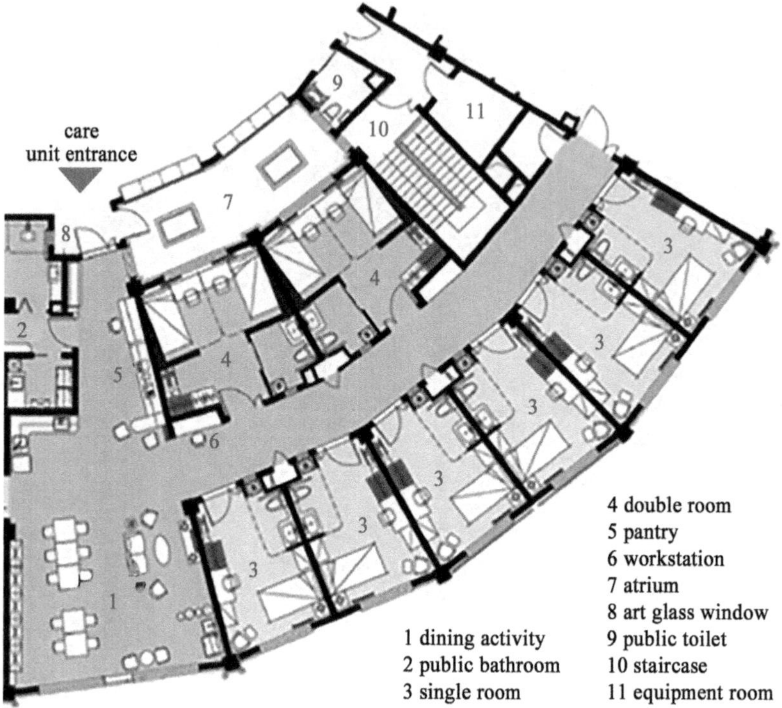

a) Single room floor plan

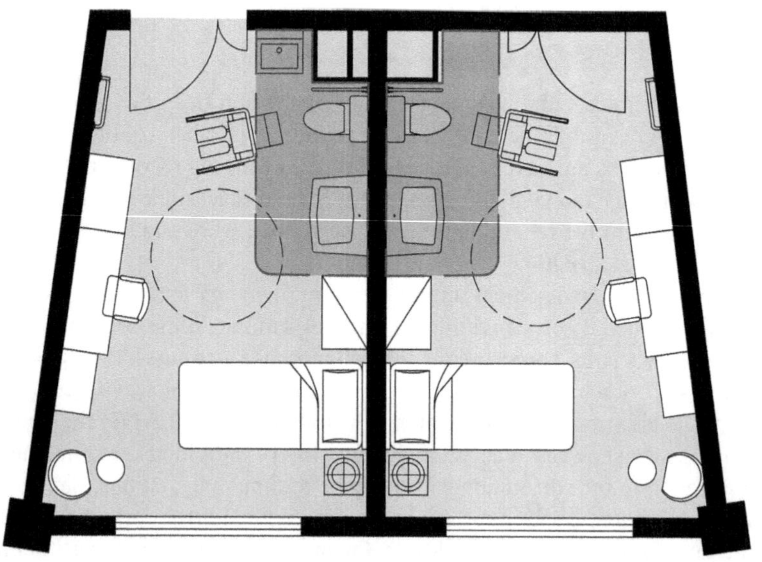

b) Double room floor plan

Figure 5.17(a-c) Care unit and elderly bedroom floor plans

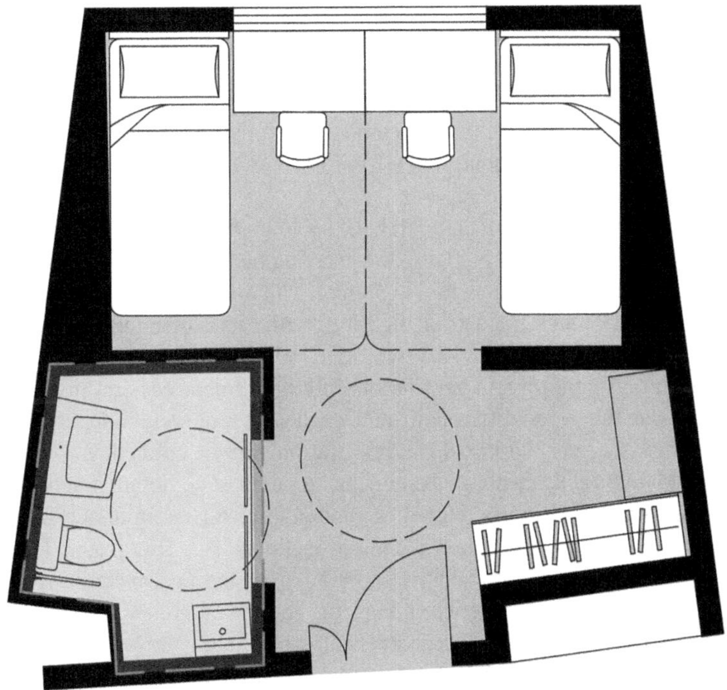

c) Floor plan of a small unit for 10 persons

Figure 5.17(a-c) (Continued)

ease. The entrance spaces of the bedrooms, owing to their fan-shaped partitions, tended to be narrow. To address this, distinct strategies were adopted for single and double rooms. Single rooms, positioned along the building's perimeter, boasted an open layout with soft curtain partitions dividing the living spaces from the adjacent bathrooms (Figure 5.17). Conversely, double rooms, nestled toward the building's interior, featured separate bathrooms partitioned by walls and sliding doors, thus meeting privacy requirements effectively. Moreover, each unit was equipped with communal bathrooms and toilets to enhance accessibility for elderly individuals with restricted mobility.

Figure 5.16 also provided glimpses of the nursing home's indoor environment, showcasing a predominance of wooden furniture. Wooden flooring graced corridors, bedrooms, and public activity areas complemented by wooden suspended ceilings in select spaces, while others remained untreated. Room walls, mostly painted with coatings or adorned with wooden veneer panels, adhered to a warm color scheme, fostering a cozy ambiance. The inherent sound-absorbing properties of wooden materials and soft furnishings, such as sofas and mattresses, contributed to an improved acoustic environment within the care homes.

5.4.2 Case 7-DCC

Case 7-DCC stands proudly on Yongji Avenue in Nanjing City's Gulou district, overlooking the serene Mu Yan Binjiang Scenic Area to the north and the majestic Yangtze River to the south, providing residents with breathtaking views. Spanning nearly 7000 square meters, this facility boasts 170 beds catering to elderly individuals across various health conditions, from those in good health to those requiring semi-self-care and cognitive support.

Once a bustling restaurant and hotel, the building fell into disuse due to mismanagement [12]. However, recognizing the pressing need for eldercare services in the region, it was revitalized into a nursing home. The original structure's considerable depth posed challenges for natural lighting, while its elongated layout hampered nursing efficiency. To remedy this, two light wells were strategically integrated to enhance internal lighting and ventilation. The building's redesign involved dividing the volume into three distinct clusters, each with relatively independent spaces, streamlining caregiver workflows and bolstering service efficiency.

With two floors at its disposal, the nursing home boasts a vibrant first floor housing commercial and leisure areas, including dining services, essential shops, children's entertainment facilities, and a versatile multifunctional hall. This ground level buzzes with activity, drawing in locals and visitors alike, fostering a dynamic environment and encouraging interaction between residents and the community. Additionally, the first floor accommodates clusters for semi-self-care and cognitive support. Mirroring this layout, the second floor houses healthy elderly living clusters above the bustling public spaces, while a laundry room and rooftop drying area add functionality to the topmost level [13]. Detailed functional zones for each floor are outlined in Figure 5.18.

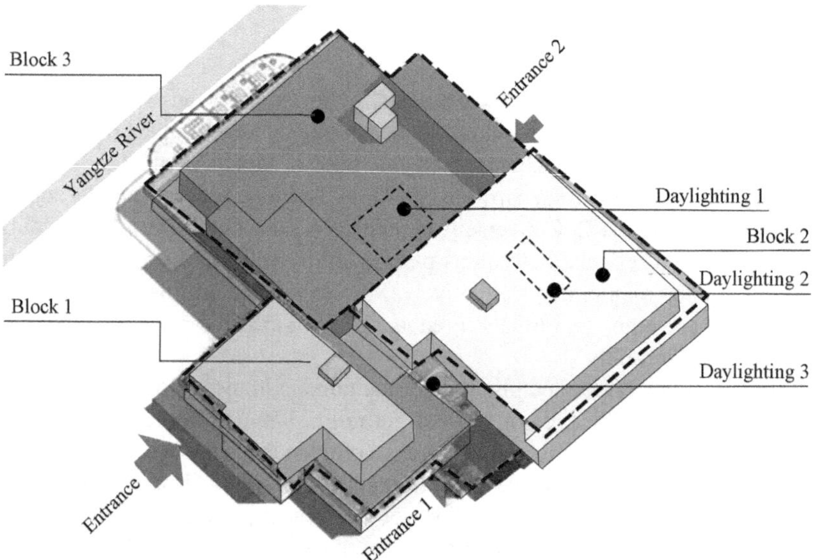

a) Building space

Figure 5.18(a-c) Functional zoning of the nursing home floors

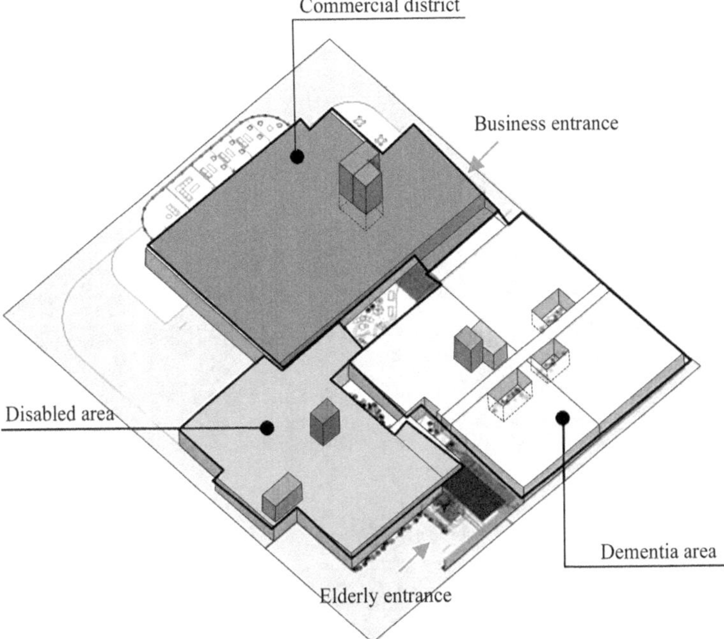

b) 1F Functional division

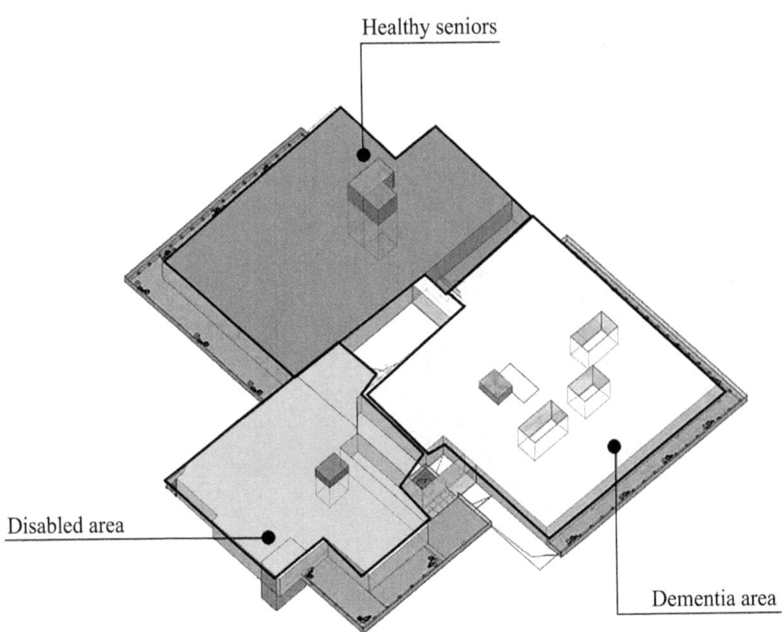

c) 2F Functional division

Figure 5.18(a-c) (Continued)

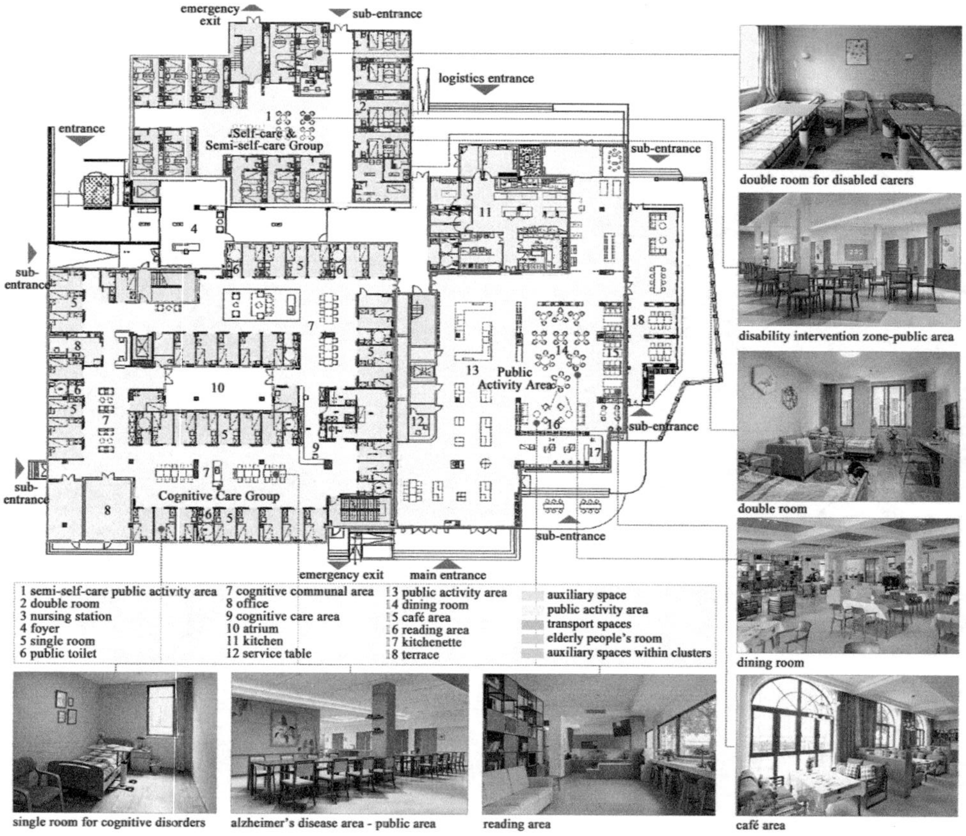

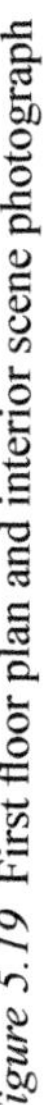

Figure 5.19 First floor plan and interior scene photograph

The cognitive care zone comprises 80 single rooms, each around 10.5 square meters in size, interconnected by three communal living rooms, promoting resident mobility (Figure 5.19). Bathrooms are thoughtfully distributed throughout the clusters, with centrally located showers. Meanwhile, the disabled care zone offers 28 double occupancy rooms, totaling 56 beds, all equipped with electric nursing beds. On the second floor, 34 beds are arranged in double rooms within the elderly living quarters, with each cluster boasting a dedicated nursing station for prompt assistance.

Figure 5.19 offers a glimpse into the indoor public spaces of the nursing home, showcasing anti-slip rubber flooring and walls adorned with colorful coatings to delineate different areas. Ceilings, predominantly painted white, feature wooden decorative suspended ceilings in some sections. Wooden furniture dominates the indoor landscape, complemented by soft furnishings like sofas known for their sound-absorbing qualities. While no specialized acoustic treatments have been implemented, the interconnected nature of the public spaces may lead to noise interference, potentially impacting the auditory experience of the elderly.

Except for the single occupancy dementia rooms, the residential clusters primarily comprise double rooms, as depicted in Figure 5.19. Wooden flooring graces all rooms, while walls and ceilings bear coatings. Minimalist wooden furniture adorns the interiors, with beds and sofas contributing to acoustic comfort. Although no specific acoustic treatments have been applied, the smaller size of the bedrooms and the presence of soft furnishings likely enhance the acoustic quality compared to the public spaces.

5.4.3 Simulation analysis

In the meticulous analysis of dementia care centers, emblematic nursing homes situated in diverse regions across China were scrutinized. Both underwent renovation, where the incorporation of atriums aimed to enhance indoor lighting and ventilation. Nevertheless, their distinct floor plans had a direct bearing on the indoor acoustic environment's quality.

Figure 5.20 delineates the sound pressure level distribution in the public spaces of the dementia care center. Case 6-DCC displays a relatively uniform sound pressure level distribution, with slightly elevated levels in activity zones and marginally lower levels at corners. Conversely, Case 7-DCC exhibits a stark variation in indoor sound pressure levels, with concentrations of the elderly witnessing higher levels and other areas experiencing lower ones. This disparity could result in significant discrepancies in the nursing home's acoustic experience, potentially affecting the elderly's comfort.

Figure 5.21 provides insights into the reverberation time within the public spaces of the care center. In Case 6, the reverberation times span from 0.9 to 2.2 seconds, with mid-frequency sounds exhibiting lengthier durations and low and high-frequency sounds experiencing shorter ones. Conversely, Case 7 presents a different scenario, with reverberation times ranging approximately from 1.6 to 2.7 seconds, gradually decreasing as sound frequency increases. This disparity may stem from a deficiency in materials absorbing mid-to-low frequency noise within indoor public spaces, resulting in excessively prolonged reverberation times. Such conditions not only

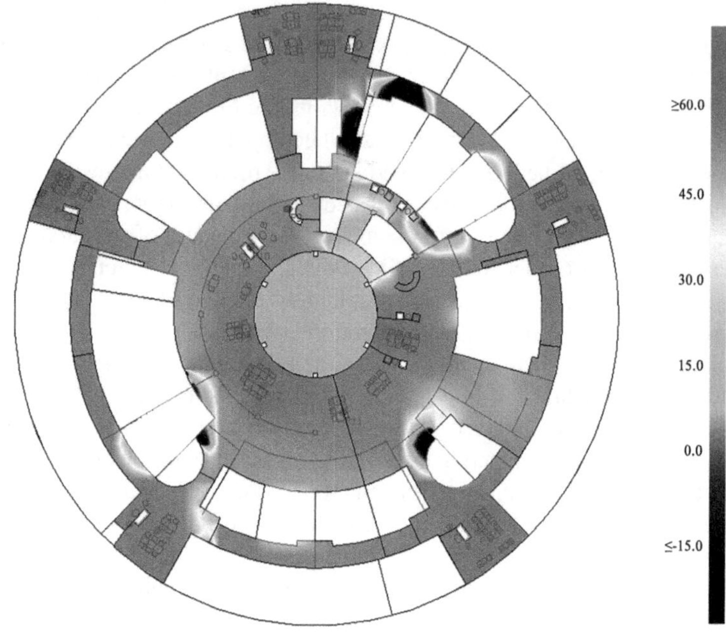

a) Case 6-DCC

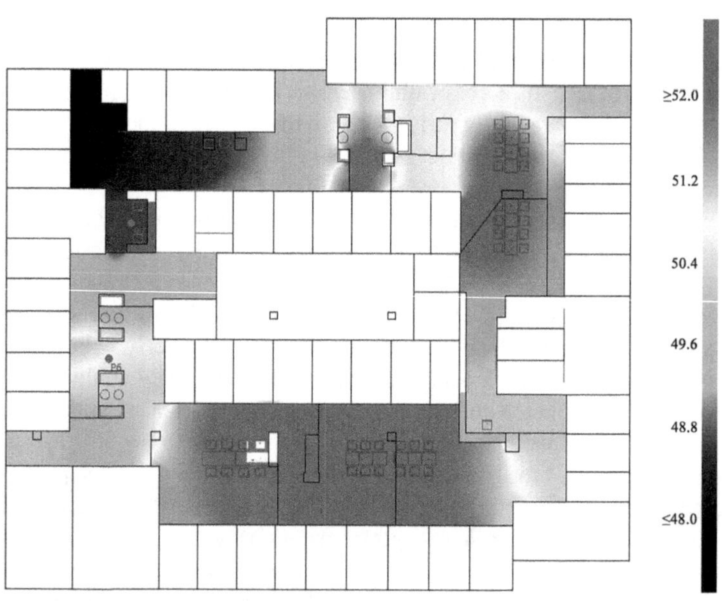

b) Case 7-DCC

Figure 5.20(a-b) Sound pressure level(dB)

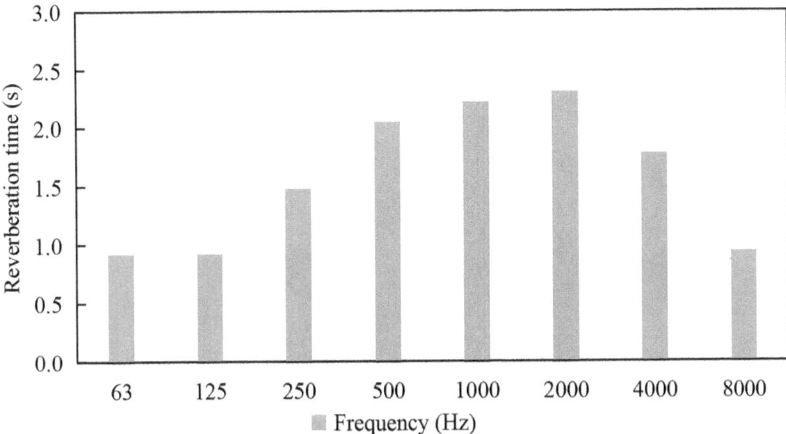

a) Case 6-DCC

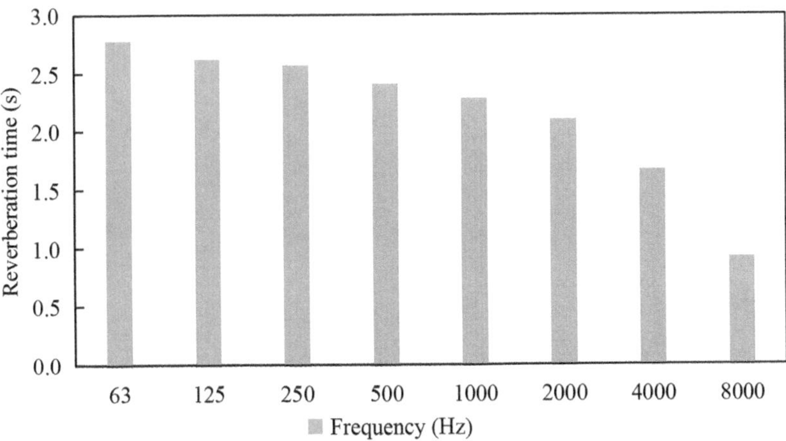

b) Case 7-DCC

Figure 5.21(a-b) Reverberation time in nursing homes

compromise speech clarity but also adversely impact the daily lives and communication of the elderly, necessitating measures to enhance the care center's acoustic quality.

Figure 5.22 delves into the spatial distribution of reverberation times in the dementia care center. With the exception of the atrium area, Case 6 displays lower indoor reverberation times compared to Case 7. Notably, the central area of Case 6 exhibits significantly higher reverberation times than its surroundings. This phenomenon may be attributed to the presence of a three-story high atrium,

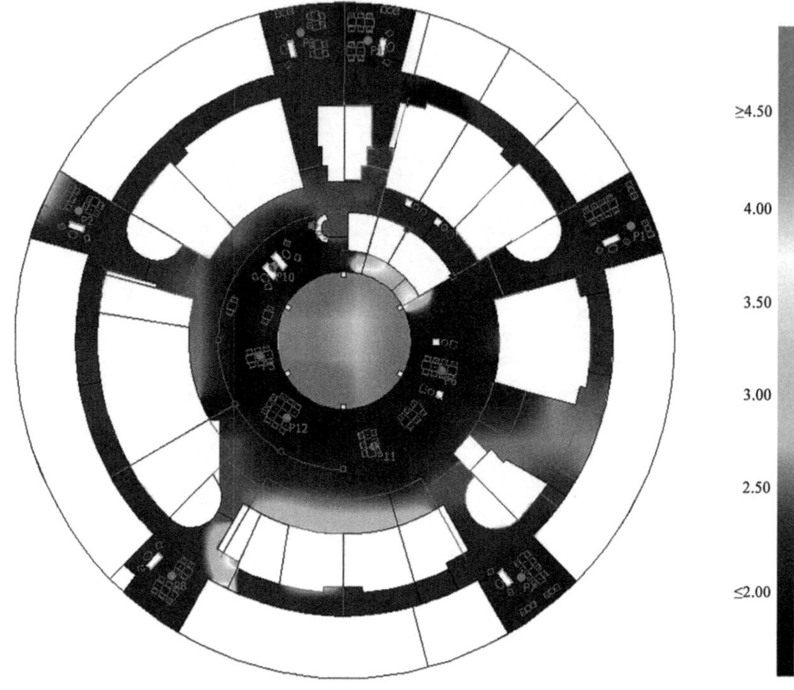

a) Case 6-DCC

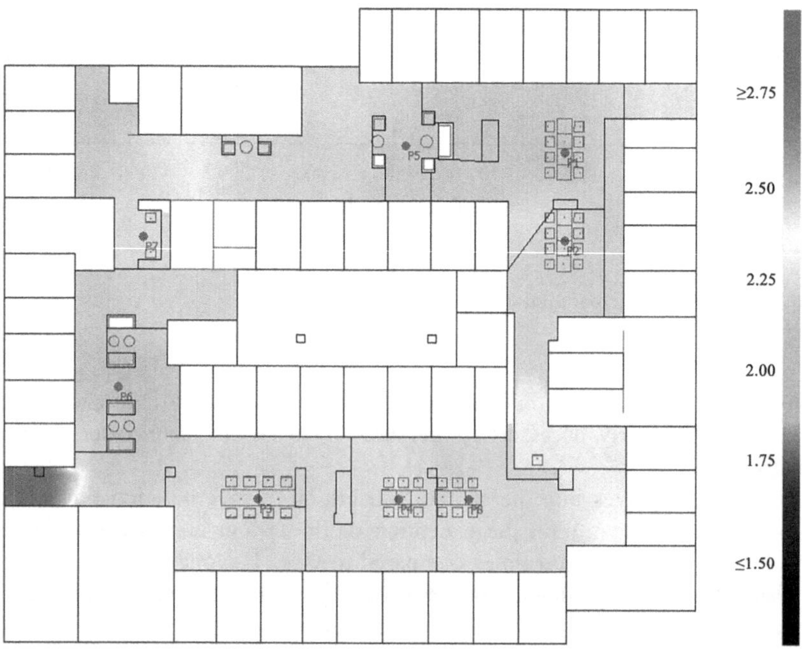

b) Case 7-DCC

Figure 5.22(a-b) Spatial distribution of reverberation time in dementia care centers

where sound waves encounter minimal obstacles or reflections during propagation, allowing for longer sound travel distances and consequently resulting in prolonged reverberation times. Conversely, in other areas of the nursing home, reverberation times remain relatively short, ensuring optimal speech clarity. Conversely, Case 7 experiences relatively longer reverberation times, possibly due to its more expansive space and the interconnected nature of various public areas, facilitating wider sound wave propagation and prolonging sound duration indoors. Furthermore, abrupt spikes in reverberation time occur in certain areas of the nursing home. Hence, targeted measures are imperative to enhance the acoustic quality and sound comfort for the elderly, thereby fostering their health and well-being.

5.5 Conclusion

This chapter endeavors to examine the current landscape of care homes in China by scrutinizing representative cases from diverse regions. The goal is to conduct a thorough investigation into their spatial arrangements and interior designs while delving into the intricacies of the indoor acoustic environment and pinpointing prevalent issues. Through meticulous case analysis, it emerged that the majority of care homes in China lack comprehensive acoustic design for their indoor spaces. Common areas within care homes, such as activity rooms and painting and calligraphy rooms, predominantly feature rubber or wooden flooring, complemented by painted ceilings and walls, with some adorned with wooden veneer panels that offer marginal sound absorption. However, the overarching spatial environments of care homes typically suffer from a dearth of acoustic treatment. Moreover, the indoor public spaces in care homes boast strong connectivity, with various functional areas seamlessly interconnected sans sound insulation measures, resulting in mutual interference between different zones. While the disruption to the elderly's living quarters remains relatively minimal, the indoor walls and ceilings primarily bear coats of paint, coupled with wooden floors, thus underscoring the prevalent lack of acoustic treatment in the indoor environment. It is evident that acoustic environment design is conspicuously deficient in the spatial environment research of care homes in China.

Nevertheless, existing studies underscore the significant impact of the acoustic environment on the physical and mental well-being of the elderly. Hence, drawing on the acoustic simulation software Odeon, this paper selected representative cases for an in-depth analysis of the indoor acoustic environment. The analysis results demonstrate that sound pressure levels and reverberation times in elderly care facilities are closely related to building form, functional layout, and interior materials. Due to these factors, there are often considerable differences in the indoor acoustic environments across different facilities. On the whole, many care homes have issues such as excessive sound pressure levels and prolonged reverberation times in public activity spaces, which do not meet regulatory standards and may even affect the daily lives and communication of the elderly. Therefore, it is necessary to take corresponding measures to improve the quality of the indoor acoustic environment, thereby promoting the health and well-being of the elderly.

References

[1] Zhou YM. *Design and interpretation of elderly care facility 1*[M]. Beijing: China Architecture & Building Press, 2018. (In Chinese)

[2] Yuan WX. *Research on the development of elderly facilities based on statistical analysis of literature*[D]. Beijing: Xi'an University of Architecture and Technology, 2023. (In Chinese)

[3] Mu J, Kang J, Wu Y. Acoustic environment of comprehensive activity spaces in nursing homes: A case study in Harbin, China[J]. *Applied Acoustics*, 2021, 177(24):107932.

[4] Mu J, Kang J, Sui Z. Effect of music in large activity spaces on the perceptions and behaviours of older adults in China[J]. *Applied Acoustics*, 2022(Jan.):188.

[5] Meng YX. *Study on the spatial design of cognitive institutions under PCC concept*[D]. Beijing: Harbin Normal University, 2023. (In Chinese)

[6] Zhou YM. *Design and interpretation of elderly care facility 3*[M]. Beijing: China Architecture & Building Press, 2020. (In Chinese)

[7] GB50176–2016. *Code for thermal design of civil building*[S]. Beijing: China Architecture & Building Press, 2017.

[8] Chen X. Beijing, China Taiyichun Care Center[J]. *Archicreation*, 2020, (5):56–65. (In Chinese)

[9] Chen Y. Foshan, Guangdong, China Leshanju nursing home[J]. *Archicreation*, 2020, 5:82–87. (In Chinese)

[10] Fang C, Zhao YQ. Noting the rebirth of a building: Reconstruction and reflection of Vanke Yi Garden Elderly Center, Tianjin[J]. *Architecture Technique*, 2020, (5):91–93. (In Chinese)

[11] Li JJ. Beijing, China Zhangyou Huiyuan memory care center[J]. *Archicreation*, 2020, 5:66–73. (In Chinese)

[12] Zhao F. Research on energy utilization of old buildings transformed into facilities for the aged-taking pension project of Langshi Ivy Wumadu as an Example[J]. *Urban Architecture Space*, 2020, 27(2):32–35. (In Chinese)

[13] Lei JW. *Study on the living space design of dementia long-term care facilities – From the perspective of daily activities*[D]. Nanjing: Southeast University, 2019. (In Chinese)

6 Strategies for improving indoor acoustic environment in care homes

6.1 The elderly's needs for indoor acoustic environment in care homes

Amidst the escalating global trend of population aging and the burgeoning consciousness surrounding health, scholarly interest in the acoustic milieu of care homes has gradually surged. Research has unveiled that subpar acoustic environments can profoundly impact the physical well-being of the elderly, potentially precipitating sleep disturbances, hypertension, and cardiovascular ailments [1]. Hence, delving into the acoustic landscape of care homes becomes imperative.

Regarding indoor acoustic requisites, older adults gravitate towards tranquil environments, yearning to attenuate noise levels within care homes. Their predilection extends to (near) silent activities [2]. Moreover, natural sounds garner preference over other auditory stimuli among the elderly, exhibiting a noteworthy positive correlation with their overarching acoustic environment preferences and the inclination towards integrating natural sounds [3].

A serene acoustic ambiance assumes a pivotal role in fostering the recuperation of the elderly from illnesses and perceptual rehabilitation. Evidence suggests that noise within care homes can perturb individuals with cognitive impairments, whereas soothing melodies can assuage agitation and enhance food intake among the elderly [4]. Additionally, adept soundscape interventions can assuage the neuropsychiatric symptoms (NPS) of dementia patients [5], underscoring the transformative potential of a comforting acoustic environment in elevating the health status of the elderly.

Studies have underscored the positive influence of music on human behavior, owing to its modulation of mood and arousal levels, wherein tempo (fast vs. slow) plays a pivotal role [6]. Despite the plethora of studies extolling the salutary effects of music on the well-being of the elderly, its impact on the daily routines and activities of residents in care homes remains nebulous [7]. Thus, this study endeavors to engineer an experimental acoustic setting to unravel the elderly's responses to divergent acoustic environments, with a primary focus on delineating the effects of varied music genres on their satisfaction and emotional states [8].

Two music settings were meticulously crafted: settings labeled 'without music' and settings adorned with the mellifluous strains of melodies. For the 'with music'

DOI: 10.1201/9781003407232-6

settings, the experiment unfolded in two distinct groups. In the first cohort, three eclectic compositions graced the airwaves: instrumental harmonies, lyrical serenades accompanied by musical instruments, and the serene symphony of natural sounds. In the second assembly, two distinct musical pieces, each imbued with a unique melody, took center stage: a lively, tempo-driven instrumental composition and a tranquil, slow-paced instrumental melody. Throughout this phase, objective acoustic parameters such as sound pressure levels were meticulously gauged in the hall to scrutinize the environmental nuances entwined with the diverse musical tapestries. Following this, individual interviews were conducted with the older adults to complete the comprehensive questionnaire survey.

The questionnaire itself comprised two distinct segments: the initial segment aimed at collating essential demographic particulars of the participants, while the subsequent section delved into their nuanced evaluation of the acoustic environment. Utilizing a seven-point Likert scale, a widely acclaimed instrument in survey methodology for eliciting subjective assessments of environmental acoustics, the respondents conveyed their impressions [9]. A trove of 302 valid questionnaires was amassed from the survey site. To delve into the psychological disposition of the participants, the evocative pleasure-arousal-dominance emotion status model took center stage [10], delineating emotional responses across three key axes: pleasure (the spectrum of positive to negative feelings), arousal (the degree of physiological activation), and dominance (the perception of control). Moreover, the findings from the questionnaire, in conjunction with insights from the pleasure-arousal-dominance model, were harnessed to discern the emotional threshold, gauging the sensitivity of emotional responses among the elderly cohort.

Descriptive statistics were meticulously computed for the questionnaire data, while analysis of variance (ANOVA) was deftly deployed to unravel the intricate interplay between the psychological disposition of elderly individuals and the manifold acoustic environments, including diverse musical stimuli. To delve deeper into the preferences of the elderly participants, a comprehensive two-way ANOVA was meticulously executed, dissecting the effects of music presence or absence, diverse rhythmic cadences, and an eclectic array of musical genres on the psychological states of distinct subsets of elderly participants. Additionally, to glean further insights into the musical predilections of the elderly cohort and their tolerance for varying volumes, Pearson's correlation coefficient was adroitly employed to quantify the intricate relationship between the satisfaction levels of the elderly participants, as expressed in the questionnaire responses, and the varying sound pressure levels across different decibel thresholds.

6.2 The influence of music on the well-being of the elderly

There existed a profound distinction in the mean emotional threshold among older adults immersed in the 'with music' ambiance ($p < 0.01$). Within this immersive setting, participants experienced an average surge of 1 in pleasure, arousal, and dominance in their emotional responses, paralleled by an impressive expansion of their emotional ranges by four-fold, two-fold, and three-fold, respectively

(Figure 6.1a-b). These findings eloquently suggest that the presence of music engenders a heightened sense of positivity among the elderly, thereby assisting them in sustaining elevated emotional states [11].

In the realm of discerning various music types, a notable divergence emerged in the mean emotional threshold with each change in musical genre ($p < 0.01$). When under the influence of slow-paced instrumental melodies, satisfaction levels experienced a notable uptick by an average of two, while the threshold range expanded by 2-fold (Figure 6.1c-d). Particularly noteworthy was the discernible variance in dominance levels between slow-paced and fast-paced instrumental music. Slow-paced instrumental melodies were found to significantly contribute to fulfilling the psychological needs of older adults and fostering a sense of dominance. Interestingly, during periods of negative mood, the elderly exhibited a marked preference for slow-paced instrumental music [12], leading to a substantial enhancement in satisfaction levels. Conversely, the dominance measure significantly diverged when compared to fast-paced instrumental music. Overall, a robust positive correlation was established between the psychological requisites of the elderly and the presence of a slow rhythm in music ($p < 0.01$), aligning seamlessly with the seminal research findings reported by Lally [13].

In the realm of comparing distinct music genres, exposure to instrumental music accompanied by lyrical content led to a notable decline in satisfaction ratings from 5 to 1, coupled with pronounced differences in approach-avoidance behaviors, pleasure, arousal, and dominance. Assessments for music with lyrical content consistently fell below those of other music genres. Conversely, evaluations for natural sounds

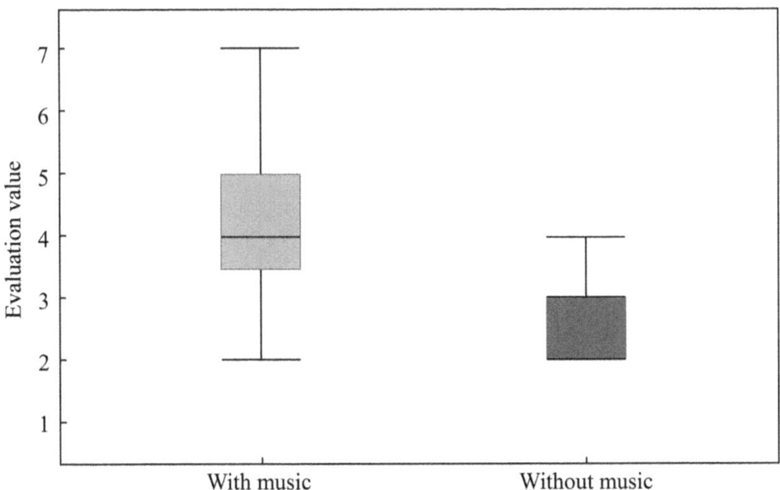

a) The evaluation value for the emotional performance of participants in with-music and without-music settings

Figure 6.1(a-f) Impact of different acoustic environments on the psychological aspects of the elderly

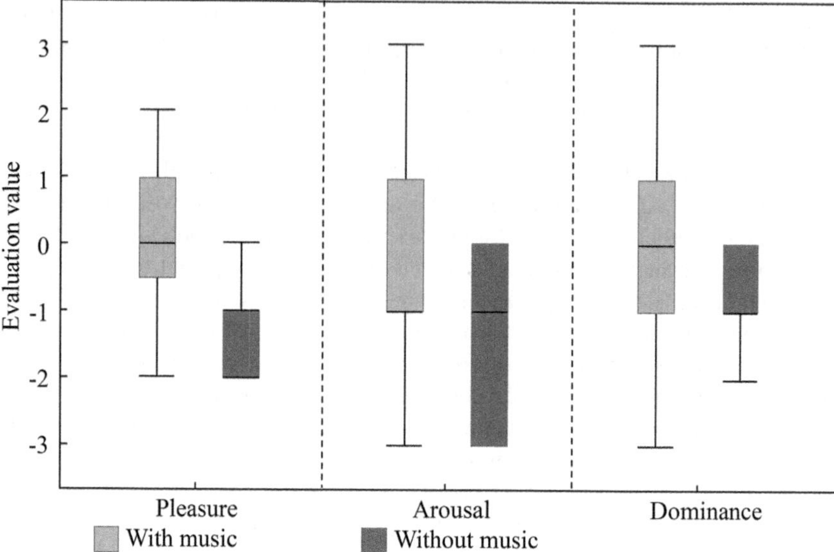

b) The evaluation values of pleasure, arousal, and domination for the emotional performance of the elderly participants in with music and without music settings

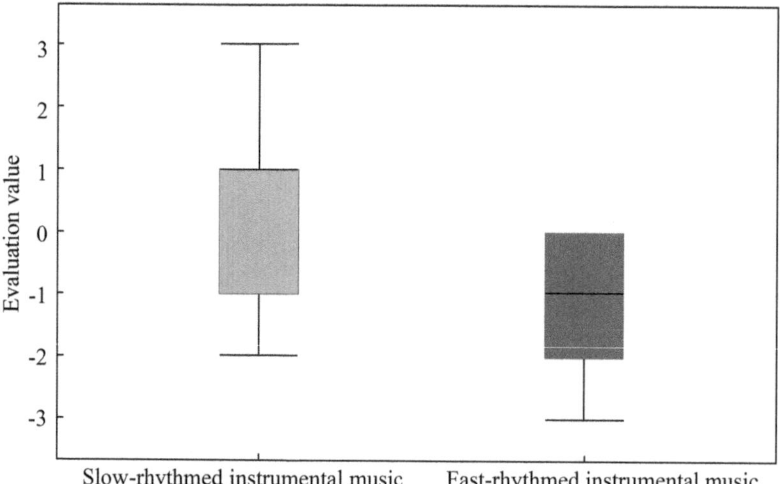

c) The elderly participants' evaluation value in slow-rhythmed instrumental music and fastrhythmed instrumental music

Figure 6.1(a-f) (Continued)

registered higher, with a statistically significant mean value of 5, echoing findings reported by Sataloff [14], underscoring the profound impact of natural sounds and music in elevating satisfaction and arousal levels. Previous scholarly investigations have also underscored that natural sounds aid in stress reduction among older adults, whereas music with lyrical content may enhance logical thinking ability, and

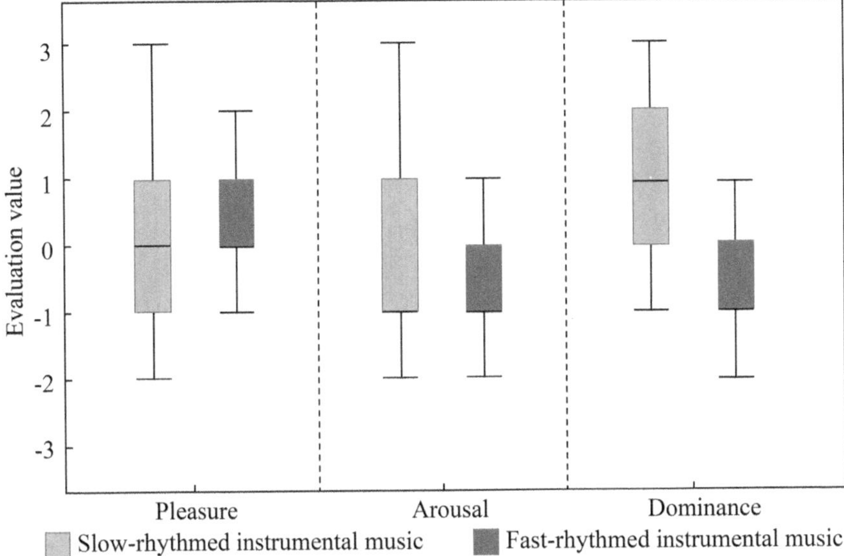

d) In the slow-rhythmed and fast-rhythmed instrumental music setting, the evaluation values of pleasure, arousal, and domination for the emotional performance of the elderly participants

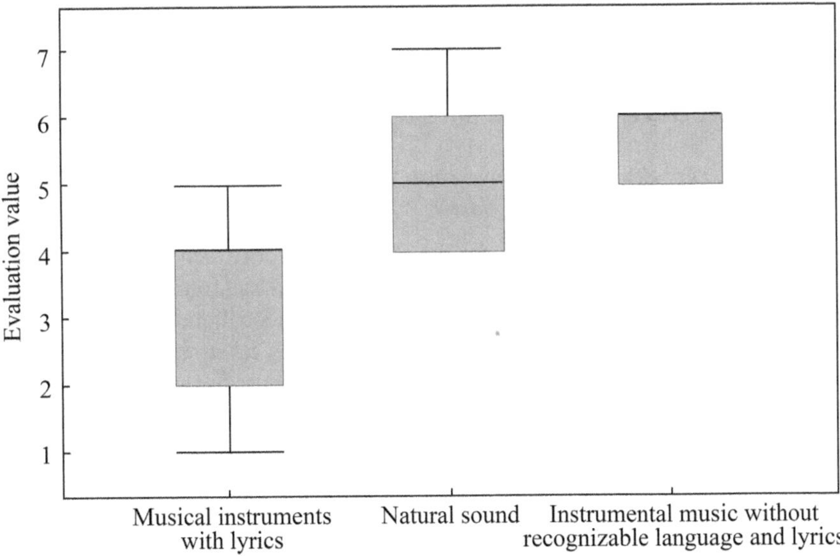

e) The elderly participants' evaluation value in the case of musical instruments with lyrics, natural sounds, and instrumental music

Figure 6.1(a-f) (Continued)

instrumental melodies can elevate aesthetic appreciation [15, 16]. Detailed statistical data are meticulously presented in Figure 6.1(e)-(f). Therefore, playing natural sounds or instrumental music without lyrics in care homes can help improve the elderly's pleasure, arousal, and dominance, promoting a positive emotional state.

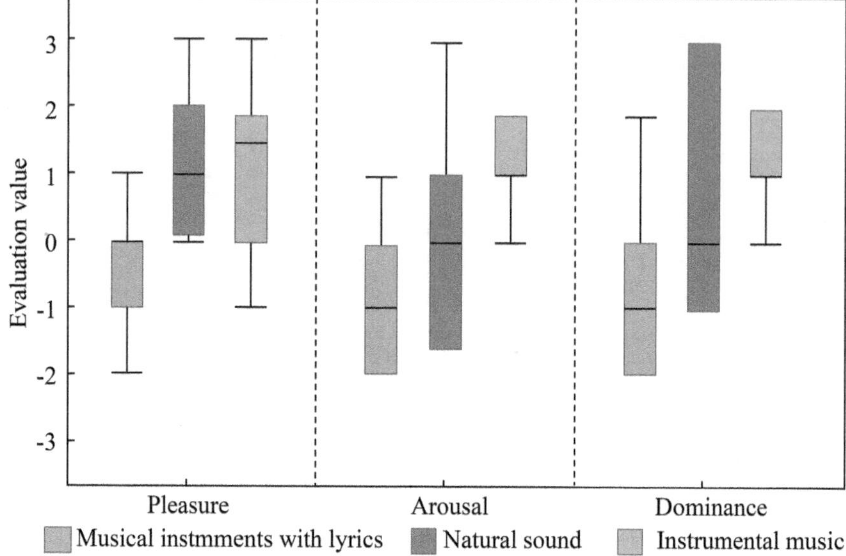

f) Evaluation values of pleasure, arousal, and domination for the emotional performance of the elderly participants in the settings of musical instruments with lyrics, natural sounds, and instrumental music

Figure 6.1(a-f) (Continued)

6.3 Positive effects of music on the elderly

6.3.1 Impact of 'with music'/'without music' surroundings on the psychological aspects of the elderly

The survey findings illuminated a profound connection between the elderly's level of cultural literacy and their perception of pleasure-arousal-dominance [8]. Within environments enhanced by music, the elderly with higher cultural literacy exhibited a heightened susceptibility to the emotive sway of musical stimuli. As depicted in Figure 6.2a, the elderly with a primary school education or lower evinced a diminished sensitivity to music compared to their more educated counterparts. Specifically, the pleasure-arousal-dominance scores of the elderly with a primary education experienced a modest increase of 1.89, regardless of music presence. Remarkably, within music-enriched environments, their values for arousal (0.21), pleasure (-0.15), and dominance (-0.31) were at their nadir. Conversely, the elderly boasting a college degree or higher showcased the loftiest pleasure-arousal-dominance values, both in the presence and absence of music, while those with intermediate education levels demonstrated intermediate pleasure-arousal-dominance values. These findings underscore a palpable correlation between the elderly's educational attainment and their capacity for musical appreciation ($p < 0.05$). Regarding arousal levels, the elderly's perceptions of music's presence remained consistent across diverse educational backgrounds, as illustrated in Figure 6.2b. Furthermore, satisfaction levels exhibited notable disparities across distinct activity conditions, with the elderly participating in the most tranquil activities expressing the utmost satisfaction with the acoustic environment.

Concerning pleasure and arousal, our findings suggest that individuals aged 60 to 80 years exhibit heightened receptivity to music, with arousal positively linked to age. Nonetheless, dominance emerged more prominently in the elderly aged 80 years and above under the sway of music (Figure 6.2c). Harmonious melodies tend to instill better moods in the elderly, thereby heightening their propensity for engagement in activities. Additionally, activities within the promenade area were associated with elevated levels of satisfaction, dominance, pleasure, and arousal in the presence of music. Solely dominance and arousal levels in the fan-shaped hall were elevated in the absence of music (Figure 6.2d). In contrast, in environments without music, the dominance and arousal levels of elderly residents in the fan-shaped hall increased, but their pleasure and satisfaction levels decreased (Figure 6.2d). Therefore, playing music in public activity spaces within elderly care facilities can help maintain positive emotional levels among the elderly residents.

6.3.2 *Impact of musical content on the psychological aspects of different subsets of the elderly*

For different music types, slow- and fast-rhythmed instrumental music was regarded as two quintessential genres and was juxtaposed across age groups, education levels, activity areas, and activity types. It became apparent that satisfaction and dominance soared notably among the elderly aged over 80 years when immersed in slow-rhythmed instrumental melodies, potentially reflecting their predilection for this genre. Conversely, the level of arousal notably diminished among the elderly aged 60 – 80years when exposed to fast-rhythmed instrumental music, as depicted in Figure 6.3a. Examination of music

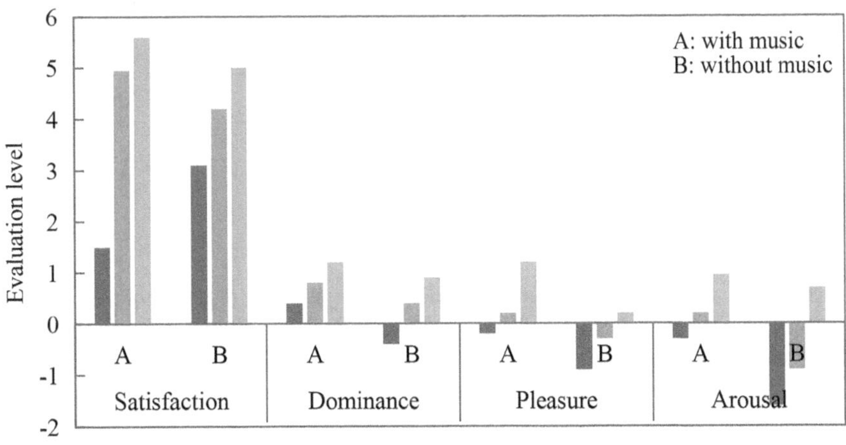

a) Education

Figure 6.2(a-d) Impact of 'with music'/'without music' surroundings on the psychology of different subsets of the elderly participants

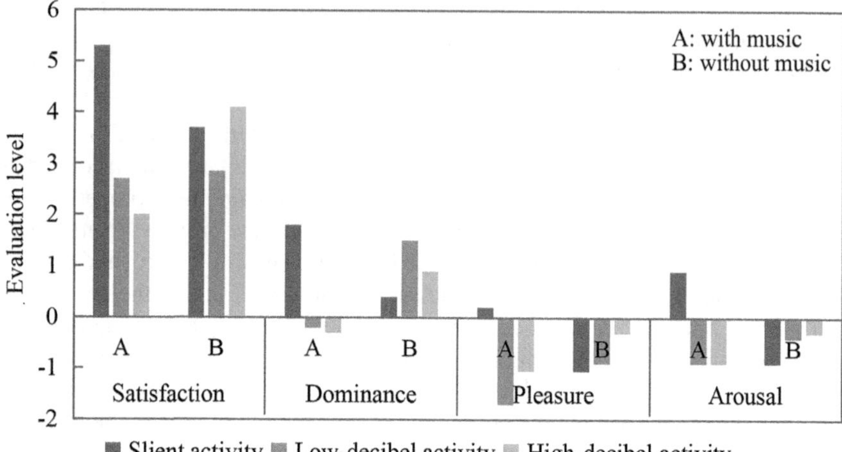

b) Activity type

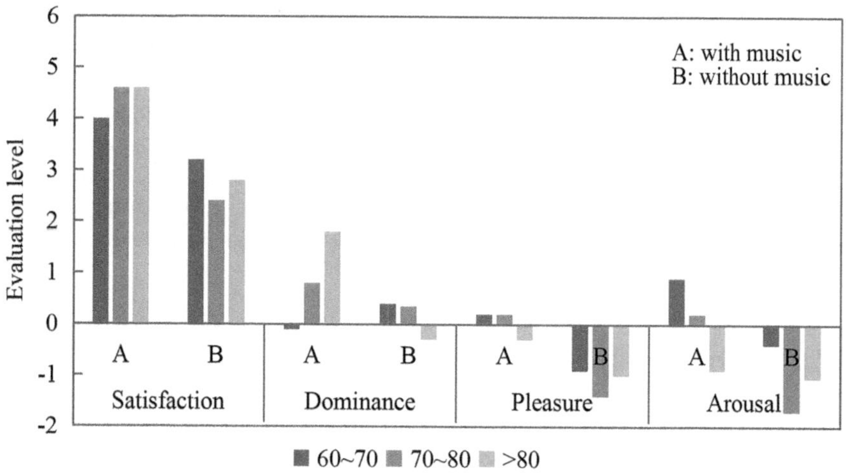

c) Age

rhythms and education levels revealed significant variations in pleasure values between the two musical cadences ($p < 0.05$), while no significant differences were noted in dominance and arousal ($p < 0.05$), as depicted in Figure 6.3b. The contentment of the elderly in each subgroup experienced an upsurge under the sway of slow-rhythmed instrumental music. Despite the preference of the elderly over 80 years for rhythmic instruments, the allure of serene, slow-paced melodies persisted overall. The elderly with higher educational backgrounds tended to lean towards slow-rhythmed instrumental music, perhaps because it induced a deeper sense of relaxation. Previous research has underscored that slow-rhythmed instrumental music can amplify therapeutic effects in the elderly [17]. Furthermore, findings in harmony with ours suggest that older adults

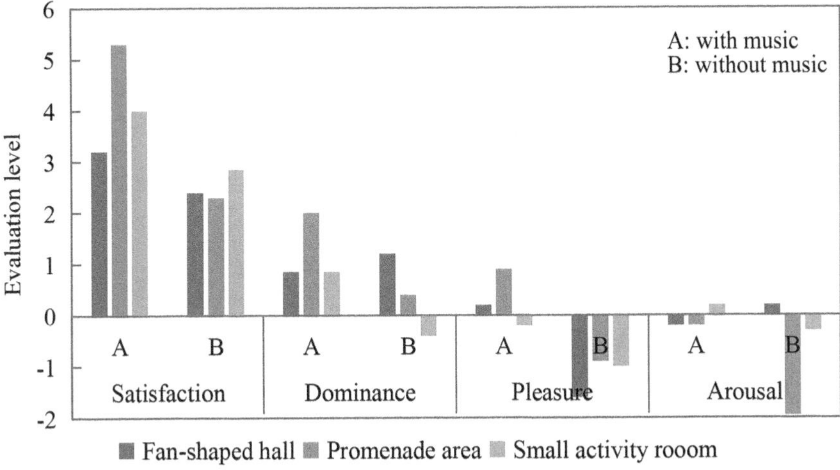

d) Activity area

Figure 6.2(a-d) (Continued)

with higher education levels gravitate towards slow-rhythmed instrumental music owing to the subtle aesthetic nuances present in the melodies [18].

Comparative analysis of music rhythms across distinct activity areas unveiled significant disparities in pleasure and dominance ($p < 0.05$), as depicted in Figure 6.3c. However, no significant difference in arousal was discerned. Figure 6.3d illustrates that the elderly exhibited heightened satisfaction when engaged in silent activities. Nonetheless, those participating in low- and high-decibel activities evinced a proclivity for fast-paced instrumental music. This inclination may stem from the music's propensity to invigorate and heighten cortical activity [19, 20]. However, slow-paced instrumental music continued to reign supreme overall, likely due to its pacifying effect [21]. Various activities exert distinct effects on different indicators [22], with slow-paced instrumental music notably augmenting arousal levels by nurturing the mental and emotional well-being of the elderly [23]. Therefore, it is necessary to play appropriate types of music based on the spatial context and the activity needs of the elderly. For example, playing fast-paced music in fitness areas and slow-paced music in public leisure areas can enhance the pleasure and emotional well-being of the elderly residents.

6.3.3 Impact of acoustic environment on the activities of the elderly

The presence or absence of lyrics directly shapes the essence of a song, delineating its classification. The elderly manifest diverse preferences, with age playing a pivotal role in how music is perceived [24]. Concerning dominance and pleasure, no significant disparity was noted between age and lyrical preference ($p < 0.05$). However, in terms of arousal, individuals aged 60–80 years seemed to be more susceptible to stimulation, especially those in the 70–80 age bracket, with a discernible discrepancy observed based on the presence of lyrics

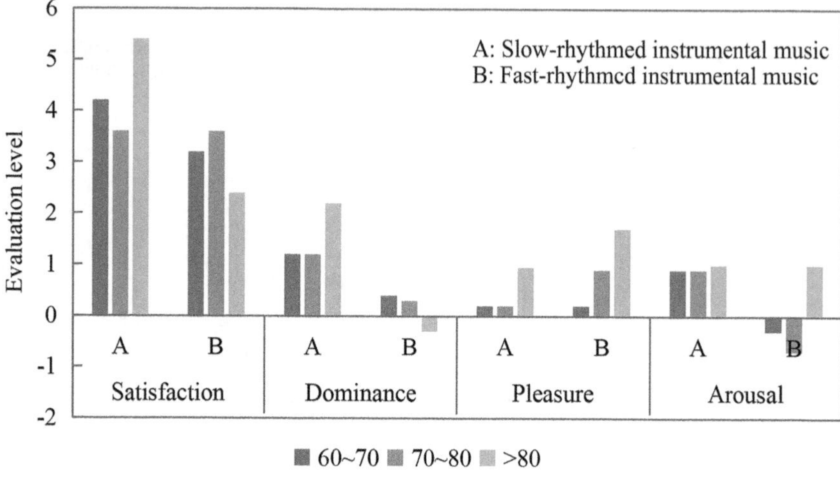

a) Age

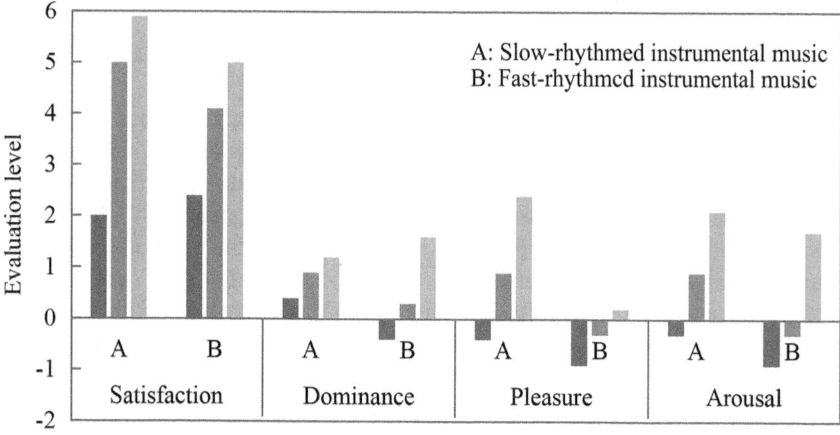

b) Education level

Figure 6.3(a-d) The impact of different music types on the psychological aspects of different subsets of the elderly participants

($p < 0.05$), as depicted in Figure 6.4a. Conversely, there was no notable difference between lyrical presence and education levels ($p < 0.05$). Figures 6.4a-b illustrate that the elderly favored natural sounds and instrumental melodies over lyrics or unintelligible languages; the elderly individuals aged between 60 and 70 years exhibited the highest satisfaction with instrumental music. Those with lower educational backgrounds derived greater satisfaction and pleasure from instrumental music, whereas those with secondary education rated natural sounds the most favorably. These findings are in concordance with prior

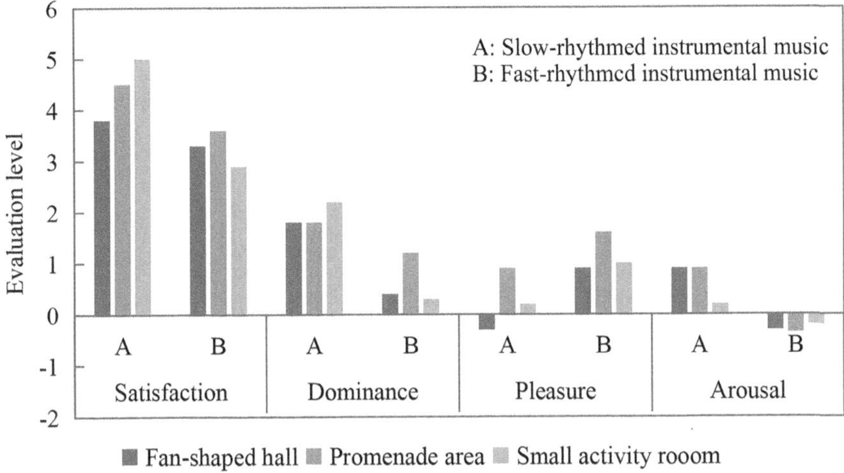

c) Activity area

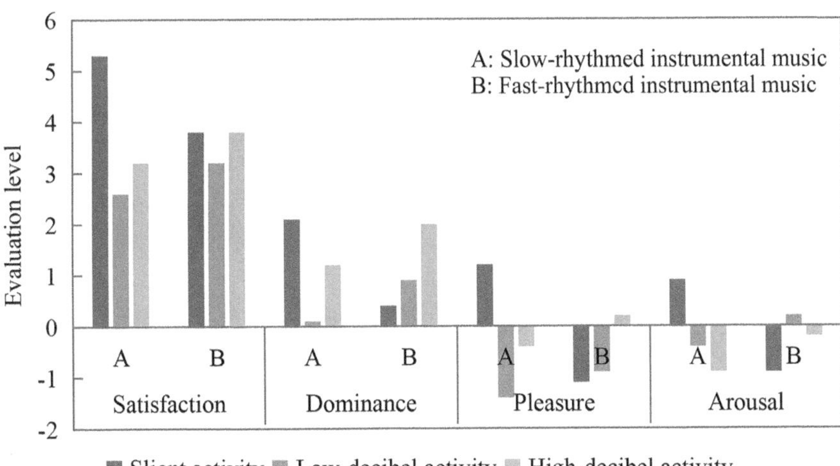

d) Activity type

Figure 6.3(a-d) (Continued)

research suggesting that educational background influences satisfaction and dominance regarding musical content [25].

Statistical outcomes unveiled significant variations in pleasure-arousal-dominance ($p < 0.05$). Nonetheless, there was no marked difference between lyrical presence, activity types and areas, and pleasure-arousal-dominance ($p < 0.05$), as portrayed in Figure 6.4c-d. Due to differences in the cost, types of services, and service levels in care homes, the elderly in these settings often share certain common characteristics in terms of age, educational background, and economic status. Therefore, it is possible to improve their emotional well-being by playing suitable types of music or natural sounds, based on these common characteristics.

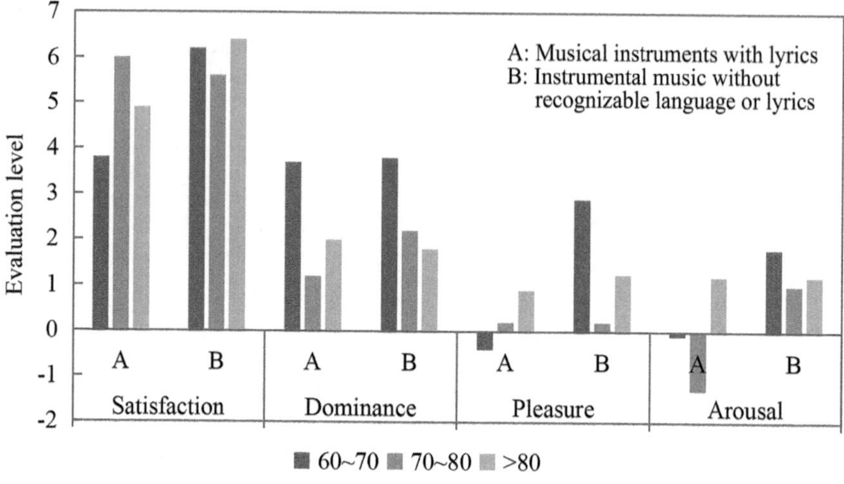

a) Age

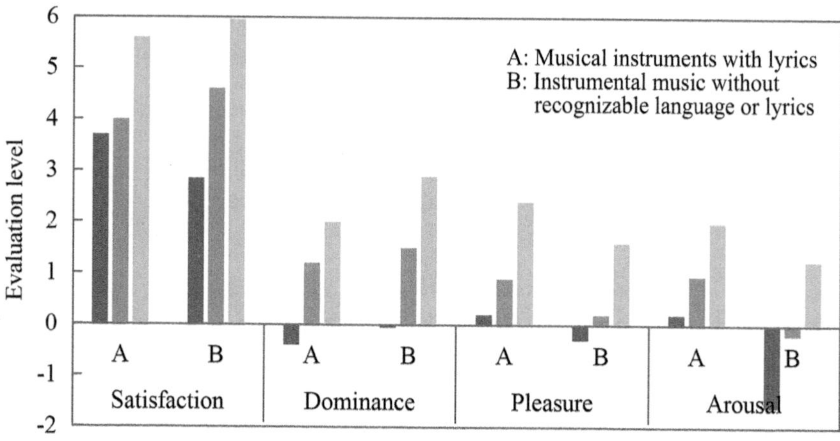

b) Education level

Figure 6.4(a-d) Impact of different music content on the psychological aspects of different subsets of older adults

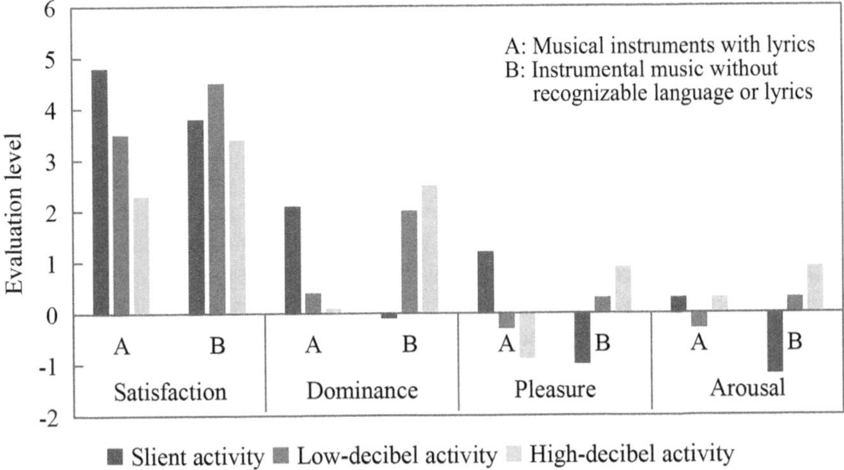

c) Activity type

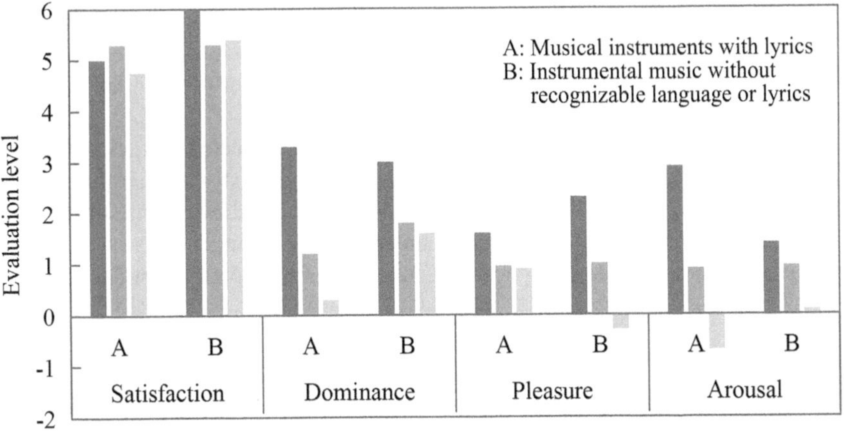

d) Activity area

Figure 6.4(a-d) (Continued)

6.4 Strategies for enhancing acoustic environment at the architectural design level

6.4.1 Overall planning

In terms of planning and design, the selection of sites for care homes should strive to steer clear of urban main thoroughfares. Urban main roads often exhibit excessively high sound pressure levels, with traffic noise, horn honking, and nocturnal truck movements all exerting adverse effects on the physiological health of the elderly. Research indicates that while the elderly generally exhibit higher tolerance for acoustic environments, they are also more sensitive to them [26]. Therefore, concerted efforts should be directed toward mitigating the detrimental effects of unfavorable acoustic environments on the elderly. For existing care homes situated close to urban thoroughfares, appropriate acoustic shielding measures should be enacted near the roads, such as planting trees and setbacks from the roadway.

In terms of sound shielding, studies have underscored that plants can diminish noise levels by absorbing sound energy, with the effectiveness of sound insulation improving with the diversity of plant layers and the density of branches and canopies [27]. Consequently, when care homes are positioned near roads, cultivating diverse layers of vegetation can yield superior sound insulation effects while also fostering a delightful visual landscape, augmenting the elderly's inclination to partake in outdoor activities.

Furthermore, owing to the susceptibility of care homes situated near urban roads to noise disturbances, particularly those buildings adjacent to external roads, bedrooms, and communal living areas for the elderly should be positioned away from street-facing positions, and architectural walls should integrate certain sound insulation measures, such as soundproof windows, to furnish a certain degree of sound isolation.

6.4.2 Layout design

The functional types within Chinese care homes encompass four primary categories: (1) Elderly activity spaces, including communal living rooms, dining rooms, card rooms, art rooms, billiard rooms, and multipurpose halls; (2) Elderly bedrooms; (3) Circulation spaces such as stairs and elevators; and (4) Auxiliary spaces like kitchens, laundry rooms, and training rooms, with some care homes integrating medical spaces such as wards and health rooms. Besides elderly living quarters, other areas often exhibit higher sound pressure levels, necessitating efforts to minimize noise disturbances on the elderly during layout planning.

In architectural layout, it's prudent to refrain from situating rooms with elevated sound pressure levels (like dining rooms, multipurpose rooms, and card rooms) adjacent to elderly living quarters. Furthermore, since elevators and equipment rooms produce noise and vibration, these spaces should be distanced from elderly living quarters. Concerning functional circulation, distinct flow paths for different groups should be delineated to prevent crossover and interference, with logistics personnel and the elderly having separate routes (Figure 6.5).

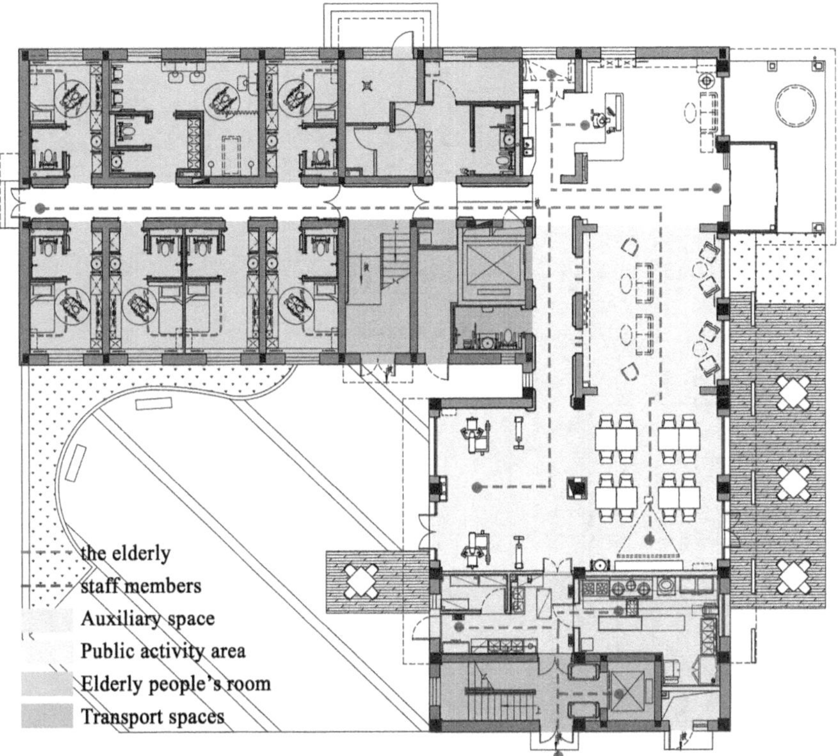

a) Small-scale care home

Figure 6.5(a-b) Examples of care home flats

6.4.3 Vertical space design

In the vertical distribution of space, it's crucial to achieve a logical separation between dynamic and static zones, guided by the principle of 'activity below, tranquility above' through vertical spatial division. Areas with high noise levels, like dining rooms, kitchens, billiard rooms, card rooms, rehabilitation fitness rooms, and multipurpose halls, are best situated on lower floors, while elderly living quarters find their place on higher floors (see Figure 6.6). Moreover, since the circulation pathways of auxiliary spaces such as medical rooms, offices, and meeting rooms differ from those of the elderly, and certain auxiliary areas like laundry rooms and training rooms may produce considerable noise, it's imperative to keep these functional spaces separate from elderly living quarters.

Presently, the treatment of vertical space design in large-scale care homes is relatively sophisticated. Some care homes opt to position service centers on lower floors and elderly living quarters on higher floors to prevent any mutual interference. However, for medium-sized and small-scale care homes, a layered design

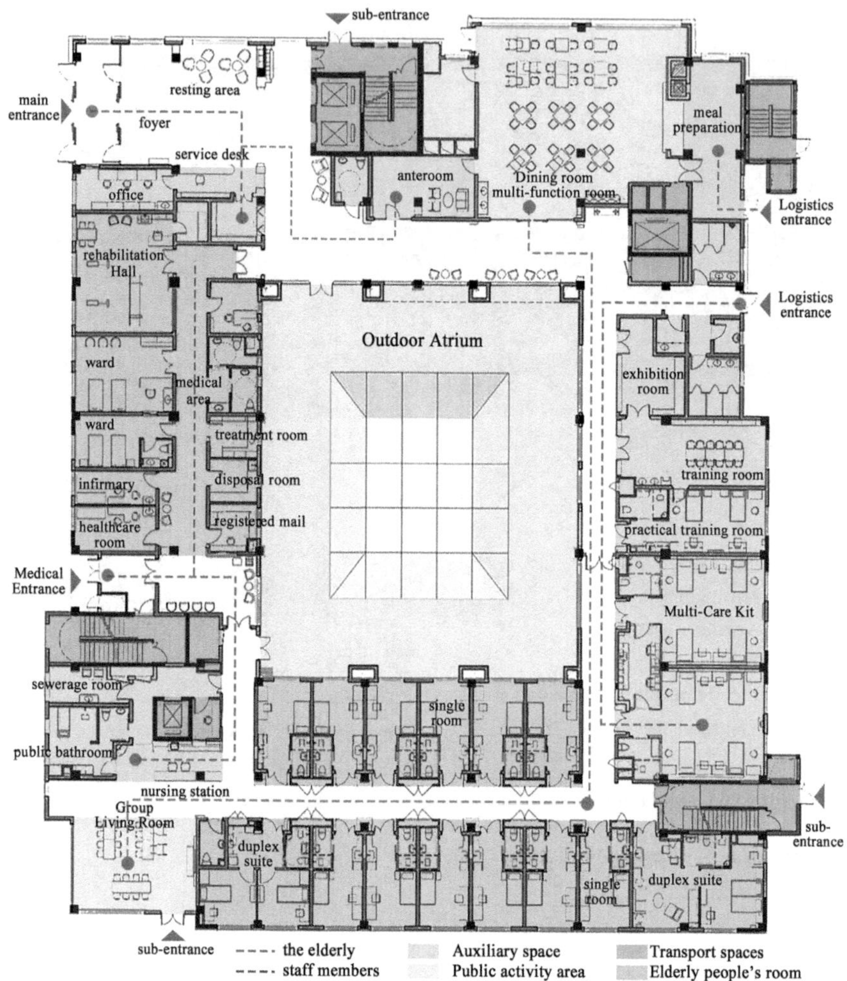

b) Large-scale care home

Figure 6.5(a-b) (Continued)

approach becomes particularly crucial. The mingling of functional spaces in some care homes has led to a negative acoustic environment experience for the elderly.

Overall, meticulous consideration and analysis of the acoustic environment quality in care homes should be a priority during the initial stages of architectural design. Currently, in the architectural design process of care homes in China, architects predominantly prioritize aspects like orientation, natural lighting, ventilation, and age-friendly design, with some attention to the visual environmental

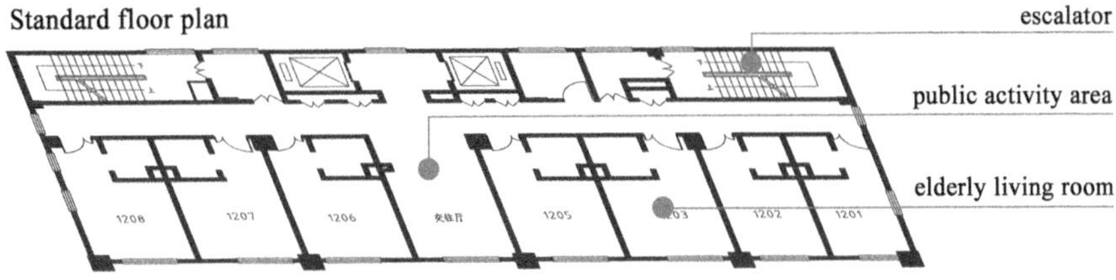

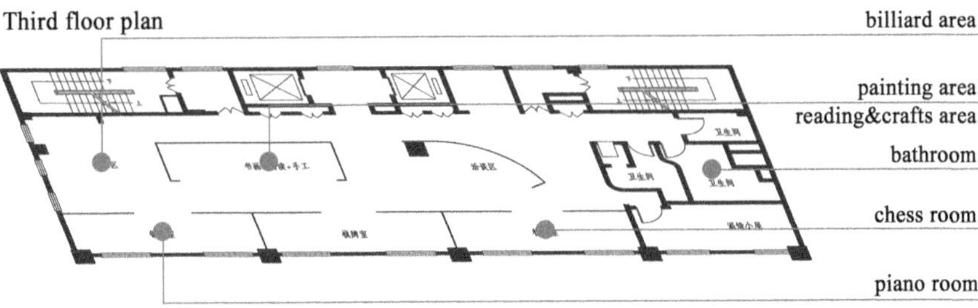

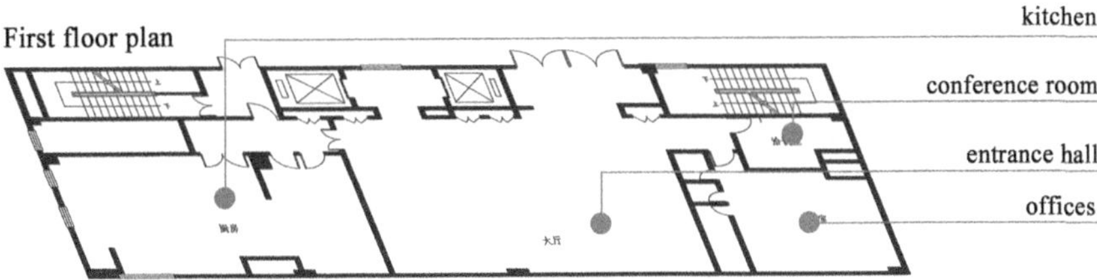

a) Small-scale care home

Figure 6.6(a-b) Vertical spatial distribution of care homes

design of care homes. However, there's a noticeable lack of focus on the acoustic environment. Yet, existing research underscores that poor acoustic environments may trigger diseases such as hypertension [1], significantly impacting individuals' physical and mental health. Therefore, integrating considerations for the acoustic environment during the design phase, such as through software simulation analysis of care home acoustic environment quality, and implementing improvements can effectively enhance auditory comfort and promote the health levels of the elderly.

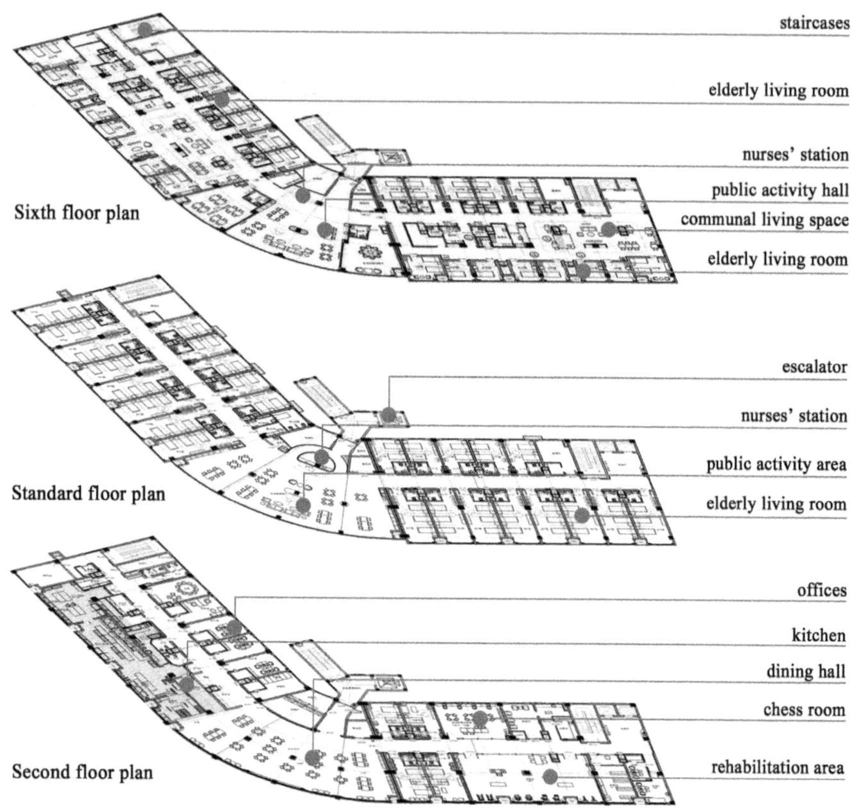

b) Medium-sized care home

Figure 6.6(a-b) (Continued)

6.5 Acoustic environment enhancement strategies at the noise control level

6.5.1 Indoor acoustic environment status of care homes

In order to better promote the physical and mental health of the elderly, relevant building regulations have established explicit standards for the quality of the indoor physical environment of care homes. According to the "Standard for design of care facilities for the aged" (JGJ450–2018) [28], the permissible noise levels in rooms for the elderly must comply with the specifications outlined in Table 6.1.

However, actual surveys indicate that meeting these regulatory noise level standards within care homes is challenging [29]. Figure 6.7 illustrates the indoor sound pressure levels in various functional rooms across different seasons. Notably, except for autumn, daytime sound pressure levels in elderly bedrooms frequently exceed 40 dB, with averages typically ranging between $50-55dB$. In activity rooms, sound pressure levels vary significantly, with peaks reaching up

Table 6.1 Permissible indoor noise levels for rooms for the elderly [28]

Room type		*Allowable noise level (equivalent continuous A sound level, dB)*	
		Daytime	*Evening*
Living quarters	Room	≤40	
	Foyer	≤40	≤30
Recreation and fitness rooms		≤45	
Rehabilitation and medical rooms		≤40	

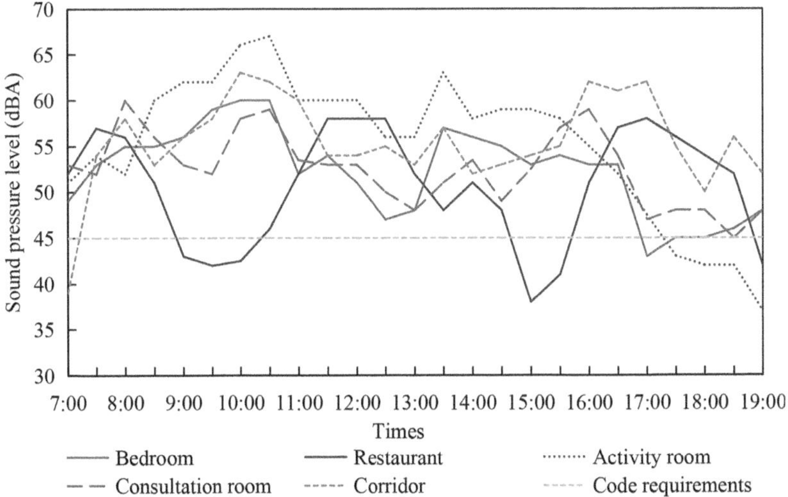

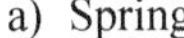
a) Spring

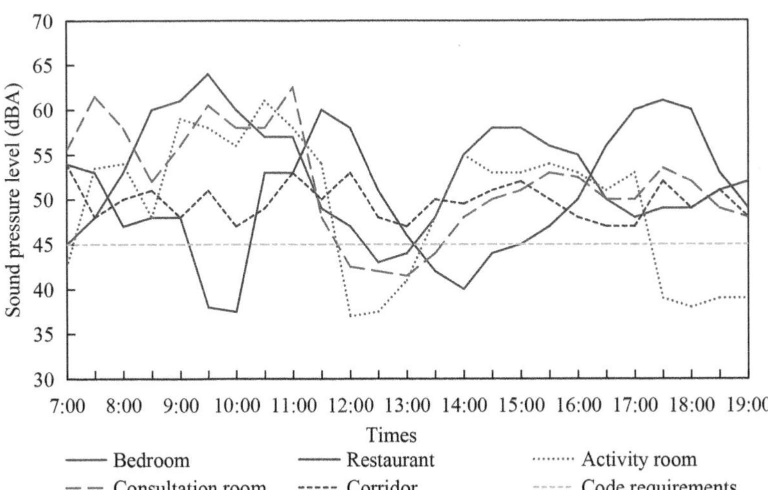

b) Summer

Figure 6.7(a-d) Sound pressure level measurement in different seasons and different rooms

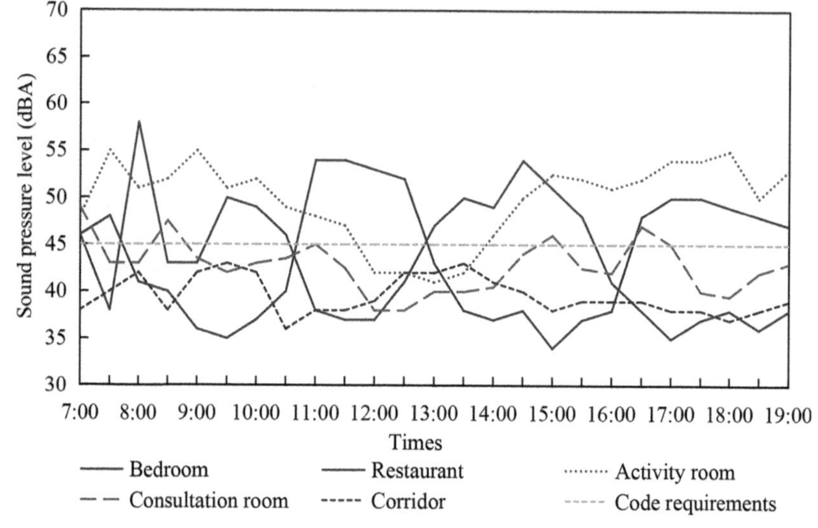

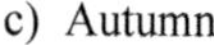
c) Autumn

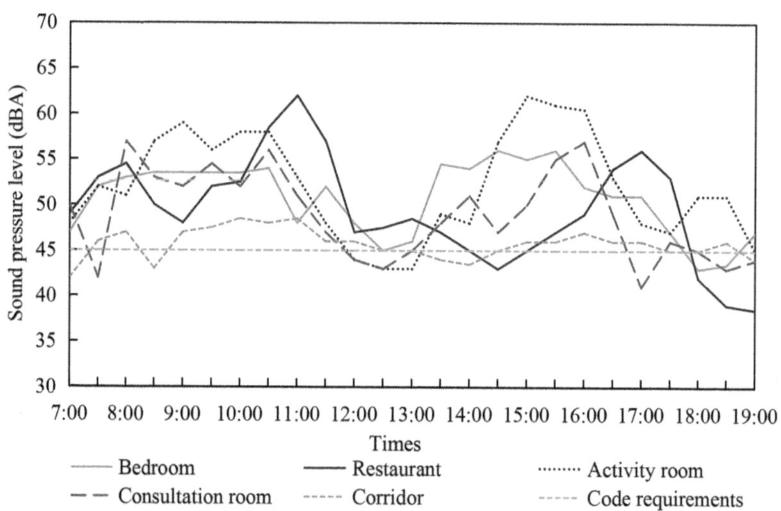

d) Winter

Figure 6.7(a-d) (Continued)

to 65 dBA. Overall, maintaining the required indoor sound pressure levels in care homes proves difficult throughout the year.

In addition to sound pressure levels, reverberation time is another crucial metric for evaluating the indoor acoustic environment of care homes. Research indicates that prolonged reverberation time can impair the elderly's ability to discern sounds, negatively impacting their daily activities and social interactions. Consequently, building regulations also set standards for indoor reverberation time, as detailed in Table 6.2.

However, in actual surveys, we similarly found it challenging for the indoor reverberation time of care homes to meet regulatory requirements. Figure 6.8 presents the measured reverberation time results of public spaces in a care home, revealing that the maximum reverberation time in the hall can reach up to 6 seconds, far exceeding the standard requirement of 1.4 seconds. Simulation results

Table 6.2 Mean values of reverberation time (octave) from 500Hz to 1000Hz in the empty field of a room for the elderly [28]

Room volume (m³)	*Reverberation time (s)*
<200	≤0.8
200~600	≤1.1
>600	≤1.4

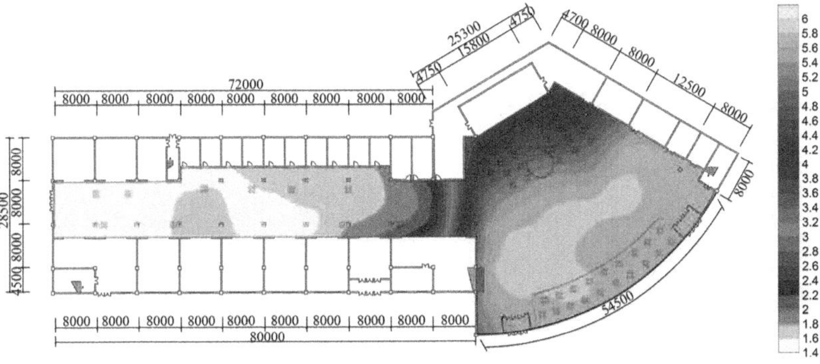

Figure 6.8 The measurement of reverberation time in the activity hall, units in mm and reverberation time in s

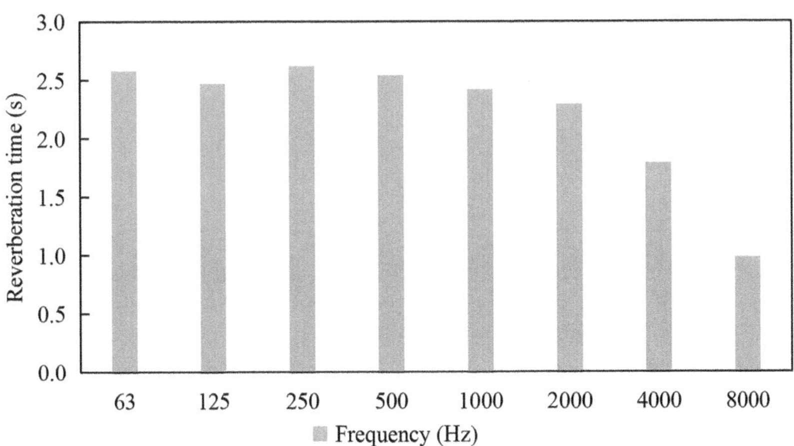

a) Nursing homes

Figure 6.9(a-c) Reverberation time simulation results for different types of care homes

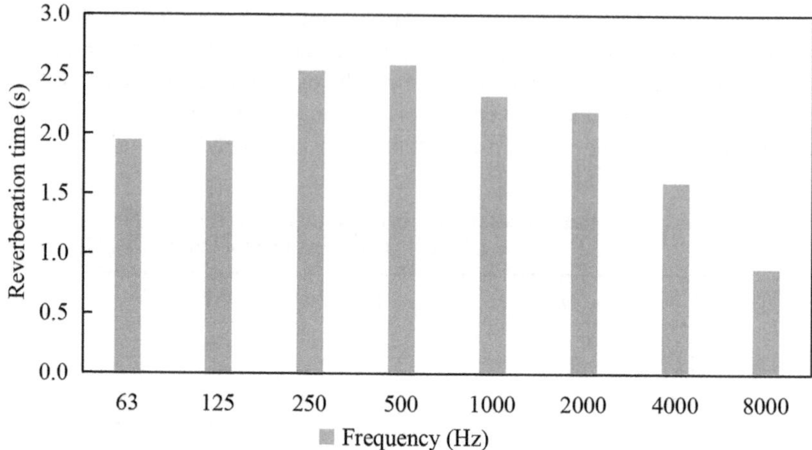

b) Service center for the elderly

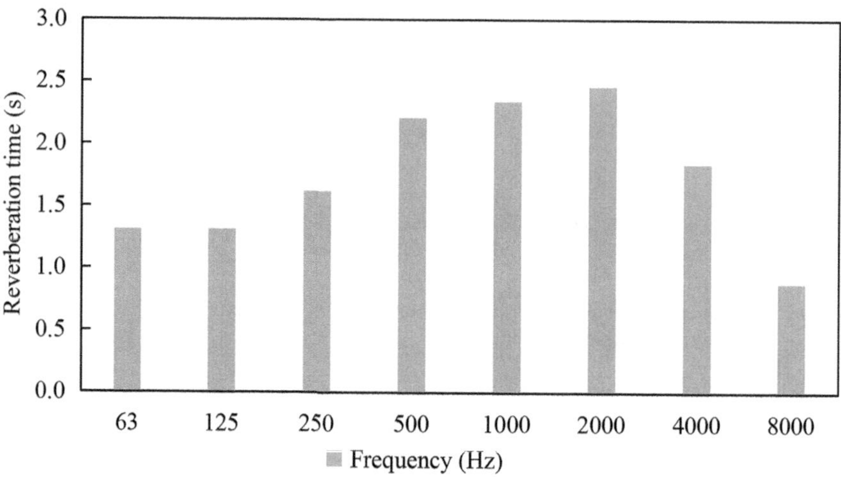

c) Cognitive care center

Figure 6.9(a-c) (Continued)

from various representative care homes also demonstrated that the average reverberation time of public spaces typically hovers around 2.4 seconds (Figure 6.9), also falling short of regulatory requirements.

Moreover, our study on the comfort and satisfaction with the acoustic environment in care homes revealed that the elderly rated the acoustic environment in quiet areas the highest, followed by corridors, rest areas, and small activity areas, with the activity areas receiving the lowest ratings. This indicates a clear preference among the elderly for quieter environments. The comfort of the elderly's acoustic environment is closely related to the sound pressure level. Research indicates that as the sound pressure level increases, the satisfaction of the elderly with their acoustic environment gradually decreases. Therefore, it is imperative to implement measures to enhance the quality of the acoustic environment of care homes.

6.5.2 Improvement of acoustic environment quality in care homes

Through preliminary research, we found that some architectural spaces' acoustic problems are difficult to solve solely through layout design in plan and vertical spaces. Therefore, it is necessary to implement sound insulation, absorption, vibration isolation, and noise reduction treatments on the building's walls, floors, ceilings, and other structures to create a comfortable indoor acoustic environment.

Sound insulation methods can be broadly categorized into wall insulation, floor insulation, and door and window insulation. For rooms with higher sound pressure levels (such as multipurpose halls and piano rooms), wall designs should be tailored accordingly. This might include thickening walls or using double-layer hollow walls or lightweight steel frame walls to reduce interference with adjacent spaces. For rooms adjacent to elderly living quarters or activity spaces on different floors, floor insulation methods are crucial. Many elderly people use canes due to mobility issues or declining vision, generating noise. Additionally, noises from dragging chairs or playing chess or piano can disturb adjacent spaces, necessitating floor insulation treatment. Special spaces with impact sound requirements should be equipped with elastic cushioning layers.

Furthermore, during the survey process, we found that most accommodation-based care homes adopt cluster-style designs (Figure 6.10), with each cluster accommodating 10–30 elderly residents and featuring a common living room where residents can chat, play cards, and watch TV. However, due to varying hearing conditions among the elderly, the sound pressure level in the common activity area is often too high, easily causing disturbances to adjacent spaces. This can be addressed through the use of soundproof doors and windows. Doors can be made of heavier materials, while windows can use glass materials with high sound insulation properties and enhanced soundproof seals.

The reverberation time in nursing homes should also be effectively controlled, as prolonged reverberation time can lead to decreased speech clarity and affect daily communication among the elderly. The use of sound-absorbing materials can effectively reduce reverberation time. When optimizing the acoustic environment design, materials or structures with good sound absorption at low, medium, and high frequencies should be used in combination according to the existing environment, fully exploiting their sound-absorbing properties.

Since most sound-absorbing materials are applied to interior surfaces and are often combined with finishing materials, material selection should consider fire resistance, durability, non-toxicity, and ease of construction [30]. Additionally, since the visual environment significantly impacts the daily lives of the elderly, studies have shown that good lighting and color combinations can effectively enhance visual comfort and spatial understanding for the elderly [31]. Therefore, when selecting sound-absorbing materials, attention should also be paid to their aesthetics and visual effects.

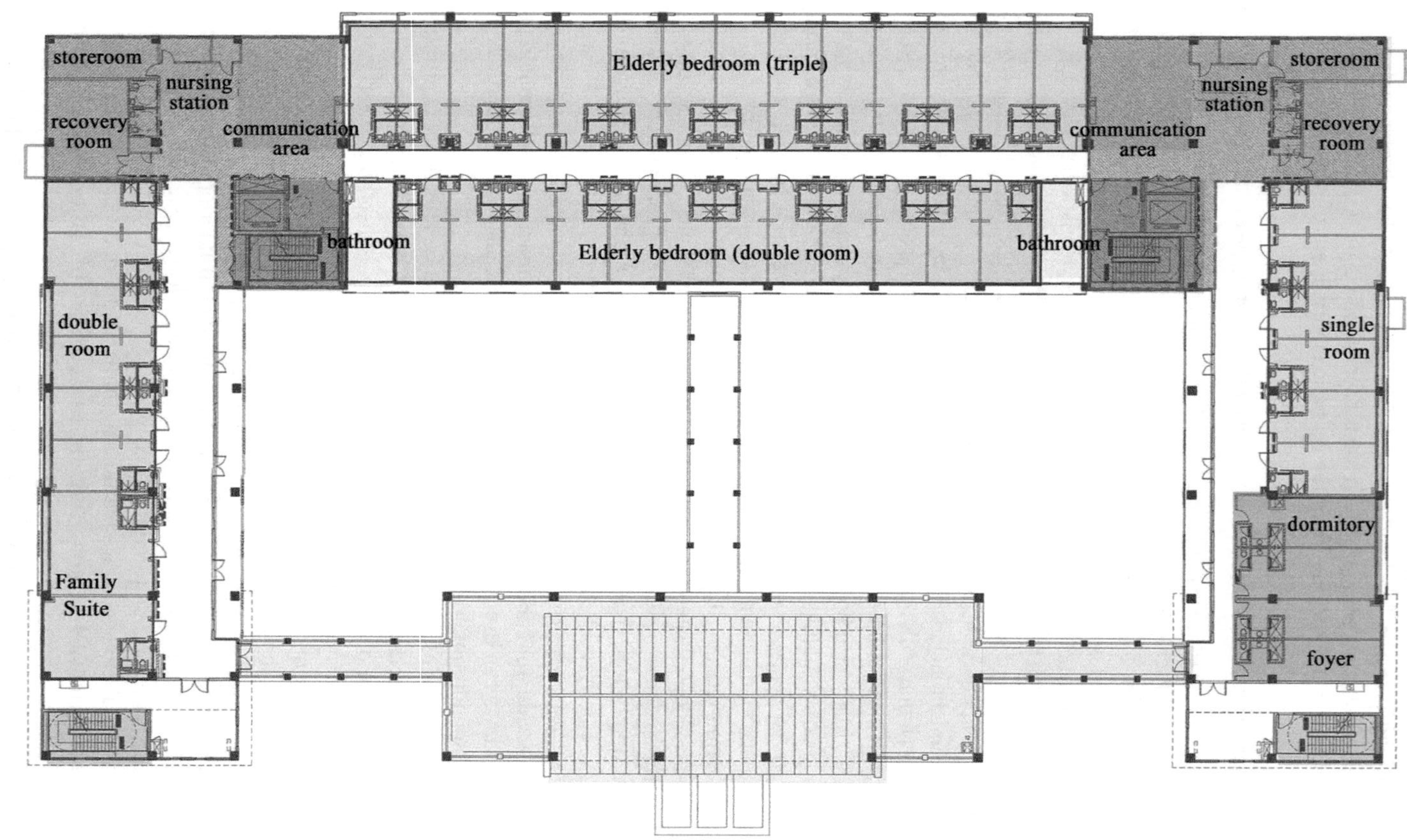

a) Datong home care center

Figure 6.10(a-b) Cluster layout of nursing homes

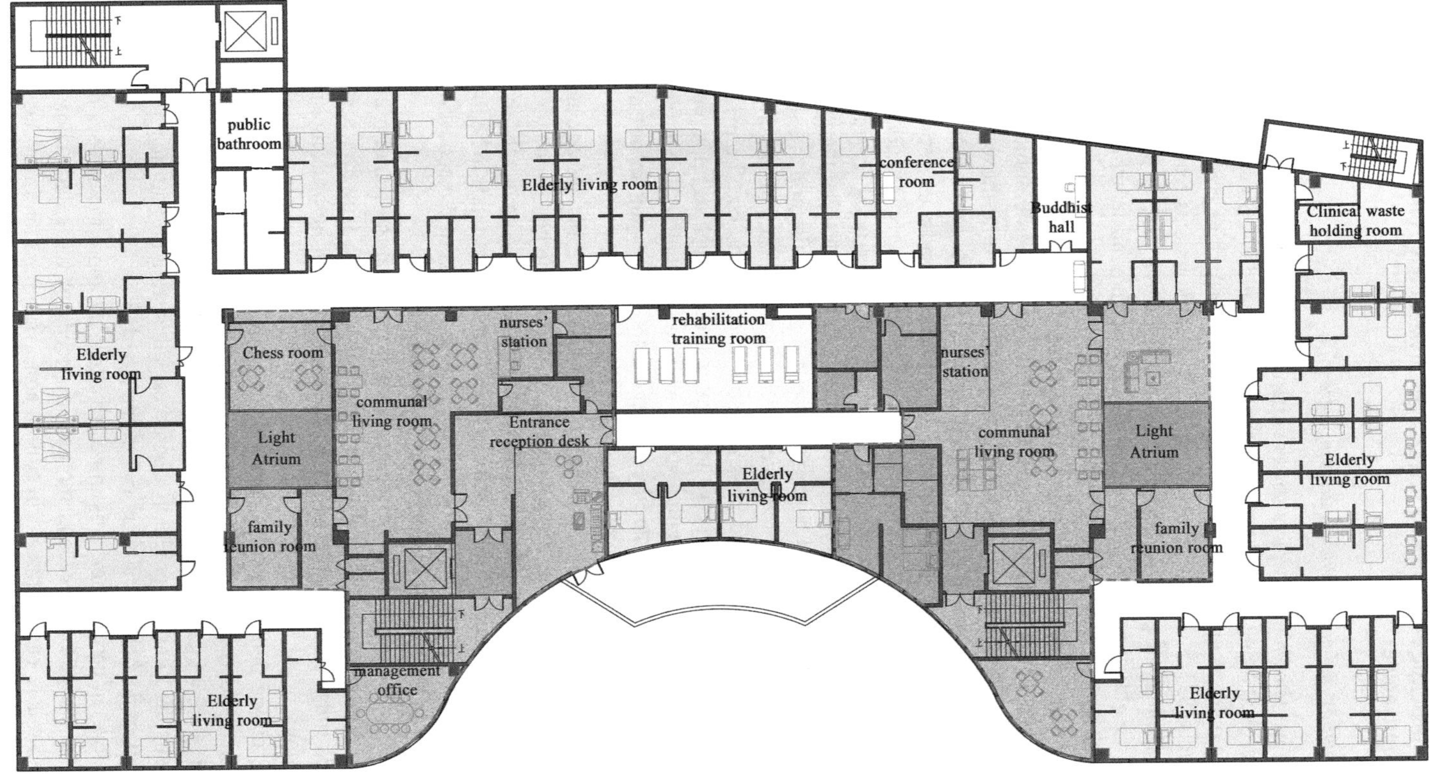

b) Leshanju nursing home

Figure 6.10(a-b) (Continued)

6.6 Soundscape creation and integrated physical environment enhancement

6.6.1 Healthy and comfortable soundscape creation

Research has shown that the acoustic environment can profoundly influence the psychological well-being and behavioral activities of the elderly. Soothing music, compared to a quiet environment, has been found to evoke positive emotions and reduce stress levels [32]. Studies have demonstrated that environments featuring music can enhance feelings of pleasure, arousal, and dominance in elderly individuals. Specifically, the elderly tend to prefer slow-paced, lyric-free music, which significantly boosts their satisfaction levels. Additionally, natural sounds are rated highest by the elderly for their stress-relieving and relaxing properties compared to music with lyrics.

The impact of sound varies among different elderly demographics. Individuals aged 60–80 are more sensitive to the effects of music, while those over 80 show the highest satisfaction with slow-paced music. There is also a notable positive correlation between the education level of the elderly and their satisfaction with slow-paced instrumental music, with highly educated elderly individuals expressing the highest levels of satisfaction. These insights are crucial for improving the acoustic environment in care homes. Our research indicates that the backgrounds of residents in different care homes show certain similarities and are significantly correlated with the nature and fee levels of the facilities. Care homes in China can be categorized into public and private institutions. Public care homes, operated by the government, primarily serve vulnerable groups, such as impoverished and disabled elderly individuals, with a strong welfare orientation. In contrast, private nursing homes, often established by entrepreneurs, offer better infrastructure and eldercare services, albeit at higher fees.

For example, in a surveyed privately-owned care home, the average age of residents was 82, with 37% having a college education or higher. Among them, 26% were former teachers and 17% were former civil servants. Conversely, the average education level of residents in welfare-oriented care homes tends to be lower. This disparity underscores the need for tailored improvements in the acoustic environment based on the specific circumstances of each facility.

In terms of behavioral activities, it was found that natural sound backgrounds encourage more low-decibel activities among the elderly. However, exposure to fast-paced music significantly increases the proportion of high-decibel activities. Observations of activity spaces indicate that music, especially natural sounds, increases crowd density. As the duration of natural sound playback extends, the proportion of elderly individuals engaging in various activities also rises. However, as crowd density increases during low or high-decibel activities, satisfaction with the acoustic environment gradually decreases, suggesting that music types significantly impact the behavioral activities of the elderly.

Therefore, in care homes, it is imperative to play appropriate types of sounds based on the type of space and the activity needs of the elderly. For instance, fast-paced music can be played in fitness areas, natural sounds or classic songs in public leisure areas, and low-decibel, slow-paced, lyric-free music or no music at all in reading rooms and calligraphy studios. By creating a comfortable indoor acoustic environment, the emotional well-being of the elderly can be enhanced, subtly improving their enthusiasm for participating in activities and exercises, and ultimately promoting their health.

6.6.2 *Comprehensive enhancement of indoor physical environment*

The subjective evaluation of the elderly towards acoustic environment may be influenced by other physical environmental factors, such as thermal environment and light environment [33]. The comprehensive physical environment of care homes also plays a significant role in the physical health and quality of life of the elderly [34]. In this study, firstly, the evaluation indicators of physical environmental factors and quality of life were comprehensively sorted out (Table 6.3). Then, SPSS and AMOS software were employed to construct a structural equation model, aiming to deeply analyze the impact of the indoor physical environment of care homes on the quality of life of the elderly.

The calculation results of the structural equation model are presented in Table 6.4 and Figure 6.11. It can be observed that the acoustic environment ($\beta = 0.288$, $p < 0.05$), light environment ($\beta = 0.234$, $p < 0.05$), thermal environment ($\beta = 0.386$, $p < 0.05$), and air quality ($\beta = 0.197$, $p < 0.05$) all have significant positive impacts on the

Table 6.3 Evaluation indicators of physical environmental factors

Environmental factors	*Specific indicators*
Acoustic environment	Overall evaluation, satisfaction level, comfort level, noise level, impact of activities, sense of relaxation
Light environment	Overall evaluation, preference, comfort level, brightness, indoor lighting, indoor color scheme, lighting fixtures
Thermal environment	Satisfaction level, comfort level, temperature evaluation, humidity evaluation, air dryness
Ventilation and air quality	Ventilation conditions, indoor air quality evaluation, indoor odor evaluation, air cleanliness
Quality of life	Physical health, mental health, social health, indoor environmental quality, residential environment evaluation, residential satisfaction

Table 6.4 Path coefficients

Influence path			*Standardized coefficient*	*Unstandardized coefficient*	*S.E.*	*C.R.*	*P*
Light environment	→	Life quality	0.234	0.244	0.023	10.398	***
Acoustic environment	→	Life quality	0.288	0.324	0.026	12.554	***
Thermal environment	→	Life quality	0.386	0.362	0.023	15.901	***
Ventilation and air quality	→	Life quality	0.197	0.201	0.022	9.036	***

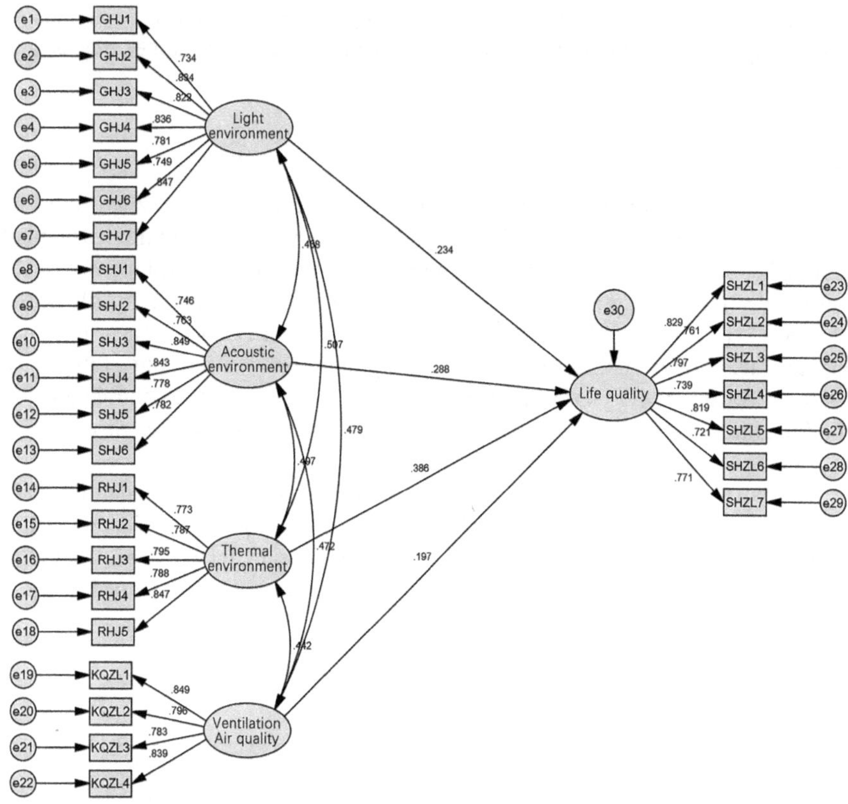

Figure 6.11 Results of structural equation modeling analysis.

quality of life of the elderly. Among these factors, the thermal environment exerts the greatest influence, followed by the acoustic environment. Comparatively, the light environment and air quality have relatively smaller impacts.

The analysis of interaction factors among environmental elements indicates that there are interrelationships between the acoustic environment and other environmental factors such as lighting, thermal conditions, and air quality. The interaction with the thermal environment was found to be the most significant, followed by interactions with lighting and air quality. This suggests that the elderly's assessments of the acoustic environment are interrelated with their evaluations of other physical environmental factors, which in turn have both direct and indirect effects on their quality of life. Therefore, in the process of improving the acoustic environment, it is essential to simultaneously enhance the overall quality of the indoor physical environment in care homes to improve acoustic comfort and overall quality of life for the elderly residents.

6.7 Conclusion

This chapter aims to propose the strategies for improving indoor acoustic environment in care homes. It begins by analyzing the influence of different types of music on individuals' satisfaction, as well as their emotional and behavioral responses, to accurately control audio variables within specific spaces. The main findings of this chapter are as follows:

(1) Behavioral Effects of Acoustic Environments: The comparative analysis of different acoustic environments on the elderly reveals that they do not exhibit a strong preference for environments with or without music. However, when it comes to music tempo, the elderly show a clear preference for slow-paced instrumental music, and regarding music types, they favor natural sounds.
(2) Correlation with Education Level: There is a significant positive correlation between the education level of the elderly and their preference for slow-paced music ($p < 0.001$). This finding indicates that the elderly with higher education levels express the highest satisfaction with slow-paced instrumental music.
(3) Psychological Impact and Behavioral Enhancement: The psychological impact of acoustic environments on the elderly is evident in how music enhances individual behavior, leading to higher perceived satisfaction with the acoustic environment compared to bystanders. Under natural sound settings, all three activity zones engaged in more low-decibel activities ($p < 0.001$). Conversely, exposure to fast-paced instrumental music resulted in a significant increase in the proportion of high-decibel activities among the elderly. These findings suggest that the elderly are more inclined to participate in activities when the music environment is appropriately tailored to their preferences.

This chapter also examines the comprehensive effects of various music types and indoor environmental quality on the psychological and physiological well-being, as well as the acoustic comfort, of the elderly in large activity spaces. The findings highlight the importance of considering the influence of different music types on the activities and social interactions of the elderly in care homes and communities.

Based on previous research, strategies for improving the acoustic environment quality of care homes are proposed from three perspectives:

(1) Architectural Design: Care homes should be situated away from major urban thoroughfares whenever possible. For existing buildings, noise interference can be mitigated through methods such as planting trees and creating setback roads. Effective dynamic and static zoning should be implemented in both plan and vertical space design to prevent placing functional rooms with high sound pressure levels adjacent to elderly living quarters. Additionally, functional circulation pathways should be clearly distinguished to avoid crossing and interference between different groups.
(2) Noise Control: Given that existing care homes often struggle to meet relevant specifications, excessively high sound pressure levels can have adverse effects on the physical and mental health of the elderly. To address this, sound insulation, absorption, vibration isolation, and noise reduction treatments should be applied to the walls, floors, ceilings, and other structural elements of buildings, thereby creating a comfortable indoor acoustic environment.

(3) Comprehensive Environmental Improvements: Creating a healthy and comfortable acoustic environment involves enhancing the overall indoor physical environment. A well-designed acoustic environment can promote the psychological health and behavioral activities of the elderly. Additionally, elements such as lighting and thermal conditions significantly impact the elderly's satisfaction with the acoustic environment. Therefore, in the process of improving the acoustic environment, pleasant acoustic settings can be achieved by incorporating music, while the overall physical environment of care homes can be upgraded to promote the health and well-being of the elderly.

In conclusion, this chapter first analyzes the impact of sound types on the mental health of the elderly. Based on this analysis, combined with the previous content, it proposes strategies to improve the indoor acoustic environment of care homes, aiming to promote the health and well-being of the elderly and provide inspiration and reference for creating a comfortable acoustic environment in such facilities.

References

[1] Kerns E, Masterson EA, Themann CL, et al. Cardiovascular conditions, hearing difficulty, and occupational noise exposure within US industries and occupations[J]. *American Journal of Industrial Medicine*, 2018, 61(6):477–491.

[2] Mu J, Kang J, Wu Y. Acoustic environment of comprehensive activity spaces in nursing homes: A case study in Harbin, China [J]. *Applied Acoustics*, 2021, 177(24):107932.

[3] Wang L, Kang J. Acoustic demands and influencing factors in facilities for the elderly [J]. *Applied Acoustics*, 2020, 170:107470.

[4] Janus SIM, Kosters J, Bosch KAVD, et al. Sounds in nursing homes and their effect on health in dementia: A systematic review [J]. *International Psychogeriatrics*, 2020:1–18.

[5] Kosters J, Janus SIM, van den Bosch KA, et al. Soundscape awareness intervention reduced neuropsychiatric symptoms in nursing home residents with dementia: A cluster-randomized trial with MoSART [J]. *Journal of the American Medical Directors Association*, 2023, 24(2):192.

[6] Bottiroli S, Rosi A, Russo R, et al. The cognitive effects of listening to background music on older adults: Processing speed improves with upbeat music, while memory seems to benefit from both upbeat and downbeat music [J]. *Frontiers in Aging Neuroscience*, 2014, 6:284.

[7] Dahms R, Haesner M, Steinhagen-Thiessen E. The effect of music on daily structures of nursing home residents [J]. *Innovation in Aging*, 2017, 1(suppl_1).

[8] Mu J, Kang J, Sui Z. Effect of music in large activity spaces on the perceptions and behaviours of older adults in China [J]. *Applied Acoustics*, 2022(Jan.):188.

[9] Yang W, Moon HJ, Jeon JY. Comparison of response scales as measures of indoor environmental perception in combined thermal and acoustic conditions[J]. *Sustainability*, 2019, 11(14):3975.

[10] Mehrabian A, Russell JA. *An approach to environmental psychology*[J]. Cambridge: MIT Press, 1974.

[11] Schubert E. The influence of emotion, locus of emotion and familiarity upon preference in music[J]. *Psychology of Music*, 2007, 35(3):499–515.

[12] Scherer KR. Which emotions can be induced by music? What are the underlying mechanisms? And how can we measure them?[J]. *Journal of New Music Research*, 2004, 33(3):239–251.

[13] Altenmüller E, Schürmann K, Lim VK, et al. Hits to the left, flops to the right: Different emotions during listening to music are reflected in cortical lateralisation patterns[J]. *Neuropsychologia*, 2002, 40(13):2242–2256.
[14] Lally E. 'The power to heal us with a smile and a song': Senior well-being, music-based participatory arts and the value of qualitative evidence[J]. *Journal of Arts & Communities*, 2009, 1(1):25–44(20).
[15] Hays T, Minichiello V. The meaning of music in the lives of older people: A qualitative study[J]. *Psychology of Music*, 2005, 33.
[16] Dhar V, Chang EA. Does chatter matter? The impact of user-generated content on music sales[J]. *Journal of Interactive Marketing*, 2009, 23.
[17] Levitt P. Peggy Levitt is associate professor in the department of sociology at Wellesley college and research fellow at Harvard University. Roots and routes: Understanding the lives of the second generation transnationally[J]. *Journal of Ethnic & Migration Studies*, 2009, 35(7):1225–1242.
[18] Wang SC, Yu CL, Chang SH. Effect of music care on depression and behavioral problems in elderly people with dementia in Taiwan: A quasi-experimental, longitudinal study[J]. *Aging & Mental Health*, 2015:1.
[19] Cohen A, Bailey B, Nilsson T. The importance of music to seniors[J]. *Psychomusicology: A Journal of Research in Music Cognition*, 2002, 18(1–2):89–102.
[20] McDowell C. Why music in schools? Students' written responses: A descriptive analysis[J]. *Gen Music Today*, 2002, 16(1):25–31.
[21] Perham N, Withey T. Liked music increases spatial rotation performance regardless of tempo[J]. *Current Psychology*, 2012, 31(2):168–181.
[22] Staum MJ, Brotons M. The effect of music amplitude on the relaxation response[J]. *Journal of Music Therapy*, 2000, 37(1):22–39.
[23] Schäfer T, Sedlmeier P, Städtler C, et al. The psychological functions of music listening[J]. *Frontiers in Psychology*, 2013, 4:511.
[24] Kumar A, Jaiswal A. Systematic literature review of sentiment analysis on Twitter using soft computing techniques[J]. *Concurrency and Computation Practice and Experience*, 2019, 32(1):e5107.
[25] Savage M. The musical field[J]. *Cultural Trends*, 2006, 15(2–3):159–174.
[26] Du X. Investigation of indoor environment comfort in large high-speed railway stations in Northern China[J]. *Indoor and Built Environment*, 2019, 29(1):1420326X1984229.
[27] Zhang RN. *Research on the restorative experience and influencing factors of soundscape of waterfront parks in cold cities*[D]. Shenyang: Shenyang Jianzhu University, 2021.
[28] JGJ450–2018. *Standard for design of care facilities for the aged*[S]. Beijing: China Architecture & Building Press, 2018.
[29] Mu JY, Kang J. Indoor environmental quality of residential elderly care facilities in northeast China[J]. *Frontiers in Public Health*, 2022, 10:860976.
[30] Kang HP. *Research on the optimal design of acoustic environment in open Chinese restaurants*[D]. Shandong: Shandong Jianzhu University, 2022.
[31] Guerry E, Caumon C, Bécheras, E, et al. Influence of chromatic and lighting on the visual environment of the elderly: A critical literature review[J]. *Color Research and Application*, 2020, 46(1).
[32] Iyendo OT. Exploring the effect of sound and music on health in hospital settings: A narrative review[J]. *International Journal of Nursing Studies*, 2016, 63:82–100.
[33] Jiang WS, Meng Q, Li MM. Research on future urban soundscape map based on facial expression analysis: A case study of harbin children's park[J]. *New Architecture*, 2022, (06):2–30. (In Chinese)
[34] Wang Q, Liu J, Zhou L, et al. Usability evaluation of mHealth apps for elderly individuals: A scoping review[J]. *BMC Medical Informatics and Decision Making*, 2022, 22(1):317.

Index

Note: Page numbers in *italic* indicate a figure and page numbers in **bold** indicate a table on the corresponding page.

For Product Safety Concerns and Information please contact our EU representative GPSR@taylorandfrancis.com Taylor & Francis Verlag GmbH, Kaufingerstraße 24, 80331 München, Germany

Batch number: 10397794

Printed by Printforce, the Netherlands